Immune Tolerance Research Developments

Immune Tolerance Research Developments

Emile B. Pontell
Editor

Nova Science Publishers, Inc.
New York

For permission to use material from this book please contact us:
Telephone 631-231-7269; Fax 631-231-8175
Web Site: http://www.novapublishers.com

Library of Congress Cataloging-in-Publication Data

Available Upon Request

ISBN 978-1-60456-209-5

Published by Nova Science Publishers, Inc. ✈ New York

Contents

Preface

Immune or immunological tolerance is the process by which the immune system does not attack an antigen. It occurs in three forms: central tolerance, peripheral tolerance and acquired tolerance. Central tolerance is immunological tolerance developed during T and B cell differentiation. Peripheral tolerance is immunological tolerance developed after T and B cells mature and enter the periphery. Acquired or induced tolerance is the immune system's tolerance for external antigens. This new book presents the latest research from around the world.

Expert Commentary I - Development of inhibitors to coagulation factors is one of the major problems faced by persons with hemophilia. Cumulative incidence of inhibitor formation in patients with severe hemophilia A is 25 % to 35 % during the course of their disease and management [1]. About 80 % of these patients are high responders with inhibitor titers exceeding 5 Bethesda Units (BU); the remainder represent low responders, and further, inhibitors developed by some patients are transient [2]. Emergence of inhibitors during hemophilia therapy has an enormous impact upon therapeutic strategies. Antibody titers of patients with inhibitors, particularly high responders, rise following exposure to factor VIII concentrate (FVIII). Consequently, larger and more frequent doses of FVIII concentrate are unable to control bleeding episodes. Instead, when bleeding occurs in patients who develop high inhibitor titers, they must be treated with bypassing agents.

A critical alternative management approach is to attempt to eradicate the inhibitor by inducing immune tolerance, aiming to restore efficacy of FVIII. Several protocols for immune tolerance induction (ITI) have been evaluated, including the Bonn protocol, the Malmo protocol, and others [3]. At present, a prospective international randomized study is in progress. Meanwhile, in the absence of any results from a randomized study comparing ITI protocols with placebo, ITI protocols such as the two mentioned above have been reported to achieve a success rate between 50 % and 80 %.

Expert Commentary II - In the 1950s surgeons demonstrated the feasibility of removing a kidney and transplanting it into another individual with the expectation of good function. (1)

This was an important stimulus to develop organ transplantation but, with the exception of grafts between identical twins, immunological difficulties were immediately apparent. A spark of optimism followed the demonstration by Medawar and his colleagues of natural tolerance in dizygotic cattle twins and experimental tolerance between inbred strains of mice (2,3). The data suggested that presentation of donor tissue to an embryo or neonate rodent before the immune system was fully developed, could result in a tolerant state. Early workers wondered if there might be strategies to render the adult immune system similar to that of the embryo for a short spell whilst a transplant was performed.

The degree of tolerance varied from acceptance of skin grafts in perfect condition long-term, to only moderate prolongation. This fact has often been neglected by subsequent workers who have repeatedly insisted that the definition of tolerance is complete graft acceptance for a natural lifetime without any need for maintenance immunosuppression.

Chapter 1 - The establishment of viral inactivation methods and recombinant technology has improved the safety of factor VIII (FVIII) concentrates for the treatment of hemophilia A. However, the reactive development of anti-FVIII alloantibodies (inhibitors) by patients undergoing this therapy remains a critical issue. Approximately 20-33% of patients with severe type hemophilia A develop inhibitor antibodies that reduce or completely negate the benefits of replacement therapy. Immune tolerance induction therapy (ITI) is the only proven strategy for the treatment for hemophilia A patients who develop inhibitors of FVIII. It has been known that ITI increases production of antiidiotypic antibodies, which prevent anti-FVIII antibodies from combining with FVIII antigens. The authors previously demonstrated that antiidiotypic antibodies are present in the patient plasma before, during, and after ITI, regardless of whether tolerance was induced. They also presented the possibility that ITI induces affinity maturation of antiidiotypic antibodies. In addition, the authors characterized the mechanism underlying the therapeutic response to ITI by investigating the effect of ITI on various inhibitors by studying a total of 79 plasma samples obtained from 17 hemophilia A inhibitor patients treated with ITI. Inhibitor levels were quantified by the Bethesda method for detection of FVIII-neutralizing antibodies, and by the immunoprecipitation (IP) method for FVIII (or A2, C2 domain, or light chain)-binding antibodies. Eleven patients were treated with plasma-derived FVIII (pdFVIII), and six were treated with recombinant FVIII (rFVIII). Immune tolerance was induced in 8 of 11 patients in the pdFVIII group and in 3 of 6 in the rFVIII group. In most of the successful patients in whom tolerance was induced, the Bethesda titer decreased to undetectable levels, whereas the IP titer remained within the detectable range. Pre-ITI inhibitor levels were lower in patients in whom immune tolerance was induced compared to those in whom immune tolerance was not induced. Antibodies from all cases in the rFVIII group and from all patients in whom immune tolerance was induced recognized three domains (A2, C2 and A3-C1). Three domain-recognizing antibodies were also present in 7 of the 11 patients in the pdFVIII group and in the group of patients in whom immune tolerance was not induced. These data indicate that FVIII-binding antibody-producing clones can persist even after successful ITI.

Chapter 2 - Adoptive T cell activation is an essential feature of allograft rejection. Two signal systems are required for T cell full activation, a first signal provided by T-cell receptor ligation and a second signal provided by engagement of co-stimulatory molecules with their respective ligands on antigen-presenting cells. Costimulatory pathways play crucial roles in regulating T cell responses. Recent investigation identifies that the members of the CD28:B7 family of costimulatory pathway play crucial roles in not only initiation of adaptive immune responses, but also regulation of effector lymphocytes. Blockade of costimulatory signals to inhibit T cell activation is thought to be one of promising strategy to prevent graft rejection and facilitate tolerance induction. In vivo, costimulation blockade was indeed shown to allow for long-term allograft survival and facilitate tolerance in several transplantation models. In this review, the authors summarize the latest developments in the CD28:B7 family costimulatory molecules about their potential interest for acute and chronic allograft rejection and tolerance induction. The role of multiple combination therapies involving blockade of costimulation in induction of long-term allograft survival are discussed.

Chapter 3 - $CD4^+$ T cells that co-express high levels of interleukin (IL)-2 receptor and the transcription factor Foxp3 ($CD4^+CD25^{high}Foxp3^+$ cells) constitute a lymphocyte subpopulation with an important role in the mechanisms of peripheral immune tolerance. The $CD4^+CD25^{high}Foxp3^+$ cells, commonly called regulatory T cells (Tregs), are capable to regulate innate and adaptive immune responses in several animal models of disease and in human diseases via mechanisms of suppression of the proliferation and cytokine production from several different types of immune cell targets. Although Tregs may not require antigen specificity for suppression, the activation of these cells seems to occur preferentially via the engagement of T-cell receptors on these cells with defined antigen specificity. Numerous data have indicated that within the intricate network of interactions among Tregs, innate and adaptive cells and soluble factors, Tregs represent crucial components of immune tolerance, both *in vitro* and *in vivo*. As a consequence of that, the reconstitution of normal numbers and/or function of Treg cells in autoimmune animals with a deficit of these can beneficially affect disease development, progression and outcome, whereas elimination of these cells can be envisioned in cancer immunotherapy. Recently, the use of Treg cells from experimental animal models into clinical applications in humans has been initiated, and promising Treg-based modalities of therapeutic immune intervention are currently under preclinical investigation.

Chapter 4 - Genetically engineered plants have emerged as an attractive alternative expression platform for the production of therapeutic proteins in order to meet the ever-increasing need for protein-based human therapeutics that would be difficult to achieve by using conventional methods. This rise is due in part to a greater understanding of disease pathogenesis that has led to the development of new therapeutic treatments. One such treatment utilizes the natural phenomena of oral immune tolerance, whereby ingested protein antigens induce a state of immunologic unresponsiveness to subsequent antigen stimulation. Oral tolerance has proven to be very effective in treating experimental autoimmune diseases including type 1 diabetes. Although still preliminary, oral tolerance has shown promising results in humans as well. However, as oral tolerance induction requires repeated administration of large amounts of protein antigens, the clinical application of oral tolerance strategy may be limited by the potentially huge cost of producing the protein. The use of transgenic plant to express and deliver protein antigens may provide a highly effective, low-cost method for inducing oral tolerance to the treatment of human autoimmune diseases as well as allergy and organ transplantation. This review will examine 1) recombinant protein biotechnology in plants; 2) oral tolerance induction in animal models using transgenic plants expressing specific antigenic proteins; and 3) future prospects for plant-based therapies against immune-mediated diseases.

Chapter 5 - The advent and successful evolution of human solid organ transplantation over the past 50 years has been a remarkable achievement that has provided thousands of patients with certain types of end stage organ disease an improved life with notably reduced morbidity and mortality. In order to achieve this success there has been the need for significant immunosuppression of the host to prevent recipient alloimmune responses from rejecting the genetically disparate donor organ. Unfortunately, the application of immunosuppression comes at a price and carries with it the potential for numerous life threatening and debilitating side effects. Since donor allograft tolerance has been extensively characterized and accomplished in animal models, transplant physicians have always attempted to achieve immunological tolerance in human transplant recipients in order to attain a state of specific nonreactivity to the donor transplant with little or no immunosuppression but without sacrificing graft function. To date, the realization of true immunological tolerance in human transplantation remains elusive; however, there have been many examples where a state of "operational" tolerance has been achieved. This chapter will describe these clinical occurrences and based upon animal models, an overview of some postulated mechanisms in immune tolerance.

Chapter 6 - The need for indefinite use of combinations of immunosuppressive drugs in organ transplantation may paradoxically impair long-term graft function. Tolerance induction may eliminate this need. One route for tolerance induction is to harness the power of dendritic cells (DCs) which are antigen presenting cells that have remarkable plasticity and the dichotomous function of directing immune responses toward either immunity or tolerance. It has also been recognized in recent years that a subtype regulatory T cells, the $CD4^{+}CD25^{+}$ T_{reg} cells, play a critical role in mediating allo-specific tolerance. More importantly, there appears to be bi-directional signaling between DCs and $CD4^{+}CD25^{+}$ T_{reg} cells. DCs mediate central as well as peripheral T_{reg} cell development and expansion. Conversely, T_{reg} cells may directly down-regulate the ability of DCs to stimulate effector T cells. Here the authors consider the specific characteristics of both DCs and $CD4^{+}CD25^{+}$ T_{reg} cells that are relevant to induction of transplant alloantigen-specific tolerance and discuss the therapeutic potential of DC or T_{reg} cell-based therapy in organ transplantation.

Chapter 7 - The burst of interest and activity in stem cell research in recent years, which foretells the dawn of regenerative therapy for many diseases, has been accompanied by a number of moral and ethical controversies. One of such issues is the strategy to use cloned human embryonic stem cells in order to avoid immune rejection by the recipient of the stem cell therapy. It had been taken for granted that the stem cells will be subjected to immune surveillance like any other cells, such that only autologous cells will be immunologically tolerated and accepted.

As it turned out, it is now known that stem cells derived from a number of sources exhibit unique immune tolerance, both in the *in vitro* and *in vivo* studies. Their ability to circumvent immune surveillance allows them to be chosen as "universal donor cells" for therapeutic use, with vast clinical and logistic advantages. Such development should be able to circumvent these ethical/moral controversies, thus accelerate the advance and realization of regenerative therapies.

Chapter 8 - More and more evidence accumulates for a defect in thymus-dependent tolerance to islet β cells as a major factor in initiation and development of the diabetogenic autoimmune response. Type 1 diabetes (T1D) results from specific and progressive β-cell destruction by auto-reactive T cells directed against three auto-antigens: Insulin (as the primary and β-cell specific auto-antigen), the 65-kDa isoform of glutamic acid decarboxylase (GAD65), and the insulinoma-associated tyrosine phosphatase 2 (IA-2). The thymus plays a prominent role in T-cell education to recognize and tolerate neuroendocrine functions through transcription by thymic epithelial cells (TEC) of genes belonging to neuroendocrine families. All members of the Insulin gene family are transcribed in the thymus according a precise hierarchy and cell topography, whereby *IGF2* (cortical [c] and medullary [m] TEC) exceeds *IGF1* (macrophages), and is much higher than *INS* (subsets of mTEC). The autoimmune regulator gene (*AIRE*) encodes a transcription factor that controls the level of intrathymic expression of genes encoding T1D-related self-antigens (including *IGF2*, *INS*, and *GAD67*), as well as many – but not all - tissue-restricted antigens. The genetic locus *IDDM2* (VNTR) determines individual susceptibility to T1D through modulation of intrathymic *INS* transcription. A defect in thymus-dependent self-tolerance results in both a progressive enrichment of the T-cell repertoire with "forbidden" islet self-reactive T cells, as well as to a decrease in the thymic generation of T1D self-antigen specific regulatory T cells (T_{Reg}). Undoubtedly, further knowledge of the thymic mechanisms responsible for central tolerance of islet Insulin-secreting β cells will lead to the development of novel therapies aiming to restore T-cell tolerance to T1D auto-antigens.

In: Immune Tolerance Research Developments
Editor: Emile B. Pontell, pp. 1-3
ISBN: 978-1-60456-209-5

Expert Commentary

Immune Tolerance Research Developments: Potential of Continuous Infusion Therapy

Kazushi Tamura*, Takashi Kanazawa and Akihiro Morikawa
Department of Pediatrics and Developmental Medicine,
Gunma University Graduate School of Medicine

Development of inhibitors to coagulation factors is one of the major problems faced by persons with hemophilia. Cumulative incidence of inhibitor formation in patients with severe hemophilia A is 25 % to 35 % during the course of their disease and management [1]. About 80 % of these patients are high responders with inhibitor titers exceeding 5 Bethesda Units (BU); the remainder represent low responders, and further, inhibitors developed by some patients are transient [2]. Emergence of inhibitors during hemophilia therapy has an enormous impact upon therapeutic strategies. Antibody titers of patients with inhibitors, particularly high responders, rise following exposure to factor VIII concentrate (FVIII). Consequently, larger and more frequent doses of FVIII concentrate are unable to control bleeding episodes. Instead, when bleeding occurs in patients who develop high inhibitor titers, they must be treated with bypassing agents.

A critical alternative management approach is to attempt to eradicate the inhibitor by inducing immune tolerance, aiming to restore efficacy of FVIII. Several protocols for immune tolerance induction (ITI) have been evaluated, including the Bonn protocol, the Malmo protocol, and others [3]. At present, a prospective international randomized study is in progress. Meanwhile, in the absence of any results from a randomized study comparing ITI protocols with placebo, ITI protocols such as the two mentioned above have been reported to achieve a success rate between 50 % and 80 %.

* E-mail address: ktamura@med.gunma-u.ac.jp. Phone: +81-27-220-8205. Fax: +81-27-220-8215. Corresponding author: Kazushi Tamura, MD, PhD; Department of Pediatrics and Developmental Medicine, Gunma University Graduate School of Medicine, 3-39-22 Showa-machi, Maebashi, Gunma, Japan

Many additional factors have been shown to affect likelihood of success in ITI, such as the dose of factor concentrate and pretreatment inhibitor titers. Unfortunately, for patients with persistently high inhibitor titers, no standard approach exist; many of these patients are left indefinitely with an inhibitor. Such patients are most in need of a broad armamentarium of safe and effective salvage strategies. Switching from recombinant concentrate to a von Willebrand factor-containing plasma-derived product has been suggested as a way to rescue some patients in whom ITI appears to be failing. If initial therapy has used a low-dose regimen, changing to a high-dose protocol should be considered, possibly with concurrent immunosuppression. In addition to such alternative approaches, a few reports have described hemophilia A inhibitor patients treated with a monoclonal mouse-human chimeric anti-CD20 antibody, rituximab [4]. The results suggest that rituximab may be beneficial for patients with severe hemophilia and high inhibitor titers in whom standard therapies have failed, but larger prospective studies are required to determine safety, efficacy, and predictors of success.

Continuous infusion of factor concentrate has been suggested to be safe and effective as preoperative care and as treatment for severe bleeding. By administering replacement factor product at a steady rate approximately equal to its clearance, circulating amounts of plasma factor concentrate will remain steady without excessive peaks. Factor replacement administered as a continuous infusion also has been shown to diminish the amount of concentrate required by some patients, as opposed to treatment with intermittent injections. Moreover, the constant antigen load provided by continuous infusion rather than intermittent injection may have a theoretical advantage in inducing immune tolerance.

We previously reported the first hemophilia A patient with high inhibitor titers to successfully undergo induction of immune tolerance by continuous infusion of recombinant FVIII (rFVIII) [5]. Our patient was a 5-year-old Japanese boy diagnosed with severe hemophilia A who had been treated with rFVIII replacement therapy. Anti-FVIII inhibitor at 7 BU was detected for the first time when he was 2 years old. ITI was begun with rFVIII at 100 units/kg/day 3 times weekly. After beginning therapy, the inhibitor increased to high titers, reaching 109 BU, but then decreased. Subsequent laboratory evaluation, however, continued to detect a high inhibitor titer for 1 year, representing ITI failures.

The patient had a sudden onset of severe neck pain accompanied by reduction of cervical spine motion, and was diagnosed with spinal hematoma. Factor replacement therapy was initiated in preparation for emergency laminectomy for evacuation of the hematoma. Since FVIII inhibitor had been detected at 15 BU 1 week before, a massive bolus rFVIII injection of 500 U/kg was given with the aim of overwhelming the inhibitor. Treatment then was continued with continuous rFVIII infusion at 6 to 12 U/kg/hr for 3 weeks. This treatment was adjusted according to monitoring results for activated partial thromboplastin time (APTT) and FVIII concentration. The postoperative course was uneventful. Following the 3 weeks of continuous infusion, the inhibitor titer became undetectable. And then, prophylactic treatment with rFVIII was initiated. The inhibitor has remained undetectable for 2 years.

Another group reported two hemophilia B patients with high inhibitor titers who underwent immune tolerance induction by continuous infusion of FIX concentrate [6]. Both patients had been treated according to the Malmo protocol without success. Factor IX concentrate was given as continuous infusion at a dose of about 300 U/kg daily for 3 weeks. The inhibitor titer declined in one patient, but tolerance was not achieved. In the second patient the inhibitor titer remained high. Despite failure of treatment by continuous infusion in their two cases, those authors suggested that continuous infusion of factor concentrate might be of greater benefit in immune tolerance induction than their experience suggested. Some studies have raised concern that continuous infusion might trigger development of inhibitors, especially in patients with mild hemophilia [7], however, their data are inconclusive. As presently reported observations are preliminary, large prospective long-term studies of continuous infusion therapy in severe hemophilia with inhibitors are needed.

Although various ITI protocols have been used for as many as 30 years, we lack a clear understanding of mechanisms responsible for downward modulation of the established antibody response and induction of durable immune tolerance. We will need to improve our understanding of the immunology of ITI in order to prevent development of inhibitors and to treat existing inhibitors. Our patient's successful ITI by continuous infusion of factor concentrate suggests an option for patients who have experienced failure of conventional ITI. Continuous factor concentrate infusion may be a potentially effective salvage therapy for inducing immune tolerance. This would be of particular importance for patients expected to fare poorly with conventional ITI regimens in addition to those whose ITI has failed.

References

[1] Ehrenforh, S., Kreuz, W. & Scharrer, I. et al. (1992). Incidence of development of factor VIII and factor IX inhibitors in haemophiliacs. *Lancet,* **339**, 594-598.

[2] Key, N.S. (2004). Inhibitors in congenital coagulation disorders. *Br J Haematol,* **127**, 379-391.

[3] Wight, J., Paisley, S. & Knight, C. (2003). Immune tolerance induction in patients with haemophilia A with inhibitors: a systemic review. *Haemophilia,* **9**, 436-463.

[4] Carcao, M., St. Louis, J. & Poon, M.C. et al. (2006). Rituximab for congenital haemophilics with inhibitors: a Canadian experience. *Haemophilia,* **12**, 7-18.

[5] Tamura, K., Kanazawa, T. & Suzuki, M. et al. (2006). Successful induction of immune tolerance by continuous infusion of recombinant factor VIII in a haemophilia A patient with high-inhibitor titres. *Haemophilia,* **12**, 100-102.

[6] Tengborn, L. & Berntorp, E. (1998). Continuous infusion of factor IX concentrate to induce immune tolerance in two patients with haemophilia B. *Haemophilia,* **4**, 56-59.

[7] Mulcahy, M., Walsh, M. & Scully, M.F. (2005). Retrospective audit of a continuous infusion protocol for haemophilia A at a single haemophilia treatment centre. *Haemophilia,* **11**, 208-215.

In: Immune Tolerance Research Developments
Editor: Emile B. Pontell, pp. 5-7

ISBN: 978-1-60456-209-5

Expert Commentary

Prope Tolerance

R.Y. Calne
Dept of Surgery, University of Cambridge

In the 1950s surgeons demonstrated the feasibility of removing a kidney and transplanting it into another individual with the expectation of good function. (1)

This was an important stimulus to develop organ transplantation but, with the exception of grafts between identical twins, immunological difficulties were immediately apparent. A spark of optimism followed the demonstration by Medawar and his colleagues of natural tolerance in dizygotic cattle twins and experimental tolerance between inbred strains of mice (2,3). The data suggested that presentation of donor tissue to a embryo or neonate rodent before the immune system was fully developed, could result in a tolerant state. Early workers wondered if there might be strategies to render the adult immune system similar to that of the embryo for a short spell whilst a transplant was performed.

The degree of tolerance varied from acceptance of skin grafts in perfect condition long-term, to only moderate prolongation. This fact has often been neglected by subsequent workers who have repeatedly insisted that the definition of tolerance is complete graft acceptance for a natural lifetime without any need for maintenance immunosuppression.

In bone marrow transplantation complete tolerance can be obtained. Initially the method used was complete ablation of the recipient's immune system and replacement with donor bone marrow. More recently non-ablative tolerance protocols have been used with success and less severe conditioning of the recipient. It is important to note that in all types of bone marrow transplantation the HLA matching of donor and recipient is of the utmost importance. The best results are obtained with full MHC matching where the donor is a sibling. Bone marrow transplantation carries with it an additional risk of graft versus host disease, which may be helpful in the case of malignant conditions, for example, graft versus leukaemia activity may provide important therapy for the patient.

Another form of tolerance is natural tolerance resulting after liver transplantation in pigs and in rodents (4). This can occur across an MHC major mismatch and usually involves an immune reaction, both biochemical and histological which subsides spontaneously. This led to the hypothesis that immunological engagement of donor and recipient was necessary to produce a tolerant state. Excessive immunosuppression might prevent tolerance from occurring and by implication suggested that natural switch-off mechanisms of the immune response which are very important in the control of infectious disease, might also result in graft acceptance. A so-called window of opportunity for immunological engagement (WOFIE) might be necessary for some forms of tolerance to be established (5). This concept is sympathetic to the important role of regulatory T cells in graft acceptance. These may be destroyed by powerful immunosuppression. Nevertheless in man immunosuppression appears to be necessary to produce a tolerant or partially-tolerant state.

It has proved difficult to design experimental protocols in which tolerance can be produced in animals for other organ transplants but in pigs donor antigen in the form of lymphoid cells together with a short course of high dose cyclosporine may result in prolonged renal and cardiac graft acceptance.

An important clinical experiment was performed by some of Dr. Starzl's liver transplant patients who, without telling their physicians, stopped immunosuppression and avoided the penalty of graft rejection. This could not always been done but a number of patients have survived with continuing good liver function for more than 20 years after stopping immunosuppressive drugs (6). Unfortunately there is no laboratory test available to provide a reliable prediction of which patients with good liver function after five years can safely stop or be weaned off immunosuppression.

There are many protocols of producing tolerance or partial tolerance in rodents but these have not so far been effective in clinical practice. Physicians instead have tended to add each new immunosuppressive agent to an already powerful regimen of drug treatment for patients with organ allografts. Excessive doses of calcinurin inhibitors can cause severe and permanent renal damage and each of the immunosuppressive drugs has its own specific side effects, separate from immunosuppression.

I feel that the tendency of maximal immunosuppression is the opposite direction in which we should be going and minimal immunosuppression consistent with good graft function is the best approach we can adopt in the next few years. Encouraging results have followed the use of the powerful lympholytic induction agent Campath 1H followed by low dose maintenance immunosuppression (7). Campath 1H monoclonal antibody is given in the perioperative phase followed by low dose cyclosporine maintenance immunosuppression as a monotherapy. Similar results have occurred, substituting cyclosporine for FK506. When Campath 1H has been followed by a non-calcinurin inhibitor, for example rapamycin, adequate immunosuppression has not been achieved, nevertheless non-calcinurin inhibitor agents might be substituted at a later stage to avoid drug induced renal damage. Definitive data on this have yet to be established.

In summary, the "*prope*" (or almost) tolerance consisting of powerful induction followed by minimal maintenance would seem to be our best current option although it falls short of the strict definition of tolerance. Perhaps it is helpful to think of tolerance by an analogy to happiness. There are various degrees of tolerance and happiness and we may not be aware of the fact when the patient has established tolerance to a graft but rejection or loss of happiness is instantly recognised, causing graft damage and returning to the analogy, acute unhappiness.

References

[1] Murray JE, Merrill JP, Harrison JH: (1955)Renal homotransplantation in identical twins. *Surg. Forum* 6: 432-436

[2] Anderson D, Billingham RE, Lampkin GH et al. (1951) The use of skin grafting to distinguish between monzygotic and dizygotic twins in cattle. *Heredity* 5. 379-397.

[3] Billingham RE, Brent L, Medawar PB (1953) Actively acquired tolerance of foreign cells. *Nature* 172: 603-606.

[4] Calne RY, Sells, RA, Pena JR et al. (1969) Induction of immunological tolerance by porcine liver allografts. *Nature* 223: 472-6

[5] Calne RY Progress towards tolerance and xenografting. *Transplant. Proc.* (1997): 29: 16-28

[6] Mazariegos GV, Reyes J. Marino I. Et al. (1997) Risks and benefits of weaning immunosuppression in liver transplant recipients: long-term follow-up. *Transp. Proc.*, 29: 1174-7

[7] Calne RY, Friend PJ, Moffatt S, Bradley A, Hale G, Firth J, Bradley J, Smith K, Waldmann H. (1998) Prope tolerance, perioperative campath IH, and low-dose cyclosporin monotherapy in renal allograft recipients. *Lancet* 351: 1701-2

In: Immune Tolerance Research Developments
Editor: Emile B. Pontell, pp. 9-26
ISBN: 978-1-60456-209-5

Chapter 1

The Longitudinal Alteration of Anti-factor VIII Alloantibodies in Hemophilia A Patients Treated with Immune Tolerance Induction Therapy

Yoshihiko Sakurai**, *Tomohiro Takeda, Midori Shima and Akira Yoshioka

Department of Pediatrics, Nara Medical University School of Medicine, 840 Shijo-cho Kashihara Nara 634-8522, Japan

Abstract

The establishment of viral inactivation methods and recombinant technology has improved the safety of factor VIII (FVIII) concentrates for the treatment of hemophilia A. However, the reactive development of anti-FVIII alloantibodies (inhibitors) by patients undergoing this therapy remains a critical issue. Approximately 20-33% of patients with severe type hemophilia A develop inhibitor antibodies that reduce or completely negate the benefits of replacement therapy. Immune tolerance induction therapy (ITI) is the only proven strategy for the treatment for hemophilia A patients who develop inhibitors of FVIII. It has been known that ITI increases production of antiidiotypic antibodies, which prevent anti-FVIII antibodies from combining with FVIII antigens. We previously demonstrated that antiidiotypic antibodies are present in the patient plasma before, during, and after ITI, regardless of whether tolerance was induced. We also presented the possibility that ITI induces affinity maturation of antiidiotypic antibodies. In addition, we characterized the mechanism underlying the therapeutic response to ITI by investigating the effect of ITI on various inhibitors by studying a total of 79 plasma samples obtained from 17 hemophilia A inhibitor patients treated with ITI. Inhibitor levels were quantified by the Bethesda method for detection of FVIII-neutralizing antibodies, and by the immunoprecipitation (IP) method for FVIII (or A2, C2 domain, or light

* E-mail address: ysakurai@naramed-u.ac.jp. Fax: +81-744-24-9222. Phone: +81-744-29-8881

chain)-binding antibodies. Eleven patients were treated with plasma-derived FVIII (pdFVIII), and six were treated with recombinant FVIII (rFVIII). Immune tolerance was induced in 8 of 11 patients in the pdFVIII group and in 3 of 6 in the rFVIII group. In most of the successful patients in whom tolerance was induced, the Bethesda titer decreased to undetectable levels, whereas the IP titer remained within the detectable range. Pre-ITI inhibitor levels were lower in patients in whom immune tolerance was induced compared to those in whom immune tolerance was not induced. Antibodies from all cases in the rFVIII group and from all patients in whom immune tolerance was induced recognized three domains (A2, C2 and A3-C1). Three domain-recognizing antibodies were also present in 7 of the 11 patients in the pdFVIII group and in the group of patients in whom immune tolerance was not induced. These data indicate that FVIII-binding antibody-producing clones can persist even after successful ITI.

Introduction

While the use of FVIII concentrates for treatment of hemophilia A has benefited from the institution of viral inactivation methods and recombinant technology [1, 2], reactive development of anti-factor VIII (FVIII) alloantibodies (inhibitors) by patients undergoing this therapy remains a significant problem. In fact, approximately 20-33% of severe type hemophilia A patients develop inhibitor antibodies that reduce or completely negate the benefits of replacement therapy [3, 4]. Of the methods to reduce inhibitor concentrations in patients with hemophilia A, immune tolerance induction to FVIII therapy (ITI) is the most promising. In 1977, a curative ITI protocol for inhibitor patients was first reported by Brackmann and Gormsen [5]. This Bonn Protocol is based on the administration of high doses of FVIII (150 IU/kg twice a day). In 1999, the outcome of 60 hemophilia A inhibitor patients treated according to the Bonn Protocol was reported: successful immune tolerance could be achieved in 52 patients (86.7%), while the therapy failed in eight patients (13.3%) [6]. Furthermore, several studies have been performed using a modified dosage scheme [7, 8] and the overall success rate of ITI in the recent registries is approximately 70±10% [9].

In general, immune tolerance is induced by several mechanisms [10, 11]: clonal deletion [12], clonal anergy, clonal ignorance, receptor editing [13], suppressor cells, and antiidiotypic antibody. However, the mechanism by which immune tolerance towards the inhibitor antibodies in hemophilia A patients with inhibitors occurs remains to be fully elucidated. In this chapter, we will present our latest findings on the action mechanism of ITI.

Longitudinal Alteration of Antiidiotypic Antibodies

An "idiotype" is a set of antigenic determinants specific to the variable region of an antibody molecule or T cell receptor defined by the unique sequences (idiotopes) of the antigen combining site (Figure.1). Interactions between idiotypes and antiidiotypic antibodies develop an idiotypic network, which exert a regulatory role that maintains the homeostasis of the immune system. Successful ITI might result from an equilibrium between anti-FVIII and corresponding antiidiotypic antibodies. In fact, normal individuals have both anti-FVIII and corresponding antiidiotypic antibodies [14, 15]. Therefore, the deletion of self-reactive B and T cells [16] only could not necessarily cause tolerance to FVIII.

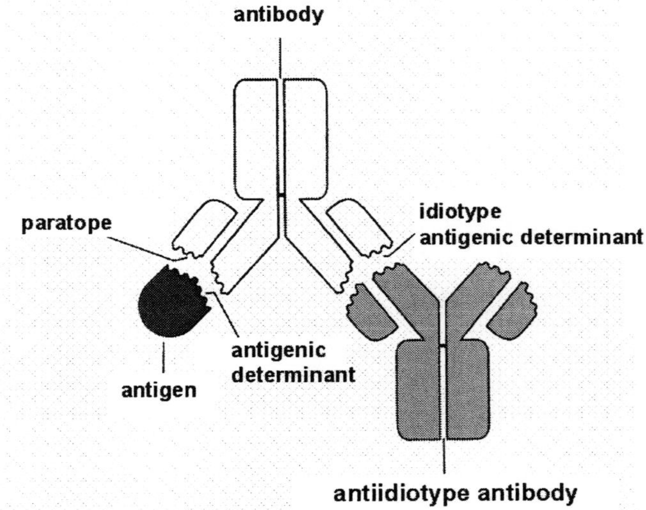

Figure 1. Antigen, antibody, and antiidiotypic antibody. Antibody recognizes the epitope (antigenic determinant) on an antigenic macromolecule. The part of an antibody that recognizes the epitope is called a paratope. The hypervariable region (also called the complementary determining region, CDR) of Ab1 consists of an antigen-recognizing site (paratope) and a non-antigen-binding site (framework). When this hypervariable region acts as an antigen, it is called an idiotype. Ab2 is an antiidiotypic antibody which recognizes the idiotype. Here, an idiotype is a shared characteristic between a group of immunoglobulin molecules based upon the antigen binding specificity and therefore the structure of their hypervariable region.

Since 1984, the presence of antiidiotypic antibodies against inhibitors has been demonstrated in intravenous immunoglobulin preparations (IVIG) [17, 18]. IVIG were reported to be therapeutically-effective for acquired hemophilia [19]. However, antiidiotypic antibodies contained in IVIG are nowadays thought to recognize naturally occurring anti-FVIII autoantibodies that healthy individuals usually possess. Thus the antiidiotypic antibodies in IVIG neutralize the inhibitors developed in acquired hemophilia A with the collapsed regulation system of natural autoantibodies, but would be ineffective for inhibitors occurring in congenital hemophilia A.

On the other hand, earlier studies have demonstrated that the ITI increase production of antiidiotypic antibodies [20-22], which prevent anti-FVIII antibodies from combining with the FVIII antigen. Furthermore, antiidiotypic antibodies may contribute to the down-regulation of anti-FVIII antibody production during ITI [22]. However, it remained unknown whether the plasma of patients who received ITI with an unsuccessful outcome contains antiidiotypic antibodies against inhibitors. Furthermore, the alteration of antiidiotypic antibody production with the course of ITI remained also unclear.

Therefore, we studied plasma samples obtained from hemophilic inhibitor patients who were treated with ITI by a novel method for detecting antiidiotypic antibodies based on a liquid phase blocking immunoprecipitation using immunoprecipitation assay (Figure 2A). The results previously reported [23] are outlined as follows. Plasma anti-FVIII antibody titer was reduced in the presence of plasma from patients who received the successful ITI (Figure 2B). This anti-FVIII antibody-neutralization activity of the plasma was abolished by the absorption treatment of IgGs (Figure 2C). In addition, the inhibitor plasma from the unsuccessful ITI patients developed an anti-FVIII antibody-neutralization activity after the depletion of FVIII-binding antibodies with the treatment of FVIII affinity beads. Furthermore, the anti-FVIII antibody-neutralization activity of 'anti-FVIII antibody-depleted plasma obtained at late period of ITI' on 'inhibitor plasmas obtained during ITI' increased in time sequence. These results provided the possibility of the presence of antiidiotypic antibodies in plasmas from the hemophilia A patients with the inhibitor who are treated with ITI whether successful or not, as well as the possibility of the affinity maturation of IgG antiidiotypic antibodies, i.e. the increase of the neutralization activity of the antiidiotypic antibody over the course of ITI.

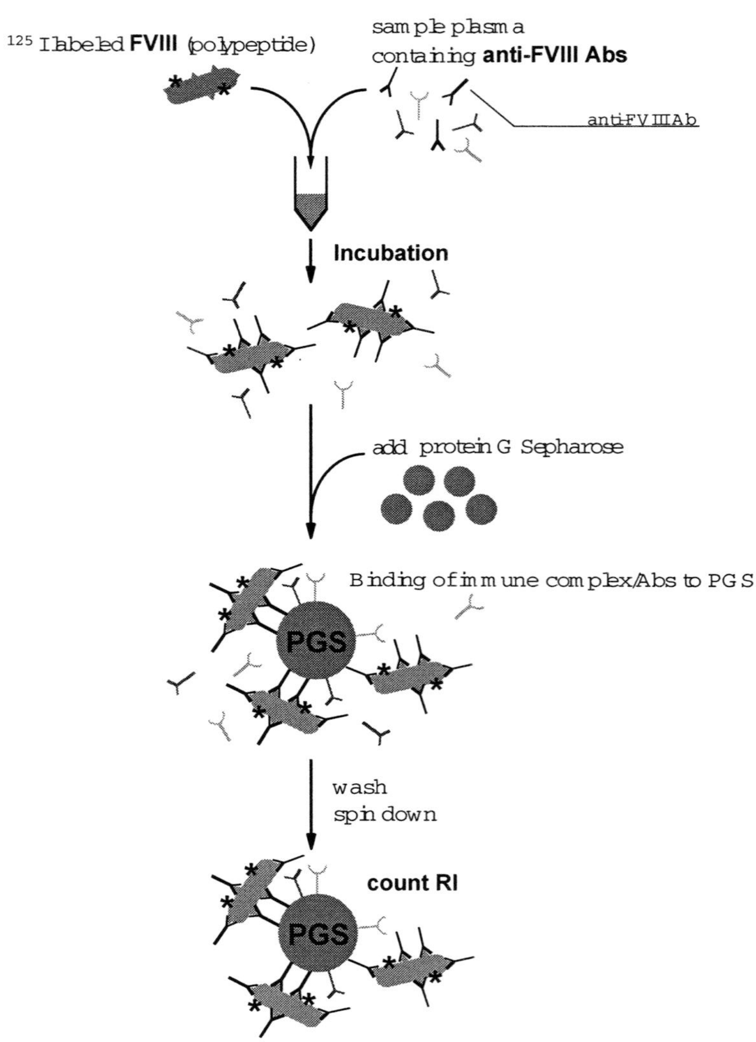

Figure 2. Continued on next page.

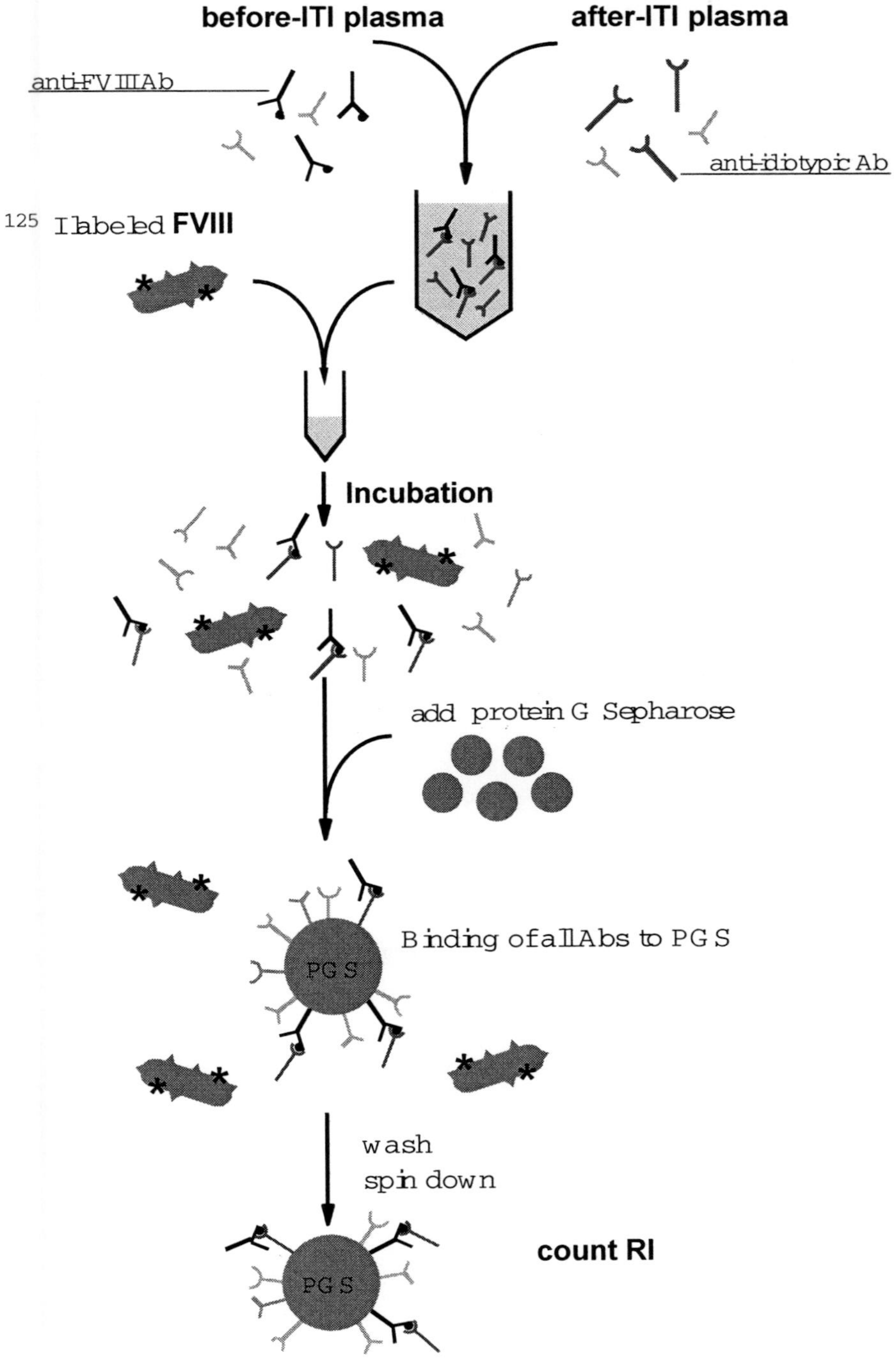

Figure 2. Continued on next page.

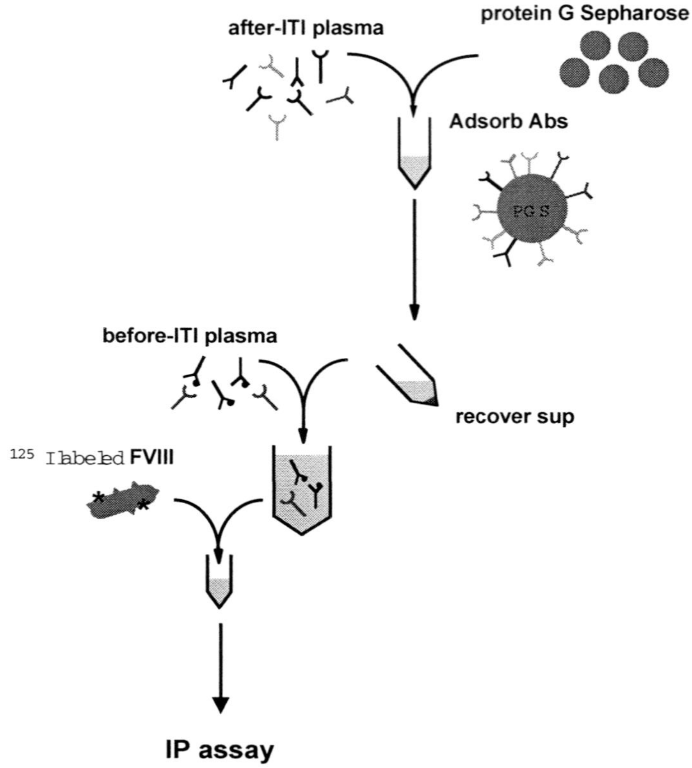

Fugure 2. Method for detecting antiidiotypic antibodies based on a liquid phase blocking immunoprecipitation. A. Conventional immunoprecipitation assay. Sample plasma is mixed with ^{125}I-labeled FVIII. After incubation, protein G Sepharose beads (PGS) are added to the tube. Since anti-FVIII IgGs (complexed with ^{125}I -labeled FVIII) are absorbed with PGS as well as the other IgGs, the radioisotope is detected from washed PGS when the sample plasma contains anti-FVIII IgGs. B. Detection of antiidiotypic antibodies based on a liquid phase blocking immunoprecipitation (I). Plasma obtained before ITI is mixed with plasma obtained after ITI. Conventional IP assay is conducted using this mixture. The IP titer of mixed plasma with plasma obtained before ITI and that from a patient who received the successful ITI, is lower than that of mixed plasma with plasma obtained before ITI and normal plasma. This indicated that plasma from a patient who received the successful ITI contains some factor(s) that can neutralize anti-FVIII IgGs. C. Detection of antiidiotypic antibodies based on a liquid-phase blocking immunoprecipitation (II). To confirm whether an anti-FVIII-neutralizing factor is included in IgG class, plasma from patients who received the successful ITI was pretreated with PGS. Plasma obtained before ITI was mixed with IgG-depleted plasma from patients who received the successful ITI, and the IP titer of the mixture was measured. This anti-FVIII antibody-neutralization activity of the plasma was eliminated by the absorption treatment of IgGs, indicating that anti-FVIII-neutralizing factor is the idiotypic antibodies.

Affinity maturation is the process by which B-cells produce antibodies with increased affinity for antigens within two weeks to several months of the antigen encounter. Similar to anti-DNA antibodies [24], anti-FVIII antibody synthesis could be regulated by an idiotype-antiidiotype network (Figure 3).

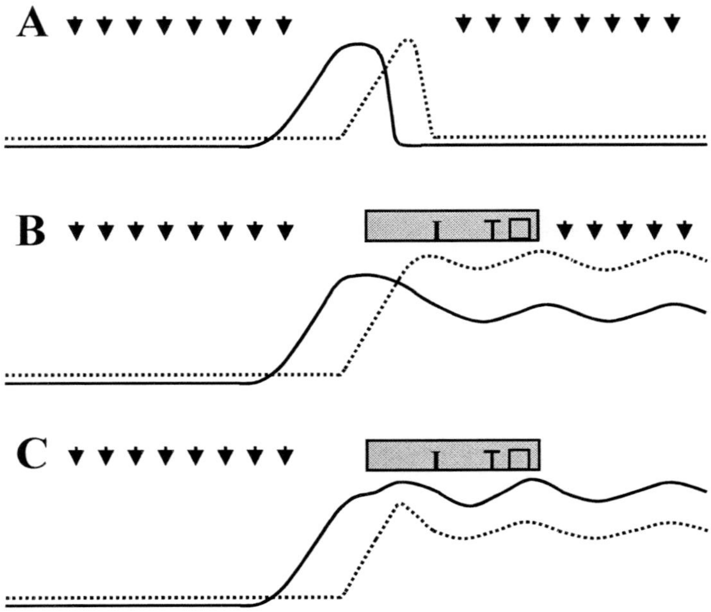

Figure 3. FVIII inhibitor-antiidiotypic antibody fluctuation model during ITI. A. Transient inhibitor: inhibitor titer (solid line) rises with the increase of total volume of infused FVIII (↓) but it falls with the increase of antiidiotypic antibody titer (dotted line). B. ITI successor: similar to A, inhibitor titer rises. Although the inhibitor titer further rises with ITI commencement, the antiidiotypic antibody titer overcomes the inhibitor. C. ITI failure: when the inhibitor further increases over antiidiotypic antibody production, ITI will be ineffective. (This model refers to the anti-DNA antibody synthesis regulation model of the idiotype-antiidiotype network.)

Longitudinal Alteration of Anti-FVIII Alloantibodies

While the role of antiidiotypic antibodies is thus being well understood, alteration of the character of inhibitors (more precisely anti-FVIII alloantibodies) during ITI has been less described [25]. Generally, anti-FVIII alloantibodies are polyclonal and highly heterogeneous, and conceived to display changes in epitope specificity over time [26]. To address this issue, we further studied the characterization of anti-FVIII alloantibodies using plasma samples obtained from hemophilia A patients with inhibitors that underwent ITI.

Patients

This study included 79 plasma samples obtained from 11 patients with hemophilia A and FVIII inhibitors that underwent ITI using highly purified FVIII concentrate derived from human plasma (pdFVIII), and from 6 patients with hemophilia A and FVIII inhibitors who were treated with ITI using recombinant FVIII (rFVIII).

Table 1. Patient characteristics

Patient group	Total no.	Historical peak (BU/mL) Range	Historical peak (BU/mL) Mean	Age at ITI start (years) Range	Age at ITI start (years) Mean
pdFVIII	11	8-500	70,5	2.0-15	5,6
rFVIII	6	5-149	117	1.2-3.7	2,1

ITI: immune tolerance therapy, pdFVIII: plasma-derived factor VIII, rFVIII: recombinant factor VIII

BU: Bethesda unit/mL, IPU: IP unit/mL

The characteristics of patients enrolled in this study are summarized in Table 1. The mean historical peak of the inhibitor titer measured by the Bethesda method (Bethesda titer) before ITI was higher in the rFVIII group than in the pdFVIII group, although this difference did not reach the level of statistical significance. Patients in the rFVIII group were significantly younger than those in the pdFVIII group ($p<0.05$).

All assessable subjects exhibited the following characteristics prior to the initiation of ITI: FVIII inhibitor $\leq$ 10 BU/mL; historical peak between 5 BU/mL and 500 BU/mL; and age $\leq$ 15-years. The dose of FVIII was 100 IU/kg, and the interval of FVIII administration was three times a week (generally every other day). In a few cases, the dose of FVIII reached approximately 150 IU/kg, depending on the patient's body weight. In this study, ITI was regarded as successful when the inhibitor titer was < 1.0 BU/mL with normal FVIII recovery. Following the infusion of FVIII concentrates, a 30-minute postinfusion recovery was assessed. The predicted FVIII recovery at the 30-minute postinfusion was calculated based on the expectation that 1 IU FVIII/kg body weight would raise plasma FVIII:C by 2%. A ratio of actual to predicted FVIII recovery $\geq$ 0.66 was considered within normal limits.

Immunoprecipitation Assay

A successful outcome after ITI is dependent on the decrease in plasma inhibitor concentration. However, the technical constraints associated with the Bethesda method [27] have limited the investigation of temporal changes in inhibitor properties, such as the ability to bind to specific FVIII regions. By contrast, the immunoprecipitation method measures the radioactivity of antibody-bound radiolabeled FVIII, and is much more sensitive for quantifying the plasma inhibitor concentration [28, 29]. Another advantage of the immunoprecipitation method is that the use of domain fragments allows for the assessment of a domain-specific inhibitor FVIII binding. Furthermore, antibody-bound FVIII is cleared at increased rates [25, 30], making the IP titer more physiologically relevant. However, as all FVIII-binding antibodies do not necessarily neutralize FVIII activity, there may be some discrepancy between the results of the IP method and the Bethesda method. Nevertheless, as described below, results from the Bethesda titer experiments generally paralleled those of the IP titer experiments.

In this study, plasma samples were characterized using the Bethesda assay for the detection of inhibitor antibodies, and using the more sensitive immunoprecipitation assay for all anti-FVIII antibodies, as previously described [31]. As for immunoprecipitation assay, in brief, 7 μg of human recombinant FVIII (kindly donated by Baxter Ltd.) in 20 μL of 0.2 M sodium acetate buffer (pH 6.8) were ^{125}I-labeled using a IODO-Gen Pre-Coated Iodination

Tube (Pierce Biotechnology, Rockford, IL), according to the manufacturer's instruction. Specific radioactivities ranged from 3.4 to 4.8 μCi/μg. Duplicates of 50 μL inhibitor plasma dilutions in 20 mM Tris, 0.15 M NaCl, pH 7.4 (TBS), and 1% bovine serum albumin (BSA) were incubated with 10 μL ^{125}I-labeled FVIII (0.75 nM, final concentration) at 4°C overnight with agitation and for two additional hours after the addition of 100 μL TBS dilution buffer and 50 μL of a suspension of protein G-Sepharose beads (Amersham Biosciences). After washing the beads three times with TBS-0.05% Tween 20, bound radioactivity was quantified in a gamma counter (ARC-380, Aloka, Tokyo, Japan). Background radioactivity without an antibody was 1% to 2%, and maximal binding with the antibody was 60% to 70%. Results were expressed as immunoprecipitation units per milliliter (IPU/mL), using the following formula: 1–(bound/total radioactivity–background)×plasma dilution×16.7.

To characterize the binding region of anti-FVIII, ^{125}I-labeled FVIII light chain (LCh), A2 domain, C2 domain, and whole FVIII were used as the antigens for the immunoprecipitation method. The FVIII LCh was obtained through the thrombin cleavage of FVIII [32]. The A2 subunit was purified from a thrombin-cleaved FVIII heavy chain by fast protein liquid chromatography, as reported previously [33]. Finally, the C2 domain was expressed in a yeast secretion system, as described elsewhere [34].

Although the specific binding of antibodies to A3-C1 domain was not directly examined, the presence or absence of A3-C1-binding antibodies can inferred by considering that FVIII LCh consists of the A3-C1 domain and the C2 domain. We determined the presence of A3-C1-binding antibodies when the IP titer for FVIII LCh is sufficiently larger than that for the C2 domain (LCh IP titer > 2×C2 IP titer at any one time point during ITI).

Inhibitory Antibody and Anti-FVIII Antibody Titers

Patients were categorized into two groups according to ITI outcome ("successful ITI" vs. "unsuccessful ITI") and to three groups based on Bethesda titer during ITI ("low responding" group: peak <5 BU/mL; "high responding" group: peak =5-100 BU/mL; and "ultra-high responding" group: peak > 100 BU/mL). Results from 11 successful cases (8 patients from the pdFVIII group, and 3 patients from the rFVIII group) are summarized in Table 2. Three of the successful patients were classified as ultra-high responders. The Bethesda titer dropped below detectable limits in all but one (Case K) of the successful cases, but the IP titer was negative in only two of the successful cases (Cases C and H). Results from 6 unsuccessful cases (3 patients from the pdFVIII group, and 3 patients from the rFVIII group) are summarized in Table 3. All the unsuccessful cases were classified as high or ultra-high responders.

Representative changes of Bethesda titer and IP titer for the whole FVIII and the regions from 5 successful cases are shown in Figure 4. The change in Bethesda titer tended to parallel the change in IP titer. Specific binding domains varied from case to case, with no one binding domain being predominant. Representative changes of Bethesda titer and IP titer for the whole FVIII and the regions from 3 unsuccessful cases are shown in Figure 5. There was no consistent pattern of change in Bethesda titer or IP titer in these patients; the inhibitor concentration followed a U-shaped curve in some patients and showed a gradual decrease in other patients. Changes in Bethesda titer generally paralleled changes in IP titer, although some patients had significant deviations in IP titers by region (Case L).

Table 2 Alterations of inhibitors in successful patients

Response	FVIII Products	Pt	Weeks after ITI start	BU/mL	IPU/mL Whole FVIII	A2	C2	LCh
Low	pdFVIII	A	0	0	1.8	1.2	0	1.4
			4	0	0.6	0	0	0
		B	0	0	45.6	1.2	0	0
			4	0	8.9	0.7	0	0
			79	0	6.4	0	0	0
		C	-1	1.1	59.1	0	32.8	105
			2	0	2.2	0	0.8	5.1
			10	0	0	0	0	0
	rFVIII	D	-2	5	34.3	NA	NA	NA
			10	0	1.7	NA	NA	NA
			25	0	6.2	0.6	2	1.2
			39	0	21.1	0.8	12.9	13.1
			62	0	10.6	0	4.8	8.1
			76	0	4.1	0	1.2	2.1
			91	0	1.4	NA	NA	NA
High	pdFVIII	E	1	26	11990	824	180	6412
			2	33	4666	728	163	4844
			12	0	77.5	1.6	7.1	57.7
			28	0	228	0.6	25.4	217
		F	1	52	NA	NA	NA	NA
			2	44	3008	1511	0	73.1
			4	23	684	332	0	5.9
			10	1.7	145	45.9	0	2.9
			52	0	3.6	1.4	0	0.4
	rFVIII	G	-9	3	26	42.3	53.5	50.3
			8	56	137	1250	90.7	54
			22	1.6	14	28.3	11.2	8.9
			34	1.9	20	54.9	4.5	12.3
			48	28	234	625	166	193
			62	2.4	46	132	21.6	22.3
			73	0.9	16	51.4	1.4	18.6
			88	NA	NA	4.5	NA	NA
			100	0	1.5	2.6	0	1.4
		H	0	1	85.6	11	30.4	38.7
			2	6	504	27.4	217	245
			7	3	262	21.1	48.9	91.4
			11	0.8	NA	NA	NA	NA
			28	0	17.8	2.4	2.5	8.7
			61	0	0	0	0	0
Ultra high	pdFVIII	I	1	12	1644	0.6	0.6	1866
			3	234	12560	0	5827	16710
			15	0	5.6	0	2.5	25.9
		J	1	284	7890	124	5847	19710
			2	756	19800	162	21850	65900
			4	178	11320	6.2	11007	28560
			30	0	14.1	2.4	31.5	46
			78	0	4.6	0.9	3.4	8
		K	0	2	14.5	0	1.3	13
			2	478	4620	2525	1437	2937
			28	1.4	21.5	19.4	14.9	25.3
			53	2.6	141	52.2	73.9	143.3
			81	0.7	58.7	41.3	3.9	55.6

pdFVIII: plasma-derived factor VIII, rFVIII: recombinant factor VIII

BU: inhibitor titer measured by Bethesda method, IPU: inhibitor titer measured by immunoprecipitation method

A2: IPU for A2 domain, C2: IPU for C2 domain, LCh: IPU for light chain

NA: not assessed

Table 3 Alterations of inhibitors in unsuccessful patients

Response	FVIII Products	Pt	Weeks after ITI start	BU/mL	IPU/mL			
					Whole FVIII	A2	C2	LCh
High	pdFVIII	L	1	49	988	1039	69.2	761
			4	12	266	318	10.9	59.6
			22	31	633	656	0.6	2.7
			26	76	NA	NA	NA	NA
Ultra high	pdFVIII	M	1	NA	9.3	5.2	2.8	6
			2	132	1780	839	278	733
			19	5.7	53.7	40.6	5.2	16.5
			38	27	NA	NA	NA	NA
		N	1	1152	NA	NA	NA	NA
			13	92	8970	15.3	2770	15760
			26	18	2542	7.7	1912	4535
			82	1.8	52.1	0	20.2	53.7
	rFVIII	O	3	103	863	202	77.8	129
			12	114	1203	590	366	1589
			49	78	1158	679	154	1277
			97	31	326	NA	NA	NA
			112	55	533	215	28.2	136
		P	0	149	2382	927	1386	8013
			4	581	10644	2177	894	20365
			54	299	4740	1343	2206	6364
			77	23	731	135	1239	2360
			91	41	1310	500	2113	5194
		Q	-1	13	15442	26580	15843	36842
			2	561	6357	5124	6920	12822
			6	112	1223	591	1993	3393
			29	22	210	12.4	277	536
			81	23	NA	NA	NA	NA

pdFVIII: plasma-derived factor VIII, rFVIII: recombinant factor VIII

BU: inhibitor titer measured by Bethesda method, IPU: inhibitor titer measured by immunoprecipitation method

A2: IPU for A2 domain, C2: IPU for C2 domain, LCh: IPU for light chain

NA: not assessed

In the present study, changes in the time course of antibody titers were generally similar when comparing the different domain-binding antibodies. Further, the type of FVIII product used during ITI generally did not affect the changes in anti-FVIII antibodies. However, there were several exceptions, including: 1) one successful case (Case E) in which IP titers of C2 and LCh remained elevated while the IP titer of A2 decreased; 2) two successful cases (Cases D and H) and one unsuccessful case (Case P) in which the IP titer increased during a certain time period after initiation of ITI; and 3) one unsuccessful case (Case O) in which IP titers of A2 and LCh remained stable while the IP titer of C2 decreased.

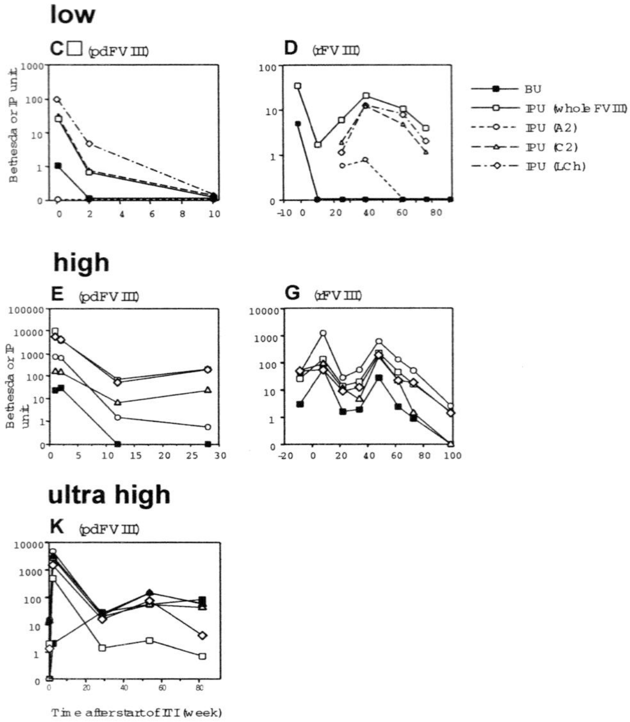

Figure 4. Changes in Bethesda and IP titers for whole FVIII and subunits during ITI: successful cases. Five representative successful cases are shown. Upper panel, low responding group (peak Bethesda titer < 10 BU/mL); middle panel, high responding group (peak Bethesda titer = 10-100 BU/mL); and lower panel, ultra-high responding group (peak Bethesda titer > 100 BU/mL).

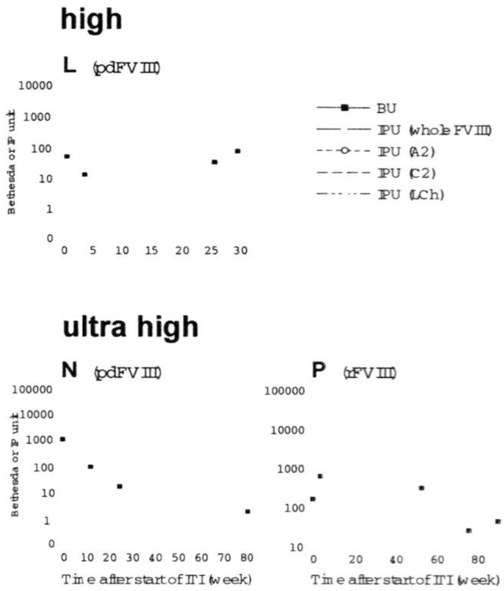

Figure 5. Changes in Bethesda and IP titers for whole FVIII and subunits during ITI: unsuccessful cases. Three representative unsuccessful cases are shown. Upper panel, high responding group (peak Bethesda titer = 10-100 BU/mL); and lower panel, ultra-high responding group (peak Bethesda titer > 100 BU/mL).

Relationship between pre-ITI IP Titer and ITI Outcome

Pre-ITI IP titer was evaluated in 9 of 17 cases. IP titer was significantly lower in the 7 successful cases (1.9 - 90.7 IPU/mL) than in the 2 unsuccessful cases (2,382 - 15,442 IPU/mL). Although limited by the small number of cases, these data suggest that low pre-ITI IP titers are associated with better ITI outcomes (Table 4).

Table 4. IP unit titer before immune tolerance therapy

	Pt	Products	Pre-ITI IP titer*	Weeks after ITI start
Successful	A	pdFVIII	1.9	0
	B	pdFVIII	43.3	0
	C	pdFVIII	59.1	-1
	D	pdFVIII	34.3	-2
	G	rFVIII	26	-9
	H	rFVIII	90.7	0
	K	pdFVIII	14.5	0
		Mean	38.5	
Unsuccessful	P	rFVIII	2382	0
	Q	rFVIII	15442	-1
		Mean	8912	

IP: immunoprecipitation, pdFVIII: plasma-derived factor VIII, rFVIII: recombinant factor VIII
*: IP unit/mL

The present study demonstrated that low pre-ITI IP titer can predict a successful ITI outcome. This is consistent with observations by Mariani et al., who reported that favorable ITI outcomes were dependent on the use of high dose protocols and the presence of low inhibitor titer at enrollment [35]. Meanwhile, DiMichele and colleagues demonstrated that successful ITI outcome parameters were related to ITI peak inhibitor titers and pre-ITI peak inhibitor titers, and were inversely related to total daily dose [36]. Regardless of the discrepancy in some parameters, both of these studies demonstrated that low pre-ITI inhibitor titer is associated with favorable ITI outcomes.

In addition, a higher success rate was observed in patients who underwent ITI with pdFVIII when compared with those who underwent ITI with rFVIII, despite the fact the previous studies suggest that inhibitor formation does not vary with the type of FVIII product [37, 38]. Since the aim of this study was not to clarify the difference of the therapeutic efficiency between rFVIII and pdFVIII in ITI, only the cases in which we could follow inhibitor titer for a certain period were analyzed, and elimination of the cases in which ITI was aborted may account for the higher success rate in the group of patients receiving pdFVIII. Discontinuation of ITI would be associated with failure of therapy.

Specificity of Binding Region

Antibodies from all six cases in the rFVIII group and from more than half of the cases (7 of 11) in the pdFVIII group recognized all three regions (Table 5). Further, antibodies from all six unsuccessful cases and from over half of the successful cases (7 of 11) recognized three regions (Table 6).

Table 5. Comparison of domain specificities of FVIII-binding antibodies

	Domain	pdFVIII (no. of cases)	rFVIII (no. of cases)
1 epitope region	A2, C2, or A3-C1	1	0
2 epitope regions	any combination	3	0
3 epitope regions	A2+C2+A3-C1	7	6
A2	alone or in combination	10	6
C2	alone or in combination	8	6
A3-C1	alone or in combination	10	6

pdFVIII: plasma-derived factor VIII, rFVIII: recombinant factor VIII

Table 6. Comparison of domain specificities of FVIII-binding antibodies

	Domain	Successes (no. of cases)	Failures (no. of cases)
1 epitope region	A2, C2, or A3-C1	1	0
2 epitope regions	any combination	3	0
3 epitope regions	A2+C2+A3-C1	7	6
A2	alone or in combination	10	6
C2	alone or in combination	8	6
A3-C1	alone or in combination	10	6

pdFVIII: plasma-derived factor VIII, rFVIII: recombinant factor VIII

FVIII consists of a sequence of domains, designated as A1-ar1-A2-ar2-B-ar3-A3-C1-C2, where "ar" indicates the acidic regions. The inhibitors that develop in hemophilia A patients typically consist of polyclonal IgG antibodies, particularly IgG_4 [39-41], which bind to the C2 domain and A2 domain [29, 42-48] and sometimes to the A3 domain [49] or to ar3 [50]. Thus, the characterization of antibody titer for these domains will be informative. In the present study, use of rFVIII for ITI resulted in the induction of antibodies against three domains (A2, C2 and A3-C1), while use of pdFVIII resulted in the induction of antibodies with relatively fewer domain-recognizing abilities. Further, antibodies against all three domains were much more frequently detected in patients with whom ITI therapy failed than in patients that developed immune tolerance in response to ITI therapy. Nonetheless, anti-FVIII antibodies from the majority of cases recognized the A2, C2, and A3-C1 domains, regardless of whether response to pdFVIII or to rFVIII or whether the ITI was successful or unsuccessful. This is consistent with previous findings that inhibitors are neutralized by the addition of A2 domain and FVIII LCh that contains the ar3-A3-C1-C2 domains [42].

We hypothesized that for polyclonal inhibitor antibodies to recognize certain binding domains evolve into oligoclonal or even monoclonal antibodies during ITI therapy. However, our results showed that polyclonal inhibitor antibodies do not necessarily converge to oligoclonal or even monoclonal antibodies. Therefore, does T cell receptor (TCR) repertoire alter during ITI? We had performed a cross-sectional T cell receptor (TCR) repertoire analysis in hemophilia patients with or without the inhibitor, and had shown that replacement therapy with a plasma-derived factor VIII concentrates induced skew in T-cell receptor usage and in the clonal expansion of CD8 T cells in HIV-seronegative hemophilia patients [51]. Recently, Misra et al. have reported the skewed TCR repertoire of CD4 T cells in severe hemophilia patients with inhibitors [52]. They also suggest that restricted β variable (BV) gene usage is evident after incubation of CD4 T cells in the presence of FVIII in vitro. Regarding this issue, we have most recently conducted a longitudinal analysis of the TCR repertoire in hemophilia A patients with inhibitor during ITI. This preliminary study included only two inhibitor patients with successful and unsuccessful ITI, but provided the possibility that an alteration profile of TCR repertoire in the early stage of ITI might have an impact on the outcome of ITI (Sakurai et al., unpublished data). Recent studies have revealed that CD4+CD25+FoxP3+ regulatory T cells play a major role in immune tolerance [53]. Further study regarding the relationship between the present results and the TCR repertoire dynamics during ITI or antigens presenting cell-regulatory T cell interactions will be required to better understand the precise mechanisms of ITI.

Conclusion

In this chapter, we discussed alteration of antiidiotypic antibodies and FVIII-binding antibodies with the course of ITI. Regarding antiidiotypic antibodies, we showed that they are present in plasmas from the hemophilia A patients with the inhibitor that underwent ITI whether successful or not, and that the affinity maturation of IgG antiidiotypic antibodies would occur. In addition, through characterization of FVIII-binding antibodies during ITI, we submitted that FVIII-binding antibody-producing clones can persist even after successful ITI. Further study with a strong immunological basis will provide profound insights into the precise mechanisms of ITI.

References

[1] Schwartz RS, Abildgaard CF, Aledort LM, Arkin S, Bloom AL, Brackmann HH, Brettler DB, Fukui H, Hilgartner MW, Inwood MJ, et al.: Human recombinant DNA-derived antihemophilic factor (factor VIII) in the treatment of hemophilia A. recombinant Factor VIII Study Group. *N Engl J Med* 1990, 323:1800-1805.

[2] Bray GL, Gomperts ED, Courter S, Gruppo R, Gordon EM, Manco-Johnson M, Shapiro A, Scheibel E, White G, 3rd, Lee M: A multicenter study of recombinant factor VIII (recombinate): safety, efficacy, and inhibitor risk in previously untreated patients with hemophilia A. The Recombinate Study Group. *Blood* 1994, 83:2428-2435.

[3] Ehrenforth S, Kreuz W, Scharrer I, Linde R, Funk M, Gungor T, Krackhardt B, Kornhuber B: Incidence of development of factor VIII and factor IX inhibitors in haemophiliacs. *Lancet* 1992, 339:594-598.

[4] Kreuz W, Escuriola-Ettingshausen C, Martinez-Saguer I, Kaiml M, Kornhuber B: Epidemiology of inhibitor development in haemophilia A patients treated with virus-inactivated plasma-derived clotting factor concentrates. Vox Sang 1999, 77 Suppl 1:3-8.

[5] Brackmann HH, Gormsen J: Massive factor-VIII infusion in haemophiliac with factor-VIII inhibitor, high responder. *Lancet* 1977, 2:933.

[6] Oldenburg J, Schwaab R, Brackmann HH: Induction of immune tolerance in haemophilia A inhibitor patients by the 'Bonn Protocol': predictive parameter for therapy duration and outcome. Vox Sang 1999, 77 Suppl 1:49-54.

[7] Mauser-Bunschoten EP, Nieuwenhuis HK, Roosendaal G, van den Berg HM: Low-dose immune tolerance induction in hemophilia A patients with inhibitors. *Blood* 1995, 86:983-988.

[8] Van Leeuwen EF, Mauser-Bunschoten EP, Van Dijken PJ, Kok AJ, Sjamsoedin-Visser EJ, Sixma JJ: Disappearance of factor VIII:C antibodies in patients with haemophilia A upon frequent administration of factor VIII in intermediate or low dose. *Br J Haematol* 1986, 64:291-297.

[9] Key NS: Inhibitors in congenital coagulation disorders. *Br J Haematol* 2004, 127:379-391.

[10] White GC, 2nd, Greenwood R, Escobar M, Frelinger JA: Hemophilia factor VIII therapy. Immunological tolerance. A clinical perspective. *Haematologica* 2000, 85:113-116.

[11] Saint-Remy JM: Hemophilia factor VIII therapy. B- and T-cell tolerance: from basic concepts to clinical practice. *Haematologica* 2000, 85:93-96.

[12] Mariani G, Kroner B: Immune tolerance in hemophilia with factor VIII inhibitors: predictors of success. *Haematologica* 2001, 86:1186-1193.

[13] Pelanda R, Schwers S, Sonoda E, Torres RM, Nemazee D, Rajewsky K: Receptor editing in a transgenic mouse model: site, efficiency, and role in B cell tolerance and antibody diversification. *Immunity* 1997, 7:765-775.

[14] Dietrich G, Algiman M, Sultan Y, Nydegger UE, Kazatchkine MD: Origin of anti-idiotypic activity against anti-factor VIII autoantibodies in pools of normal human immunoglobulin G (IVIg). *Blood* 1992, 79:2946-2951.

[15] Gilles JG, Saint-Remy JM: Healthy subjects produce both anti-factor VIII and specific anti-idiotypic antibodies. *J Clin Invest* 1994, 94:1496-1505.

[16] Algiman M, Dietrich G, Nydegger UE, Boieldieu D, Sultan Y, Kazatchkine MD: Natural antibodies to factor VIII (anti-hemophilic factor) in healthy individuals. *Proc Natl Acad Sci U S A* 1992, 89:3795-3799.

[17] Sultan Y, Kazatchkine MD, Maisonneuve P, Nydegger UE: Anti-idiotypic suppression of autoantibodies to factor VIII (antihaemophilic factor) by high-dose intravenous gammaglobulin. *Lancet* 1984, 2:765-768.

[18] Rossi F, Sultan Y, Kazatchkine MD: Anti-idiotypes against autoantibodies and alloantibodies to VIII:C (anti-haemophilic factor) are present in therapeutic polyspecific normal immunoglobulins. *Clin Exp Immunol* 1988, 74:311-316.

[19] Sultan Y, Kazatchkine MD, Nydegger U, Rossi F, Dietrich G, Algiman M: Intravenous immunoglobulin in the treatment of spontaneously acquired factor VIII:C inhibitors. *Am J Med* 1991, 91:35S-39S.

[20] Saint-Remy JM, Jacquemin MG, Gilles JG: Anti-idiotypic antibodies: from regulation to therapy of factor VIII inhibitors. *Vox Sang* 1999, 77 Suppl 1:21-24.

[21] Kazatchkine MD, Lacroix-Desmazes S, Moreau A, Kaveri SV: Idiotypic regulation of anti-factor VIII antibodies. *Haematologica* 2000, 85:97-99.

[22] Gilles JG, Desqueper B, Lenk H, Vermylen J, Saint-Remy JM: Neutralizing antiidiotypic antibodies to factor VIII inhibitors after desensitization in patients with hemophilia A. *J Clin Invest* 1996, 97:1382-1388.

[23] Sakurai Y, Shima M, Tanaka I, Fukuda K, Yoshida K, Yoshioka A: Association of anti-idiotypic antibodies with immune tolerance induction for the treatment of hemophilia A with inhibitors. *Haematologica* 2004, 89:696-703.

[24] Sugishima H, Minoda M: Effect of anti-idiotypic antibody on production of anti-DNA antibodies by splenocytes in lupus prone mice. *Japanese Journal of Allergology* 1991, 40:711-718

[25] Scandella D, Reyes H, Felch M, Sakurai Y: Characterization of antibodies to factor VIII in hemophilia A patients treated by immune tolerance therapy. *Haematologica* 2000, 85:86-88.

[26] Saint-Remy JM, Lacroix-Desmazes S, Oldenburg J: Inhibitors in haemophilia: pathophysiology. *Haemophilia* 2004, 10 Suppl 4:146-151.

[27] Kasper CK, Aledort L, Aronson D, Counts R, Edson JR, van Eys J, Fratantoni J, Green D, Hampton J, Hilgartner M, et al: Proceedings: A more uniform measurement of factor VIII inhibitors. *Thromb Diath Haemorrh* 1975, 34:612.

[28] Scandella D, Mondorf W, Klinge J: The natural history of the immune response to exogenous factor VIII in severe haemophilia A. Haemophilia 1998, 4:546-551.

[29] Scandella D, Mattingly M, Prescott R: A recombinant factor VIII A2 domain polypeptide quantitatively neutralizes human inhibitor antibodies that bind to A2. *Blood* 1993, 82:1767-1775.

[30] Dazzi F, Tison T, Vianello F, Radossi P, Zerbinati P, Carraro P, Poletti A, Girolami A: High incidence of anti-FVIII antibodies against non-coagulant epitopes in haemophilia A patients: a possible role for the half-life of transfused FVIII. *Br J Haematol* 1996, 93:688-693.

[31] Scandella D, DeGraaf Mahoney S, Mattingly M, Roeder D, Timmons L, Fulcher CA: Epitope mapping of human factor VIII inhibitor antibodies by deletion analysis of factor VIII fragments expressed in Escherichia coli. *Proc Natl Acad Sci U S A* 1988, 85:6152-6156.

[32] Fay PJ, Anderson MT, Chavin SI, Marder VJ: The size of human factor VIII heterodimers and the effects produced by thrombin. *Biochim Biophys Acta* 1986, 871:268-278.

[33] Koszelak Rosenblum ME, Schmidt K, Freas J, Mastri M, Fay PJ: Cofactor activities of factor VIIIa and A2 subunit following cleavage of A1 subunit at Arg336. *J Biol Chem* 2002, 277:11664-11669.

[34] Takeshima K, Smith C, Tait J, Fujikawa K: The preparation and phospholipid binding property of the C2 domain of human factor VIII. *Thromb Haemost* 2003, 89:788-794.

[35] Mariani G, Kroner B: International immune tolerance registry, 1997 update. *Vox Sang* 1999, 77 Suppl 1:25-27.

[36] DiMichele DM, Kroner BL: The North American Immune Tolerance Registry: practices, outcomes, outcome predictors. *Thromb Haemost* 2002, 87:52-57.

[37] Scharrer I, Bray GL, Neutzling O: Incidence of inhibitors in haemophilia A patients--a review of recent studies of recombinant and plasma-derived factor VIII concentrates. *Haemophilia* 1999, 5:145-154.

[38] Kreuz W, Ettingshausen CE, Zyschka A, Oldenburg J, Saguer IM, Ehrenforth S, Klingebiel T: Inhibitor development in previously untreated patients with hemophilia A: a prospective long-term follow-up comparing plasma-derived and recombinant products. *Semin Thromb Hemost* 2002, 28:285-290.

[39] Fulcher CA, de Graaf Mahoney S, Zimmerman TS: FVIII inhibitor IgG subclass and FVIII polypeptide specificity determined by immunoblotting. *Blood* 1987, 69:1475-1480.

[40] Shima M, Sawamoto Y, Nakai H, Kamisue S, Murakami T, Morichika S, Tanaka I, Hayashi K, Yoshioka A: Measurement of anti-factor VIII IgG, IgG4 and IgM alloantibodies in previously untreated hemophilia A patients treated with recombinant factor VIII. Kogenate Japanese Clinical Study Group. *Int J Hematol* 1995, 62:35-43.

[41] Gilles JG, Jacquemin MG, Saint-Remy JM: Factor VIII inhibitors. *Thromb Haemost* 1997, 78:641-646.

[42] Scandella D, Mattingly M, de Graaf S, Fulcher CA: Localization of epitopes for human factor VIII inhibitor antibodies by immunoblotting and antibody neutralization. *Blood* 1989, 74:1618-1626.

[43] Fulcher CA, de Graaf Mahoney S, Roberts JR, Kasper CK, Zimmerman TS: Localization of human factor FVIII inhibitor epitopes to two polypeptide fragments. *Proc Natl Acad Sci U S A* 1985, 82:7728-7732.

[44] Shima M, Scandella D, Yoshioka A, Nakai H, Tanaka I, Kamisue S, Terada S, Fukui H: A factor VIII neutralizing monoclonal antibody and a human inhibitor alloantibody recognizing epitopes in the C2 domain inhibit factor VIII binding to von Willebrand factor and to phosphatidylserine. *Thromb Haemost* 1993, 69:240-246.

[45] Suzuki H, Shima M, Arai M, Kagawa K, Fukutake K, Kamisue S, Nakai H, Morichika S, Tanaka I, Inoue M, et al: Factor VIII Ise (R2159C) in a patient with mild hemophilia A, an abnormal factor VIII with retention of function but modification of C2 epitopes. *Thromb Haemost* 1997, 77:862-867.

[46] Sawamoto Y, Shima M, Tanaka I, Nakai H, Kamisue S, Scandella D, Yoshioka A: Anti-factor VIII inhibitor alloantibodies recognizing the A2 domain in the human factor VIII heavy chain poorly bind to porcine factor VIII. *Int J Hematol* 1997, 65:151-158.

[47] Sawamoto Y, Prescott R, Zhong D, Saenko EL, Mauser-Bunschoten E, Peerlinck K, van den Berg M, Scandella D: Dominant C2 domain epitope specificity of inhibitor antibodies elicited by a heat pasteurized product, factor VIII CPS-P, in previously treated hemophilia A patients without inhibitors. *Thromb Haemost* 1998, 79:62-68.

[48] Nogami K, Shima M, Nakai H, Tanaka I, Suzuki H, Morichika S, Shibata M, Saenko EL, Scandella D, Giddings JC, Yoshioka A: Identification of a factor VIII peptide, residues 2315-2330, which neutralizes human factor VIII C2 inhibitor alloantibodies: requirement of Cys2326 and Glu2327 for maximum effect. *Br J Haematol* 1999, 107:196-203.

[49] Fijnvandraat K, Celie PH, Turenhout EA, ten Cate JW, van Mourik JA, Mertens K, Peters M, Voorberg J: A human alloantibody interferes with binding of factor IXa to the factor VIII light chain. *Blood* 1998, 91:2347-2352.

[50] Barrow RT, Healey JF, Gailani D, Scandella D, Lollar P: Reduction of the antigenicity of factor VIII toward complex inhibitory antibody plasmas using multiply-substituted hybrid human/porcine factor VIII molecules. *Blood* 2000, 95:564-568.

[51] Matsutani T, Sakurai Y, Yoshioka T, Tsuruta Y, Suzuki R, Shima M, Yoshioka A: Replacement therapy with plasma-derived factor VIII concentrates induces skew in T-cell receptor usage and clonal expansion of CD8+ T-cell in HIV-seronegative hemophilia patients. *Thromb Haemost* 2003, 90:279-292.

[52] Misra N, Bayry J, Pashov A, Kaveri SV, D'Oiron R, Stieltjes N, Roussel-Robert V, Kazatchkine MD, Boyer O, Lacroix-Desmazes S: Restricted BV gene usage by factor VIII-reactive CD4+ T cells in inhibitor-positive patients with severe hemophilia A. *Thromb Haemost* 2003, 90:813-822.

[53] Sakaguchi S: Naturally arising Foxp3-expressing CD25+CD4+ regulatory T cells in immunological tolerance to self and non-self. *Nat Immunol* 2005, 6:345-352.

In: Immune Tolerance Research Developments
Editor: Emile B. Pontell, pp. 27-49

ISBN: 978-1-60456-209-5

Chapter 2

The CD28:B7 Family Costimulatory Molecules in Allograft Rejection and Tolerance

Guo Lei[1,2*]***, Masatoshi Makuuchi***[2] ***and Shin Enosawa***[1]

[1]Department of Innovative Surgery, National Research Institute for Child Health and Development.

[2]Artificial Organ and Transplantation Division, Department of Surgery, Graduate School of Medicine and Faculty of Medicine, University of Tokyo, Japan

Abstract

Adoptive T cell activation is an essential feature of allograft rejection. Two signal systems are required for T cell full activation, a first signal provided by T-cell receptor ligation and a second signal provided by engagement of co-stimulatory molecules with their respective ligands on antigen-presenting cells. Costimulatory pathways play crucial roles in regulating T cell responses. Recent investigation identifies that the members of the CD28:B7 family of costimulatory pathway play crucial roles in not only initiation of adaptive immune responses, but also regulation of effector lymphocytes. Blockade of costimulatory signals to inhibit T cell activation is thought to be one of promising strategy to prevent graft rejection and facilitate tolerance induction. In vivo, costimulation blockade was indeed shown to allow for long-term allograft survival and facilitate tolerance in several transplantation models. In this review, we summarize the latest developments in the CD28:B7 family costimulatory molecules about their potential interest for acute and chronic allograft rejection and tolerance induction. The role of multiple combination therapies involving blockade of costimulation in induction of long-term allograft survival are discussed.

* Address correspondence to: Guo Lei, MD, PhD. Artificial Organ and Transplantation Division, Department of Surgery, Graduate School of Medicine and Faculty of Medicine, University of Tokyo. 7-3-1 Hongo, Bunkyo-ku, Tokyo, Japan; Tel: +81-3-5800-8654; Fax: +81-3-5684-3989; E-mail; leiguo12@hotmail.com

Introduction

T cell immune responses are initiated following recognition of specific antigen and resultant acquisition of effector function after proliferation and differentiation. This response is orchestrated by the two major pathways of signal transduction and expression of growth factor receptors. Immune responses against alloantigens appear to follow these same rules. Currently, it is generally accepted that two signals are required for an effective T cell response. Signal 1 is delivered following the ligation of the highly polymorphic T cell receptor [1] by peptide/MHC complexes. Signal 2 is delivered by costimulation through non-polymorphic receptors, of which there are two main groups represented by the CD28 and tumor necrosis factor receptor (TNFR) families, both of which have been extensively investigated in recent years.

Combined TCR and costimulatory signaling can induce growth factor production by activated T cells. Two important functions of such growth factors are the promotion of cell-cycle progression and proliferation, and differentiation into effector cells. Blockade of growth factor binding to their receptors significantly reduces alloreactive clonal expansion in vivo and can prevent acute graft rejection [2-4].

On activation, naïve T cells can produce different cytokines, although interleukin-2 (IL-2] predominates. However, later in the response, some T cells differentiate into Th1 or Th2 effector cells which mediate different types of immune responses.[5, 6]. Th1 cells produce interferon-γ (IFN-γ) and tumor necrosis factor-α (TNF-α), whereas Th2 cells secrete IL-4, IL-5, IL-9, IL-10, and IL-13. In addition to effector cytokine expression, Th1 and Th2 cells gain the ability to migrate into inflamed tissues in order to mediate tissue-specific responses. To control cell division by costimulation blockade during an alloimmune response would not only reduce the number of alloreactive T cells but would also limit the differentiation of these cells into effectors, and prevent them from producing the proinflammatory cytokines which mediate immunopathology.

In the transplant setting, blockade of co-stimulatory pathways has proven very effective in inhibiting T cell activation and inducing allograft acceptance and tolerance induction. This review focuses on the co-stimulatory molecules CD28/CTLA-4, ICOS, PD-1 and their ligands B7, ICOS-L and PD-L, respectively, and discusses their potential impact on the effector response and possible mechanisms contributing to allograft acceptance during costimulatory signal blockade.

CD28/CTLA-4:B71/B72 Co-stimulatory Pathways

The CD28:B7 pathway is probably the best investigated co-stimulatory system. It includes CD28 and CTLA-4 which interact with the same two ligands B7.1 [7-9] and B7.2. [10-12].

Characteristic Expression of CD28/CTLA-4 and B7.1/B7.2

CD28 is constitutively expressed by naïve and activated T cells [13], whereas CTLA-4 is not expressed on naïve T cells, but is rapidly up-regulated following activation [14]. CTLA-4 is induced under similar conditions and with similar kinetics following activation of either Th1 or Th2 clones. However, the pattern of expression on these two T cell clons is different because CTLA-4 expression is much higher in Th2 than Th1 clones[1]. CD28 and CTLA-4 competitively bind to the two ligands termed B7.1 and B7.2. B7.2 is constitutively expressed at low levels on APC. B7.1 is absent on resting T cells. After activation, B7.1 and B7.2 are up-regulated but with different kinetics. B7.1 up-regulation is slower and expression remains at a low level, but B7.2 is rapidly up-regulated and expressed at a high level [15]. B7.1 and B7.2 can both bind to their receptors CD28 and CTLA-4 and contribute to positive as well as inhibitory costimulation. Because of their different expression characteristics, B7.2 could be more important for induction of immune responses through interactions with constitutively expressed CD28. In contrast, B7.1 and CTLA-4 are both absent on resting APC and naïve T cells and are up-regulated only after activation. Thus, B7.1 might play a more important role in delivering negative signals[16]

Role in T Cell Activation and Clonal Expansion

The main effects of CD28 signaling are to augment and sustain T cell responses initiated by the antigen-receptor and to promote T cell survival [17], thereby enabling cytokines to initiate T cell clonal expansion and differentiation [18, 19] [20-22]. Ligation of CD28 has been reported to reduce the time necessary for naïve T cells to become activated, as well as to augment the magnitude of response of both naïve and primed T cells [23]. This is consistent with the kinetics of CD28 expression on naïve and activated T cells. Activated T cells require growth factors for cell division, without which they not only fail to divide but also undergo programmed cell death [24, 25]. TCR binding in the absence of CD28 ligation results in either apoptosis or the induction of a state of anergy. Such anergic T cells are incapable of producing IL-2 and proliferating in an autocrine manner. In vitro studies using mixed lymphocyte reactions as a model of alloreactivity in humans have demonstrated that blockade of the B7 pathway using antibody specific for B7.1 and B7.2 or CTLA-4-Ig can prevent T cell activation and result in anergy [26, 27] (compare with blockade of primary MLR with CsA which results only in a delayed secondary response). More potent MLR inhibition was observed with anti-B7.2 than with anti-B7.1, and combining both completely abrogated the alloresponse [28]. The predominant effect of preventing CD28 costimulation using CTLA-4-Ig is to reduce the number of alloreactive naïve T cells recruited into the pool of proliferating cells and to limit the size of the alloreactive effector cell population, whereas their antigen-specific proliferative capacity remains relatively intact. [29]. This finding is consistent with the fact that CD28 costimulation functions to lower the activation threshold of T cells receiving signals through the T cell receptor [30, 31]

CTLA-4 is the higher affinity receptor for B7 [32-34]. CTLA-4 engagement delivers a negative signal, inhibiting TCR- and CD28-mediated signal transduction thereby inhibiting IL-2 synthesis and terminating the T cell response. T cells over-expressing a tailless mutant form of CTLA-4 were defective in their ability to secrete IL-2, survive and proliferate in response to antigen stimulation in vitro [35]. However, it is not completely clear whether CTLA-4-mediated inhibition is due to out-competing CD28 for the same ligands or to direct antagonization of CD28- or TCR-mediated signaling.

Gene-knockout and antibody blocking studies have revealed a critical role for CTLA-4 in maintaining peripheral tolerance. Mice deficient in CTLA-4 display polyclonal T cell activation and a lymphoproliferative disorder that results in neonatal lethality[36, 37]. Blockade of the CD28-B7 pathway with CTLA-4-Ig prolongs the survival of allografts in several vascularized organ transplant models. Recently, a study by Ariyan et al indicated that augmenting CTLA-4 expression can directly promote allograft survival [38].

Role in T Cell Help for Effector Function

CD28 signals promote T cell differentiation towards both Th1 and Th2 subsets via production of the growth factor IL-2. CD28 also optimizes the responses of previously activated T cells, promoting IL-2 production and T cell survival, but is not involved in the effector response[39]. This suggests that Th1 and Th2 effector responses are CD28 independent.

CTLA-4 has been reported to influence the polarization of naïve CD4+ T cells towards the Th1 subset and to inhibit Th2 cell differentiation [40-42]. In contrast, Alegre et al. showed that CTLA-4 stimulation suppresses both Th1 and Th2 cytokine production, and they suggested that CTLA-4 indeed transmits a negative signal irrespective of the Th1 and Th2 status of the cells, leading to a suppression of activity and to a reduced cytokine production. Further, they suggested that CD28-dominated signaling results in a shift to Th1 but not Th2 cytokine production, whereas CTLA-4-dominated signaling skews the response towards Th2 cytokine production [1]. CTLA-4 blockade prevents this Th2 polarization in both priming and effector phases, but Th1 responses can only be inhibited in the early phase [43]. In a Th2-dominant autoimmune disease model, whole anti-CTLA-4 antibody exacerbates the disease with an exaggerated Th2 response, while anti-CTLA-4 Fab ameliorates the disease and engenders a Th1-type response [44]. Similar results have been reported in acute and chronic graft-versus-host disease (GVHD) models, in that early blocking of CD28-B7 T-cell costimulation by CTLA-4-Ig suppresses the development of both acute and chronic GVHD by preventing the activation of donor T cells. Delayed CTLA-4-Ig administration was unable to alter acute GVHD but did reverse chronic GVHD. These results together with others in the literature indicate an important role of CTLA-4 in determining the course of the immune response, and suggest that alloantigen-driven Th1 or Th2 responses are equally susceptible to costimulatory blockade at the onset of disease; however, once effector mechanisms become established, only Th2-driven responses have a requirement for further costimulation [45]. In agreement with that notion, in an allograft transplant model, CTLA-4-Ig treatment was found to inhibit Th1, but to spare Th2 cytokine production [46].

Targeting the CD28:B7 Pathway in Allograft Acceptance and Tolerance

During allograft rejection, B7.2 is strongly expressed on endothelial cells and graft-infiltrating mononuclear cells. In contrast, B7.1 expression is not seen until 72 hours after engraftment [47]. Indeed, either B7.1 and B7.2 alone is sufficient to support vigorous allograft rejection, whereas blocking both molecules, even transiently, greatly prolongs allograft survival. However, consistent with their up-regulation after grafting, antibody blockade of B7.1 appears to be less potent than B7.2.[47-49]

Blocking interactions between CD28 and it ligands using either recombinant fusion proteins or mAb results in the inhibition of a variety of cell-mediated and humoral immune responses including allograft and xenograft rejection [50-59]. Treatment with CTLA-4-Ig significantly prolongs allograft survival and even induces tolerance under conditions where CD28:B7 interactions are preferentially blocked (thereby favoring CTLA-4:B7 interactions) and blockade of CTLA-4 with antibody prevents the prolongation of allograft survival mediated by CTLA-4 [60]. This finding suggests that B7 interactions with CTLA-4 are essential for achieving tolerance even when CD28:B7 interactions are prevented with CTLA-4-Ig. Therefore, a strategy by which the T cell is targeted at the level of the CD28 receptor, rather than targeting its ligands, would theoretically allow the inhibitory consequences of the CTLA-4:B7 interactions to be retained. Anti-CD28 mAb treatment is indeed demonstrated to be effective at preventing acute rejection and prolonging allograft survival in a fully allogeneic rat cardiac transplantation model [61]. A recent study by Dong et al showed that anti-CD28 antibody treatment prevents acute allograft rejection in a major mismatch model, and is as effective as CTLA-4-Ig in protecting against chronic allograft rejection in a minor mismatch model. A synergistic effect of a short course of cyclosporine together with the anti-CD28 antibody was also observed [53]. The actual pathway involved in targeting CD28 is not clear, but the fact that CD28 signaling is essential for the inhibition of acute allograft rejection suggests a possible mechanism. In this model, anti-CD28 mAb transmits a positive signal to the T cells, resulting in the up-regulation of CTLA-4, so that the B7:CTLA-4 interaction can then down-regulate the alloimmune response. This hypothesis was confirmed in a transplant model with CD28-deficient mice, where blockade of the inhibitory CTLA-4 signal results in accelerated allograft rejection [62]. Administration of donor splenocytes has been reported to synergize with CTLA-4-Ig to promote long-term engraftment [63, 64], but this is not the case with anti-CD28 antibody treatment [53]. These data suggest that the mechanisms of action of CD28 targeting with anti-CD28 antibody are different from B7 blockade with CTLA-4-Ig in vivo.

CTLA-4-Ig has been previously reported to prevent the development of chronic rejection or to slow its progression in a partially-mismatched allogeneic transplantation model [65] [66]. Recent data from B7-deficient animals and selective B7 blockade indicate that B7.1 appears to be the critical molecule responsible for progression of chronic allograft vasculopathy, indicating the importance of CD28:B7.1 interactions for its progression [53, 67, 68].

Since the discovery of the cross-regulating Th1 and Th2 phenotypes and the elucidation of the immunoregulatory effects of Th2 in autoimmunity and infectious disease, it has been anticipated that Th1 to Th2 immune deviation may be critical in the acquisition of transplantation tolerance. It is generally accepted that the Th1 differentiation and effector response is responsible for acute allograft rejection. Immunosuppressive agents targeting prevention of Th1 differentiation (such as cyclosporine A) or inhibiting Th1 effector responses (for example, antibody deletion of effector T cells) prevent acute allograft rejection, but do not induce immune tolerance. Immunosuppressive treatment in some animal models often skewed immune activation toward a Th2-dominated response [45, 69], or the manifestation of a Th2 type response during the treatment period [4, 45, 69-71]. Thus, induction of intragraft Th2 cytokine production is thought to be the result of the temporary blockade of acute rejection, eventually leading to an immune tolerant phenotype. However, studies over the last decade have demonstrated that Th1 to Th2 immune deviation does not uniformly permit the acquisition of transplantation tolerance [4, 69, 72]. IL-2-knockout mice do reject allografts, despite a strong expression of IL-4 [73]. Both Th1 and Th2 effector responses can result in allograft rejection. Attempts to induce Th2 cytokine or immune deviation via the application of IL-12 antagonists also failed to induce permanent engraftment or to create a state of allograft tolerance [4]. It is reasonable to conclude that induction of Th2-dominated responses might shift the immune response from acute to chronic allograft rejection.

We have preciously reported that combined treatment with CTLA-4-Ig and anti-ICOS antibody induced allograft tolerance across a major mismatch. In that study, we attempted to induce permanent engraftment or create a state of allograft tolerance through blockade of both CD28:B7 and ICOS:ICOSL pathways with CTLA-4-Ig and anti-ICOS mAb [74]. Although the actual mechanism is not yet clear, blockade of both the CD28:B7 and ICOS:ICOSL pathways indeed induced a state of stable immune tolerance, and prevented chronic rejection. We postulate that the stable immune tolerance induced in this model is caused by simultaneously blocking both Th1 (by CTLA-4-Ig) and Th2 (by anti-ICOS mAb) effector responses as illustrated in Figure 1, which are responsible for acute and chronic rejection respectively.

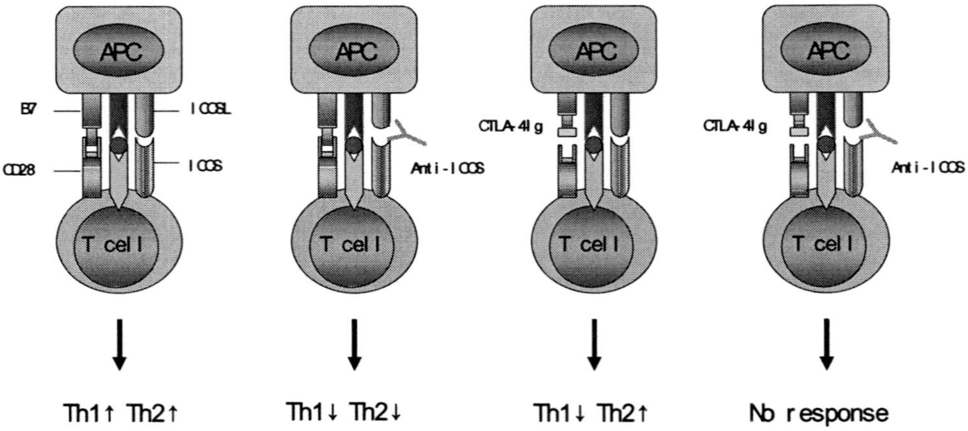

Figure 1. Effect of blockade of costimulation on T cell differentiation following alloantigenic stimulation. Alloantigenic stimuli result in T cell activation and Th1 and Th2 differentiation. Blockade of ICOS signaling with specific antibody partially down-regulates both Th1 and Th2 effector responses; blockade of CD28 signaling with CTLA-4-Ig down-regulates the Th1 effector response but spares the Th2 response. Simultaneous blockade of both signals completely prevents T cell activation and differentiation into effector cells.

Because CTLA-4 has an important role in regulating peripheral T cell tolerance, and inhibiting peripheral T cell proliferation, this makes it a useful tool for regulating immune tolerance in a transplant setting. It has been demonstrated that CTLA-4 expression on CD4+CD25+ regulatory T cells acts to maintain peripheral allograft tolerance [75]. We also reported that combined treatment with CTLA-4-Ig and anti-ICOS antibody induced CD4+CD25+ regulatory T cell development, and suggested that this played a critical role in the maintenance of peripheral tolerance [74].

The ICOS:ICOSL Co-stimulatory Pathway

Recently, an additional CD28-B7-independent costimulatory receptor termed ICOS, and its ligand ICOSL, have been found to instruct further T cell activation and differentiation programs.

Characteristic Expression of ICOS and ICOSL

ICOS is not expressed constitutively on naïve T cells but is induced rapidly after TCR engagement [76-81]. This suggests that ICOS might provide co-stimulatory signals to activated T cells. ICOS expression is influenced by both TCR and CD28 signaling [78-81]. Regulation of ICOS expression is in both a CD28-dependent and independent manner [82]. ICOS is up-regulated on both Th1 and Th2 cells during the initial phase of differentiation, then decreases on Th1 cells, but remains high on Th2 cells, suggesting a role for ICOS in Th2 cell differentiation and function.

Previous studies demonstrated that ICOSL has an interesting expression profile compared to B7. ICOSL is expressed not only by lymphoid tissues and APCs but also non-lymphoid cells, such as fibroblasts and endothelial cells, in heart, lung, lung, kidney and testis, whereas B7 is restricted to lymphoid cells and APCs [83]. Recently, Khayyamin et al reported that ICOSL on human umbilical vein endothelial cells costimulated Th1 and Th2 cytokine production by memory CD4+ T cells stimulated by superantigen, and suggested that it might have an important physiological role in mediating memory/effector T cell responses [84]. The functional significance of ICOSL expression and up-regulation on non-lymphoid cells is not yet clear. Which stimuli are most important for regulating ICOSL expression and which cell types are most important for delivering the ICOSL co-stimulatory signal need further study.

Role in T Cell Activation and Clonal Expansion

Work in the past 5 years using agonistic antibodies, blocking antibodies, or fusion proteins and gene-targeting of animals has revealed ICOS as an essential regulator in T cell activation, differentiation and effector function.

Hutloff and Yoshinaga et al first reported that ICOS signaling could enhance human and mouse T cell proliferation and IL-2 production, although not as potently as CD28 signaling [76, 77]. Furthermore, over-expression of ICOS ligand on tumor cells led to a greater immune response against them [85, 86]. ICOS-deficient mice manifest a proliferation defect after activation which can be rescued by the addition of exogenous IL-2 [87]. Engagement of ICOS, like CD28, can mediate potent costimulation of T cells [76, 85], and promote T cell proliferation at levels similar to those observed after CD28 triggering but without the accompanying increase of IL-2 production [76, 81]. This is consistent with our in vitro data that anti-ICOS antibody completely inhibited T cell proliferation after alloantigenic stimulation [88], and suggests that, at least in vitro, ICOS play a critical and non-dispensable role in T cell activation and proliferation.

Role in T Cell Help for Effector Function

Recent reports suggest that CD28 and ICOS play disparate roles in T cell differentiation, where CD28 signaling is responsible for T cell priming and ICOS signaling for regulating the effector response [89-91]. Th1 cells express lower levels of ICOS compared with Th2 cells. This difference appears to be functionally relevant in regulating effector cell function, suggesting an important role for ICOS in Th2-mediated immune events. ICOS-deficient animals have defects in their ability to produce IL-4, IL-10 and IL-13, but not IFN-γ [87, 92, 93]. This is consistent with in vivo and in vitro studies showing that blocking ICOS decreased IL-4 production, while enhancing IFN-γ production during the priming phase [81, 90]. Blocking ICOS in vivo prevents development of Th2-mediated chronic graft-versus-host disease by decreasing both IL-4 and antibody production [94]. These results suggest that ICOS signaling is critical for production of IL-4, but not IFN-γ. In the absence of ICOS, the Th1-mediated disease EAE is exacerbated by a more robust Th1 response [87]. However, if ICOS is blocked during the effector phase of the disease, Th1-mediated cytokine production is reduced to levels comparable to non-immunized animals [91]. These studies suggest that although ICOS is important for Th2 mediated immune events, in addition it has an important role for regulating Th1 effector functions. Kopf et al also reported that ICOS signaling is important for both Th1 and Th2 responses following pathogenic challenge, and ICOS signaling may compensate for the absence of CD28 [82]. Although blocking either CD28 or ICOS inhibits Th2-mediated mucosal inflammatory infiltration, the timing of the blockade seems to be important for the effect. ICOS appears to be crucial for the effector phase, whereas CD28 is important for the priming phase. There is no effect if CD28 is blocked during the effector phase [90].

Reportedly, the interaction of ICOS and ICOSL on endothelial cells has an important physiological role in the reactivation of memory/effector responses and the control of memory/effector T cell entry into inflamed tissue sites in peripheral areas [83, 84]. This T cell / endothelial cell interaction mediated through ICOS signaling induced morphological polarization of memory and Th1 cells, but not Th2 cells [95], suggesting important physiological roles for ICOS signaling in the regulation of Th1 cells, but not Th2 cells at the endothelium, and the control of the selective entry of Th1 cells into inflamed peripheral tissue [95].

Taken together, current data suggest that ICOS:ICOSL interactions represent an important pathway in T cell activation and differentiation. ICOS signaling is important in both Th1 and Th2 differentiation, although it appears to be more crucial for the latter. In inflamed peripheral tissue, ICOS signaling is also involved in the homing of T cells and the generation of effector T cell responses. Further studies on the contribution of ICOS-mediated migration and polarization during inflammation will provide valuable information for understanding the role of the ICOS/ICOSL pathway in regulating T cell effector functions.

Targeting the ICOS:ICOSL Pathway in Allograft Acceptance and Tolerance

Despite CD28 signaling being critical for allograft rejection, ICOS signaling remains an important mechanism for T cell activation during alloimmune responses, because even in the absence of the former, allografts can still be rejected, strong evidence for the existence of alternative T cell activation pathways [42, 96]. Indeed, in vitro studies, addition of anti-ICOS antibody or ICOS-Ig to the MLR resulted in inhibition of T-cell proliferation, which was more effective with ICOS-Ig plus CTLA4-Ig than with ICOS-Ig alone [88, 97].

Hancock's group first reported the intragraft presence of ICOS+ T cells amongst graft-infiltrating cells and the up-regulation of ICOSL during acute rejection in a murine cardiac transplant model. Blockade of the ICOS pathway with anti-ICOS antibody and/or ICOS-Ig suppressed intragraft T cell activation and cytokine expression [98]. This is consistent with our observations in a rat liver transplant model [88]. In that study, during allograft rejection, graft-infiltrating mononuclear cells were found to express high levels of ICOS. However, anti-ICOS mAb treatment did not completely abrogate mononuclear cell infiltration, but did reduce the number of ICOS+ T cells and prolong allograft survival [88]. Certainly, blocking the ICOS-ICOSL pathway with anti-ICOS monoclonal antibody is less effective for prolonging allograft survival than blocking the CD28-B7 pathway with CTLA-4-Ig. It is postulated that this is due to the failure to inhibit IL-2 production.

In contrast to CD28 signal blockade, ICOS inhibition at different stages of the immune response results in disparate outcomes in some autoimmune models [91, 99]. Similar results were also obtained in a murine vascularized cardiac allograft model, in that in major histocompatibility-mismatched recipients, ICOS blockade prolonged allograft survival both early and following delayed blockade. By contrast, in minor histocompatibility-mismatched recipients early blockade accelerated rejection and delayed blockade prolonged graft survival [96]. It remains unclear whether this discrepancy reflects differences between Th1 and Th2 effector responses triggered by the different target antigens. According to these data, we postulate that a possible mechanism is that with a weak antigen stimulation in minor histocompatibility-mismatched combinations, early blockade of ICOS signaling inhibits Th2 development and skews the response towards a stronger Th1 reaction, which results in the accelerated activation of Th1-mediated allograft rejection. In contrast, blockade delayed until the effector phase directly inhibits Th2 effector function, thus preventing Th2 -mediated allograft rejection, and improving allograft survival. In a major histocompatibility-mismatched combination, because of stronger allostimulation, activated T cells differentiate more readily towards a Th1 effector response. Early blockade of ICOS signaling could limit T cell activation and differentiation to either Th1 or Th2 effectors; delayed blockade of the ICOS signal would directly contribute to the inhibition of Th1 effector function. Data from our own studies and those of others suggest that in major-mismatched recipients, both early and delayed ICOS blockade prolongs allograft survival, although delayed blockade does appear to be more effective [74, 96].

Another important observation is that ICOS signal blockade significantly reduces the development of chronic rejection in cardiac transplantation. Hancock's group first reported that ICOS:B7RP-1 costimulation is required for the development of chronic rejection, because the combination of anti-ICOS therapy and cyclosporin A led to permanent engraftment with no chronic rejection of cardiac allografts. These data imply a key role for the ICOS:B7RP-1 pathway in acute and chronic rejection and highlight the benefits of targeting this pathway in combination with the use of conventional immunosuppressive agents [98]. Later, several published studies showed that combined blocking of ICOS signaling together with other costimulatory pathways, such as CD28:B7 or CD40L:CD40 (with anti-CD40L monoclonal antibody), or using conventional immunosuppressive agents, such as FK506 and Rapamycin, indeed facilitated the long-term acceptance of allografts and even induced stable antigen-specific tolerance in heart, liver and islet transplant models [88, 100-103]. Although the actual mechanism is not clear, anti-ICOS treatment together with FK506 clearly does limit intragraft lymphocyte infiltration.

Four possible mechanisms involving ICOS are thought to be responsible for the prevention of chronic allograft rejection. 1) blocking ICOS signaling directly to inhibit memory/effector T cells which express high ICOS and mediate graft rejection; 2) inhibition of recruitment of lymphocytes (Th1 cells) and migration into the inflamed tissue; 3) prevention of chronic rejection due to the disruption of the interactions between B and T cells, as it was recently confirmed that alloantibody production was significantly decreased by ICOS blockade [96]; 4) direct inhibition of Th2 effectors at suboptimal doses of immunosuppressive agents such as CsA or FK506, which results in less potent TCR signaling and induction of Th2 effector responses [104].

ICOS and CD28 have markedly different costimulatory effects on IL-10 secretion. In contrast to the modest stimulatory capacity of CD28, costimulation by ICOS routinely induced several-fold greater secretion of IL-10 [76], which is an important factor inducing terminal differentiation of B cells into memory cells and antibody-secreting plasma cells. Among T cell co-stimulatory signals, CD40 and ICOS play critical roles in T cell-dependent B cell responses, for which two signals are required for germinal center formation and antibody isotype class switching. The ICOS ligand is constitutively expressed on rat B cells [76], and is down-regulated following antigen-receptor signaling. CD40 signaling can rescue the expression of ICOS. ICOS-deficient mice cannot produce antibody, but stimulating via CD40 rescues antibody production. Indeed, ICOS signaling can itself induce CD40L expression on T cells [76, 93]. These studies illustrate the critical roles of ICOS and CD40 signaling in regulating T-B cell collaboration. In a major-mismatch allograft transplantation model, blockade of CD40-L signaling with anti-CD40-L antibody combined with blockade of ICOS with anti-ICOS antibody or ICOS-Ig prevents chronic allograft rejection and induces immune tolerance. Although the actual mechanism is not clear here either, prevention of chronic rejection by anti-ICOS therapy clearly establishes the importance of this pathway in the progression and development of chronic rejection [98].

PD-1:PD-L1/PD-L2 Pathway

Different from the classical costimulatory molecules CD28/CTLA4 and their ligands B7-1/B7-2, which are critical in the primary activation of naïve T cells, the recently described PD-1/PD-L1 and PD-L2 moieties have been implicated in the regulation of effector T cell function, especially in inflamed peripheral tissue [83].

Characteristic Expression of PD-1 and PD-L

PD-1 was isolated by subtractive hybridization of a T cell hybridoma undergoing programmed cell death. It is expressed by activated, but not by unstimulated T cells, B cells and myeloid cells [105]. Natural killer T cells also express low levels of PD-1 [106].

PD-L1 and PD-L2, the ligands of PD-1, are expressed on both lymphocytes and in non-lymphoid organs [107-109]. In humans, PD-L1 and PD-L2 are up-regulated upon activation or IFN-γ treatment of monocytes or dendritic cells [107-110]. Human and murine T cells also express PD-L1 after TCR or mitogenic stimulation, whereas PD-L2 was not detected or was only marginally expressed after stimulation [108]. Immunohistochemistry showed that human endothelial cells in the myocardium and the cardiomyocytes themselves also express PD-L1. It is expressed constitutively on the surface of a microvascular endothelial cell line and is strongly upregulated by IFN-α, β and γ [111]. This suggests that PD-L1 might play a more general role in down-regulating activated T cells in the periphery. PD-L1 and PD-L2 are also expressed on a variety of tumor cells [109]. PD-L2 expression is much more restricted and can be highly up-regulated by IL-4 only on inflammatory macrophages, whereas PD-L1 is easily inducible on a number of different cell types [112]. The differential expression of PD-L1 and PD-L2 suggests differential contributions of these two ligands to PD-1-mediated immune regulation in vivo.

In a cardiac allograft transplant setting, alloresponses initiated by the graft up-regulated both PD-1 and its ligands PD-L1 and PD-L2 during rejection. PD-1 and PD-L1 were readily detectable on infiltrating leukocytes, whereas PD-L2 staining was somewhat more restricted with regard to the numbers of mononuclear cells stained. Immunosuppression (high dose) with CsA and rapamycin decreased the intragraft expression of these three molecules. Anti-154 mAb with or without DST suppressed intragraft expression of PD-1 and PD-L2 completely, and markedly decreased PD-L1. Anti-ICOS mAb administration also resulted in suppression of PD-1 and nearly complete suppression of PD-L1 expression [113].

Role in T Cell Activation and Clonal Expansion

Studies on PD-1-deficient mice provided direct evidence for an important role of PD-1 as a negative regulator of immune responses in vivo for the maintenance of peripheral tolerance and prevention of autoimmunity [114, 115]. PD-1-deficient mice develop splenomegaly and autoimmunity in the form of arthritis, nephritis, or cardiomyopathy [114, 115], which is consistent with it's expression pattern. Therefore, it has been suggested that the PD-1 pathway may serve as an important regulator of peripheral tolerance [116].

Both PD-1:PD-L1 and PD-1:PD-L2 signals inhibit T cell proliferation by blocking cell cycle progression but not by increasing cell death. PD-L2 appeared to be slightly less potent than PD-L1 at inhibition [109]. PD-1 signals can antagonize TCR-CD28 signals depending on the strength of the TCR signal. PD-1 signals inhibit T cell activation in part by reducing IL-2 and other cytokines at the level of mRNA synthesis [109]. CD8+ T cells appear to be more sensitive to this effect than CD4+ T cells [117].

In in vitro studies, at low antigen concentrations, engagement of PD-1 by PD-L1 and PD-L2 inhibited proliferation of T cells previously activated via the TCR and reduced the production of cytokines such as IFN-γ, IL-10, IL-4, and IL-2. By contrast, at high antigen concentrations, PD-L1 and PD-L2 failed to inhibit T cell proliferation but markedly reduced cytokine production [107, 109].

Although the autoimmune phenotype of PD-1-deficient mice, as well as other in vitro data, suggest that the PD-1 pathway is inhibitory, conflicting data on its role do exist. Some studies have indicated that PD-1 can enhance T cell proliferation and IL-10 production [108, 118], and that PD-L2 can promote proliferation of naïve T cells and Th1 cytokine production [110]. Three possible explanations may be suggested to explain these disparate data: 1) there might be a second receptor for PD-1 ligands with the capacity to deliver a stimulatory signal; 2) PD-1 might act to transmit a positive signal to naïve T cells but a negative signal to resting and activated T cells; 3) PD-L1 and PD-L2 ligands might deliver different signals to their receptor PD-1 according to their relative abundance, for instance, positive signals from PD-L1 interactions, but negative from PD-L2. A recent study by Takanori seems to support this explanation. They demonstrated a differential effect on PD-1 signal blockade. Anti-PD-L1 antibody treatment prevented the development of experimental colitis associated with decreased expansion of pathogenic T cells and down-regulated Th1 cytokine production (IFN-γ, IL-2 and TNF-α), whereas, in contrast, anti-PDL-2 mAb augmented the disease [119].

Role in T Cell Help for Effector Function

Loke et al has reported that PD-L1 and PD-L2 might have different roles in regulating type (Th1) and type (Th2) responses in the periphery[112]. They found that Th1 cells induced expression of PD-L1 whereas Th2 induced PD-L2 on activated macrophages. They also suggested a possible positive feedback loop (higher PD-L1 levels on macrophages preferentially stimulate Th1 and inhibit Th2 cell function) and a negative feedback loop (PD-L1 inhibits Th1 and stimulates Th2 function). This might be an explanation for the disparate results on PD-1 function reported by different groups.

In an asthma model, which is driven by a Th2 response, Ezogelin et al reported that Th2 cytokines specifically induced PD-L2 expression on BM-DC while other B7 family members such as CD80 and CD86 were not affected, and therefore suggested that PD-L2 induction is specific to Th2-polarized immune responses. This study thus indicates a potential role for PD-L2 in Th2-mediated disease [120]. In a study on a Th1-dependent experimental autoimmune encephalomyelitis (EAE) model, Salama et al showed that the PD-1 costimulatory pathway plays a critical role in regulating peripheral tolerance in murine EAE and appears to be a major contributor to disease induction resistance in CD28-deficient mice. PD-1 and PD-L1 but not PD-L2 expression was up-regulated within the central nervous system in EAE after immunization. PD-1 blockade resulted in disease augmentation with an accelerated lymphocyte infiltration of the central nervous system by an increased frequency of IFN-γ-producing T cells, increased delayed-type hypersensitivity responses, and higher serum levels of antibody [121]. Taken together, the available data on the PD-1 signaling pathway in animal models of autoimmune disease create the strong impression that PD-1:PD-L1 interactions facilitate the development of Th1 responses, whereas, in contrast, PD-1:PD-L2 interactions skew T cell differentiation towards Th2 responses.

CD4+CD25+ regulatory T cells inhibit CD4+CD25- T cell proliferation and IFN-γ and IL-13 production in response to anti-CD3 plus anti-CD28 antibody and accessory cells. This inhibitory effect is prevented by blocking with anti-PD-L1 monoclonal antibody, although CD4+CD25+ regulatory T cells do not constitutively express PD-L1[122]. These results thus suggest that the PD-1:PD-L1 pathway might nonetheless have a role in the function CD4+CD25+ regulatory T cells. PD-L1 expression on non-lymphoid tissues and its potential interaction with PD-1 may subsequently determine the extent of immune responses at sites of inflammation. Nancy et al reported that PD-L1 is expressed on IFN-γ-stimulated cultured human and mouse endothelial cells, while PD-L2 was found on stimulated human but not mouse endothelial cells. Expression was further up-regulated by TNF-α. Antibody blockade of mouse endothelial cell PD-L1 enhanced both IFN-γ secretion and cytolytic activity of CD8+ T cells in response to endothelial cell antigen presentation. These results demonstrated that IFN-α-activated endothelial cells can also inhibit T cell activation via expression of immunoinhibitory PD-L1 and PD-L2 molecules [123].

Targeting the PD-1:PD-L1/PD-L2 Pathways in Allograft Acceptance and Tolerance

Hancock's group recently reported that targeting the PD-1:PD-L1 pathway using PD-L1-Ig and PD-L2-Ig fusion proteins can promote allograft survival. Although neither PD-L1-Ig nor PD-L2-Ig prolong cardiac allograft survival alone, a synergistic effect was obtained when PD-L1-Ig (but not PD-L2-Ig) was combined with a suboptimal dose of CsA. PD-L1-Ig synergy with rapamycin induced permanent engraftment. Combined PD-L1-Ig and CsA treatment suppressed both IFN-γ production and that of IFN-γ- induced chemokines and their receptors, but provided no evidence of immune deviation such as up-regulation of intragraft IL-4 and IL-10 expression. Moreover, supplementing CTLA-4 mAb therapy with PD-L1-Ig administration suppressed development of transplant arteriosclerosis and other hallmarks of chronic rejection in long-surviving cardiac allografts [113]. In agreement with these data, Gao et al also reported a synergistic effect of PD-L1-Ig plus anti-CTLA-4 mAb in an islet allograft transplant model [124].

There is growing evidence that PD-L1 expression contributes to the maintenance of host unresponsiveness in the periphery as well as at sites of inflammation [113, 121, 125, 126]. Blockade of the MCP-1/CCR2 pathway together with rapamycin therapy prolonged islet allograft survival, associated with infiltration by mononuclear cells expressing PD-1; accordingly, anti-PD-L1 mAb abrogated prolongation of islet allograft survival [127]. These data imply that the PD-1:PD-L1 pathway might be involved in the induction and maintenance of long-term allograft acceptance.

Induction of regulatory cells for allograft acceptance is a critically important mechanism. In vitro studies by Niimi's group showed that the PD-1:PD-L1 interaction was involved in the induction of proliferative hyporesponsiveness to donor alloantigen, the enhancement of IL-10 production, and the suppression of IFN-γ production by recipient T cells after intratracheal delivery of donor splenocytes. In agreement with the in vitro data, they also showed that PD-1 blockade with anti-PD-1 or anti-PD-L1 prevents tolerance induction in a murine cardiac allograft model, whereas anti-PD-L2 had no effect. They therefore suggested that PD-1:PD-L1 interactions might be preferentially involved in regulatory cell induction in this tolerance induction model. [128].

In summary, the PD-1:PD-L1 pathway has a profound effect on inhibition of T cell alloreactivity, and when combined with other costimulatory signal modulation approaches or conventional immunosuppression could significantly prolong allograft survival and even prevent chronic rejection, inducing long-term allograft acceptance. Although the actual mechanisms for this effect remain unclear, together with their inducibility and-widespread expression pattern, members of the PD-1 system might be involved in attenuation of inflammatory responses in peripheral tissues. Further characterization of this pathway would provide novel avenues for manipulation of cell-mediated immune responses in cancer, autoimmune diseases, viral infection, and transplant rejection.

Conclusion

The potential of costimulatory blockade for allograft acceptance opens a new therapeutic avenue for clinical transplantation. However, targeting of individual co-stimulatory interactions is unlikely to be sufficient for complete abrogation of T cell alloactivation; therefore, combination therapy may be more attractive as a therapeutic strategy. It is now becoming clear that these costimulatory pathways are intimately linked to one another. For example, ICOS up-regulation by T cells is reduced in the absence of B7, but is restored following CD28 stimulation [81], whereas CTLA-4 ligation blocks ICOS costimulation [129]. Moreover, ICOS signaling is dependent on the CD40L:CD40 pathway for its function in immunoglobulin class switching [93]. Therefore, it is important to clarify the interactions between the different pathways, and the phenotypic and functional changes not only of T cells but also APC.

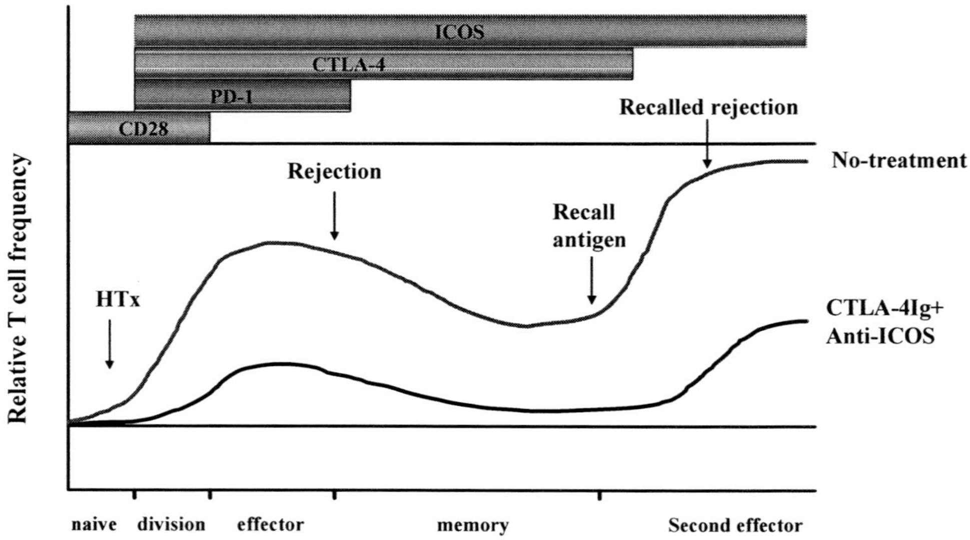

Figure 2. A possible model of how CD28 family members regulate the priming of T cells and the development of the effector response and memory after allostimulation. CD28 signaling contributes to naïve T cell activation and division, followed by up-regulation of CTLA-4, ICOS and PD-1 expression, which are involved in the effector response and memory T cell development. Recall antigen stimuli result in a rapid increase in T cell number which appears to be at least partially dependent on ICOS signaling. Simultaneous blockade of both co-stimulatory signals, CD28 and ICOS, in the early phase of transplantation, inhibits T cell activation and development of effector/memory T cells, and results in a markedly reduced frequency of secondary effector T cells during secondary responses to recall antigen.

Over the past few years, studies on the CD28:B7 superfamily have made it clear that they have a critical role in naïve T cell activation, promoting clonal expansion and differentiation into effector cells. Co-stimulation can simply promote more efficient engagement of TCR molecules to enhance the initial activation, or induce effector functions, such as cytokine secretion, cytotoxicity or help for antibody production. They might also be crucial for the generation and maintenance of T cell memory. Certainly, on the basis of the available data, a possible model of how CD28:B7 pathway superfamily interactions regulate the priming of T cells and the development of T cell memory can be put forward as depicted in Figure 2. CD28 potentates initial T cell clonal expansion and growth factor production, whereas ICOS and PD-1 signaling participate in effector function. Constitutive ICOS expression on memory T cells suggests that it might be important for secondary effector function. Many questions remain, including the true contributions of CTLA-4 and CD28 blockade to tolerance induction and maintenance. How ICOS and PD-1 signaling are involved in the effector phase, and whether they also contribute to maintaining the reactivity of effector T cells by constitutively providing survival signaling requires further investigation. More in-depth studies are required to differentiate between effects on cell survival versus proliferation and the time of action of novel ICOS and PD-1 signaling pathways. Finally, animal transplant models, using gene-deficient mice or specific monoclonal antibody blockade will be helpful to dissect which molecules are therapeutically relevant and will be crucial for clinical success.

References

[1] Alegre ML, Shiels H, Thompson CB, Gajewski TF. (1998). Expression and function of CTLA-4 in Th1 and Th2 cells. *J Immunol*, 161, 3347-3356.

[2] Brazelton TR, Morris RE. Molecular mechanisms of action of new xenobiotic immunosuppressive drugs: tacrolimus (FK506), sirolimus (rapamycin), mycophenolate mofetil and leflunomide. (1996). *Curr Opin Immunol*, 8, 710-720.

[3] Li XC, Demirci G, Ferrari-Lacraz S, Groves C, Coyle A, Malek TR, et al. IL-15 and IL-2: a matter of life and death for T cells in vivo. (2001). *Nat Med,* 7, 114-8.

[4] Li XC, Zand MS, Li Y, Zheng XX, Strom TB. (1998). On histocompatibility barriers, Th1 to Th2 immune deviation, and the nature of the allograft responses. *J Immunol*, 161, 2241-2247.

[5] Murphy KM, Reiner SL. (2002). The lineage decisions of helper T cells. *Nat Rev Immunol,* 2, 933-944.

[6] Openshaw P, Murphy EE, Hosken NA, Maino V, Davis K, Murphy K, et al. (1995). Heterogeneity of intracellular cytokine synthesis at the single-cell level in polarized T helper 1 and T helper 2 populations. *J Exp Med,* 182, 1357-1367.

[7] Freeman GJ, Gray GS, Gimmi CD, Lombard DB, Zhou LJ, White M, et al. (1991). Structure, expression, and T cell costimulatory activity of the murine homologue of the human B lymphocyte activation antigen B7. *J Exp Med,* 174, 625-31.

[8] Freedman AS, Freeman G, Horowitz JC, Daley J, Nadler LM. (1987). B7, a B-cell-restricted antigen that identifies preactivated B cells. *J Immunol*, 139, 3260-3267.

[9] Yokochi T, Holly RD, Clark EA. (1982). B lymphoblast antigen (BB-1) expressed on Epstein-Barr virus-activated B cell blasts, B lymphoblastoid cell lines, and Burkitt's lymphomas. *J Immunol,* 128, 823-827.

[10] Freeman GJ, Gribben JG, Boussiotis VA, Ng JW, Restivo VA Jr, Lombard LA, et al. (1993). Cloning of B7-2: a CTLA-4 counter-receptor that costimulates human T cell proliferation. *Science*, 262, 909-911.

[11] Freeman GJ, Borriello F, Hodes RJ, Reiser H, Gribben JG, Ng JW, et al. (1993). Murine B7-2, an alternative CTLA4 counter-receptor that costimulates T cell proliferation and interleukin 2 production. *J Exp Med*, 178, 2185-2192.

[12] Azuma M, Ito D, Yagita H, Okumura K, Phillips JH, Lanier LL, et al. (1993). B70 antigen is a second ligand for CTLA-4 and CD28. *Nature*, 366, 76-79.

[13] Gross JA, Callas E, Allison JP. (1992). Identification and distribution of the costimulatory receptor CD28 in the mouse. *J Immunol*, 149, 380-388.

[14] Linsley PS, Bradshaw J, Greene J, Peach R, Bennett KL, Mittler RS. (1996). Intracellular trafficking of CTLA-4 and focal localization towards sites of TCR engagement. *Immunity*, 4, 535-543.

[15] McAdam AJ, Schweitzer AN, Sharpe AH. (1998). The role of B7 co-stimulation in activation and differentiation of CD4+ and CD8+ T cells. *Immunol Rev*, 165, 231-247.

[16] Chitnis T, Najafian N, Abdallah KA, Dong V, Yagita H, Sayegh MH, et al. (2001). CD28-independent induction of experimental autoimmune encephalomyelitis. *J Clin Invest*, 107, 575-583.

[17] Boise LH, Gonzalez-Garcia M, Postema CE, Ding L, Lindsten T, Turka LA, et al. (1993). bcl-x, a bcl-2-related gene that functions as a dominant regulator of apoptotic cell death. *Cell*, 74, 597-608.

[18] Thompson CB, Lindsten T, Ledbetter JA, Kunkel SL, Young HA, Emerson SG, et al. (1989). CD28 activation pathway regulates the production of multiple T-cell-derived lymphokines/cytokines. *Proc Natl Acad Sci U S A*, 86, 1333-1337.

[19] Lucas PJ, Negishi I, Nakayama K, Fields LE, Loh DY. (1995). Naive CD28-deficient T cells can initiate but not sustain an in vitro antigen-specific immune response. *J Immunol,* 154, 5757-5768.

[20] Shahinian A, Pfeffer K, Lee KP, Kundig TM, Kishihara K, Wakeham A, et al. (1993). Differential T cell costimulatory requirements in CD28-deficient mice. *Science*, 261, 609-612.

[21] Sperling AI, Auger JA, Ehst BD, Rulifson IC, Thompson CB, Bluestone JA. (1996). CD28/B7 interactions deliver a unique signal to naive T cells that regulates cell survival but not early proliferation. *J Immunol*, 157, 3909-3917.

[22] Boise LH, Minn AJ, Noel PJ, June CH, Accavitti MA, Lindsten T, et al. (1995). CD28 costimulation can promote T cell survival by enhancing the expression of Bcl-XL. *Immunity*, 3, 87-98.

[23] Iezzi G, Karjalainen K, Lanzavecchia A. (1998). The duration of antigenic stimulation determines the fate of naive and effector T cells. *Immunity*, 8, 89-95.

[24] Van Parijs L, Ibraghimov A, Abbas AK. (1996). The roles of costimulation and Fas in T cell apoptosis and peripheral tolerance. *Immunity*, 4, 321-28.

[25] Van Parijs L, Biuckians A, Abbas AK. (1998). Functional roles of Fas and Bcl-2-regulated apoptosis of T lymphocytes. *J Immunol,* 160, 2065-2071.

[26] Van Gool SW, Vermeiren J, Rafiq K, Lorr K, de Boer M, Ceuppens JL. (1999). Blocking CD40 - CD154 and CD80/CD86 - CD28 interactions during primary allogeneic stimulation results in T cell anergy and high IL-10 production. *Eur J Immunol*, 29, 2367-2375.

[27] Koenen HJ, Joosten I. (2000). Blockade of CD86 and CD40 induces alloantigen-specific immunoregulatory T cells that remain anergic even after reversal of hyporesponsiveness. *Blood*, 95, 3153-3161.

[28] Jonker M, Ossevoort, Ma, Vierboom M. (2002). Blocking the CD80 and CD86 costimulation molecules: lessons to be learned from animal models. *Transplantation,* 73, S23-26.

[29] Wells AD. (2003). Cell-cycle regulation of T-cell responses--novel approaches to the control of alloimmunity. *Immunol Rev*, 196, 25-36.

[30] Wells AD, Gudmundsdottir H, Turka LA. (1997). Following the fate of individual T cells throughout activation and clonal expansion. Signals from T cell receptor and CD28 differentially regulate the induction and duration of a proliferative response. *J Clin Invest,* 100, 3173-3183.

[31] Viola A, Lanzavecchia A. (1996). T cell activation determined by T cell receptor number and tunable thresholds. *Science*, 273, 104-106.

[32] Peach RJ, Bajorath J, Brady W, Leytze G, Greene J, Naemura J, et al. (1994). Complementarity determining region 1 (CDR1)- and CDR3-analogous regions in CTLA-4 and CD28 determine the binding to B7-1. *J Exp Med*, 180, 2049-2058.

[33] Linsley PS, Greene JL, Tan P, Bradshaw J, Ledbetter JA, Anasetti C, et al. (1992). Coexpression and functional cooperation of CTLA-4 and CD28 on activated T lymphocytes. *J Exp Med*, 176, 1595-1604.

[34] Linsley PS, Greene JL, Brady W, Bajorath J, Ledbetter JA, Peach R. (1994). Human B7-1 (CD80) and B7-2 (CD86) bind with similar avidities but distinct kinetics to CD28 and CTLA-4 receptors. *Immunity*, 1, 793-801.

[35] Mao Y, Brigham D, Chen D. (2004). Overexpression of a mutant CTLA4 inhibits T-cell activation and homeostasis-driven expansion. *Exp Hematol*, 32, 735-747.

[36] Chambers CA, Kuhns MS, Egen JG, Allison JP. (2001). CTLA-4-mediated inhibition in regulation of T cell responses: mechanisms and manipulation in tumor immunotherapy. *Annu Rev Immunol,* 19, 565-594.

[37] Sharpe AH, Freeman GJ. (2002). The B7-CD28 superfamily. *Nat Rev Immunol*, 2, 116-126.

[38] Ariyan C, Salvalaggio P, Fecteau S, Deng S, Rogozinski L, Mandelbrot D, et al. (2003). Cutting edge: transplantation tolerance through enhanced CTLA-4 expression. *J Immunol*, 171, 5673-5677.

[39] Alegre ML, Frauwirth KA, Thompson CB. (2001). T-cell regulation by CD28 and CTLA-4. *Nat Rev Immunol*, 1, 220-228.

[40] Chan BM, Zheng H, Wang H, Uniyal S, Garcia B, Wang J, et al. (1998). Treatment of cardiac allografts with established leukocyte infiltration by modulation of alpha4 (CD49d) and leukocyte function-associated antigen-1 (CD11a/CD18) integrin function. *Transplantation*, 66, 277-283.

[41] Kato T, Nariuchi H. (2000). Polarization of naive CD4+ T cells toward the Th1 subset by CTLA-4 costimulation. *J Immunol,* 164, 3554-3562.

[42] Kawai K, Shahinian A, Mak TW, Ohashi PS. (1996). Skin allograft rejection in CD28-deficient mice. *Transplantation*, 61, 352-355.

[43] Via CS, Rus V, Nguyen P, Linsley P, Gause WC. (1996). Differential effect of CTLA4Ig on murine graft-versus-host disease (GVHD) development: CTLA4Ig prevents both acute and chronic GVHD development but reverses only chronic GVHD. *J Immunol*, 157, 4258-4267.

[44] Saha B, Chattopadhyay S, Germond R, Harlan DM, Perrin PJ. (1998). CTLA4 (CD152) modulates the Th subset response and alters the course of experimental Leishmania major infection. *Eur J Immunol*, 28, 4213-4220.

[45] Chen N, Gao Q, Field EH. (1996). Prevention of Th1 response is critical for tolerance. *Transplantation*, 61, 1076-1083.

[46] Akalin E, Chandraker A, Russell ME, Turka LA, Hancock WW, Sayegh MH. (1996). CD28-B7 T cell costimulatory blockade by CTLA4Ig in the rat renal allograft model: inhibition of cell-mediated and humoral immune responses in vivo. *Transplantation*, 62, 1942-1945.

[47] Hancock WW, Sayegh MH, Zheng XG, Peach R, Linsley PS, Turka LA. (1996). Costimulatory function and expression of CD40 ligand, CD80, and CD86 in vascularized murine cardiac allograft rejection. *Proc Natl Acad Sci U S A*, 93, 13967-13972.

[48] Zheng XX, Sayegh MH, Zheng XG, Li Y, Linsley PS, Peach R, et al. (1997). The role of donor and recipient B7-1 (CD80) in allograft rejection. *J Immunol*, 159, 1169-1173.

[49] Lenschow DJ, Zeng Y, Hathcock KS, Zuckerman LA, Freeman G, Thistlethwaite JR, et al. (1995). Inhibition of transplant rejection following treatment with anti-B7-2 and anti-B7-1 antibodies. *Transplantation*, 60, 1171-1178.

[50] Chiffoleau E, Beriou G, Dutartre P, Usal C, Soulillou JP, Cuturi MC. (2002). Induction of donor-specific allograft tolerance by short-term treatment with LF15-0195 after transplantation. Evidence for a direct effect on T-cell differentiation. *Am J Transplant*, 2, 745-757.

[51] Vanhove B, Laflamme G, Coulon F, Mougin M, Vusio P, Haspot F, et al. (2003). Selective blockade of CD28 and not CTLA-4 with a single-chain Fv-alpha1-antitrypsin fusion antibody. *Blood*, 102, 564-570.

[52] Rifle G, Mousson C. (2002). Dendritic cells and second signal blockade: a step toward allograft tolerance? *Transplantation*, 73, S1-2.

[53] Dong VM, Yuan X, Coito AJ, Waaga AM, Sayegh MH, Chandraker A. (2002). Mechanisms of targeting CD28 by a signaling monoclonal antibody in acute and chronic allograft rejection. *Transplantation*, 73, 1310-1317.

[54] Xiao Y, Zhu Y, Chen L, Wang S, He X. (1999). CD28/B7-mediated costimulation is required for parathyroid gland allograft rejection in rats. Chin Med Sci J, 14, 158-162.

[55] Wilson JL, Proud G, Forsythe JL, Taylor RM, Kirby JA. (1995). Renal allograft rejection. Tubular epithelial cells present alloantigen in the presence of costimulatory CD28 antibody. *Transplantation*, 59, 91-97.

[56] Guo L, Li X, Enosawa S, Harihara Y, Funeshima N, Kimura H, et al. (2003). Prolongation of liver xenograft survival by adenovirus vector-mediated CTLA-4Ig gene transfer. *Transpl Immunol*, 11, 155-162.

[57] Costa C, Pizzolato MC, Shen Y, Wang Y, Fodor WL. (2004). CD86 blockade in genetically modified porcine cells delays xenograft rejection by inhibiting T-cell and NK-cell activation. *Cell Transplant*, 13, 75-87.

[58] Benda B, Ljunggren HG, Peach R, Sandberg JO, Korsgren O. (2002). Co-stimulatory molecules in islet xenotransplantation: CTLA4Ig treatment in CD40 ligand-deficient mice. *Cell Transplant*, 11, 715-720.

[59] Feng S, Quickel RR, Hollister-Lock J, McLeod M, Bonner-Weir S, Mulligan RC, et al. (1999). Prolonged xenograft survival of islets infected with small doses of adenovirus expressing CTLA4Ig. *Transplantation*, 67, 1607-1613.

[60] Judge TA, Wu Z, Zheng XG, Sharpe AH, Sayegh MH, Turka LA. (1999). The role of CD80, CD86, and CTLA4 in alloimmune responses and the induction of long-term allograft survival. *J Immunol*. 162, 1947-1951.

[61] Dengler TJ, Szabo G, Sido B, Nottmeyer W, Zimmerman R, Vahl CF, et al. (1999). Prolonged allograft survival but no tolerance induction by modulating CD28 antibody JJ319 after high-responder rat heart transplantation. *Transplantation*, 67, 392-398.

[62] Greenwald RJ, Boussiotis VA, Lorsbach RB, Abbas AK, Sharpe AH. (2001). CTLA-4 regulates induction of anergy in vivo. *Immunity*, 14, 145-155.

[63] Lin H, Bolling SF, Linsley PS, Wei RQ, Gordon D, Thompson CB, et al. (1993). Long-term acceptance of major histocompatibility complex mismatched cardiac allografts induced by CTLA4Ig plus donor-specific transfusion. *J Exp Med*, 178, 1801-1806.

[64] Pearson TC, Alexander DZ, Hendrix R, Elwood ET, Linsley PS, Winn KJ, et al. (1996). CTLA4-Ig plus bone marrow induces long-term allograft survival and donor specific unresponsiveness in the murine model. Evidence for hematopoietic chimerism. *Transplantation*, 61, 997-1004.

[65] Azuma H, Chandraker A, Nadeau K, Hancock WW, Carpenter CB, Tilney NL, et al. (1996). Blockade of T-cell costimulation prevents development of experimental chronic renal allograft rejection. *Proc Natl Acad Sci U S A*, 93, 12439-12444.

[66] Russell ME, Hancock WW, Akalin E, Wallace AF, Glysing-Jensen T, Willett TA, et al. (1996). Chronic cardiac rejection in the LEW to F344 rat model. Blockade of CD28-B7 costimulation by CTLA4Ig modulates T cell and macrophage activation and attenuates arteriosclerosis. *J Clin Invest*, 97, 833-838.

[67] Kim KS, Denton MD, Chandraker A, Knoflach A, Milord R, Waaga AM, et al. (2001). CD28-B7-mediated T cell costimulation in chronic cardiac allograft rejection: differential role of B7-1 in initiation versus progression of graft arteriosclerosis. *Am J Pathol*, 158, 977-986.

[68] Furukawa Y, Mandelbrot DA, Libby P, Sharpe AH, Mitchell RN. (2000). Association of B7-1 co-stimulation with the development of graft arterial disease. Studies using mice lacking B7-1, B7-2, or B7-1/B7-2. *Am J Pathol*, 157, 473-484.

[69] Takeuchi T, Lowry RP, Konieczny B. (1992). Heart allografts in murine systems. The differential activation of Th2-like effector cells in peripheral tolerance. *Transplantation*, 53, 1281-1294.

[70] Onodera K, Hancock WW, Graser E, Lehmann M, Sayegh MH, Strom TB, et al. (1997). Type 2 helper T cell-type cytokines and the development of "infectious" tolerance in rat cardiac allograft recipients. *J Immunol*, 158, 1572-1581.

[71] Sayegh MH, Akalin E, Hancock WW, Russell ME, Carpenter CB, Linsley PS, et al. (1995). CD28-B7 blockade after alloantigenic challenge in vivo inhibits Th1 cytokines but spares Th2. *J Exp Med*, 181, 1869-1874.

[72] Zheng XX, Steele AW, Hancock WW, Stevens AC, Nickerson PW, Roy-Chaudhury P, et al. (1997). A noncytolytic IL-10/Fc fusion protein prevents diabetes, blocks autoimmunity, and promotes suppressor phenomena in NOD mice. *J Immunol*, 158, 4507-4513.

[73] Steiger J, Nickerson PW, Steurer W, Moscovitch-Lopatin M, Strom TB. (1995). IL-2 knockout recipient mice reject islet cell allografts. *J Immunol*, 155, 489-498.

[74] Guo L, Fujino M, Kimura H, Funeshima N, Kitazawa Y, Harihara Y, et al. (2003). Simultaneous blockade of co-stimulatory signals, CD28 and ICOS, induced a stable tolerance in rat heart transplantation. *Transpl Immunol*, 12, 41-48.

[75] Hara M, Kingsley CI, Niimi M, Read S, Turvey SE, Bushell AR, et al. (2001). IL-10 is required for regulatory T cells to mediate tolerance to alloantigens in vivo. *J Immunol*, 166, 3789-3796.

[76] Hutloff A, Dittrich AM, Beier KC, Eljaschewitsch B, Kraft R, Anagnostopoulos I, et al. (1999). ICOS is an inducible T-cell co-stimulator structurally and functionally related to CD28. *Nature*, 397, 263-266.

[77] Yoshinaga SK, Whoriskey JS, Khare SD, Sarmiento U, Guo J, Horan T, et al. (1999). T-cell co-stimulation through B7RP-1 and ICOS. *Nature*, 402, 827-832.

[78] Beier KC, Hutloff A, Dittrich AM, Heuck C, Rauch A, Buchner K, et al. (2000). Induction, binding specificity and function of human ICOS. *Eur J Immunol*, 30, 3707-3717.

[79] Coyle AJ, Lehar S, Lloyd C, Tian J, Delaney T, Manning S, et al. (2000). The CD28-related molecule ICOS is required for effective T cell-dependent immune responses. *Immunity*, 13, 95-105.

[80] Mages HW, Hutloff A, Heuck C, Buchner K, Himmelbauer H, Oliveri F, et al. (2000). Molecular cloning and characterization of murine ICOS and identification of B7h as ICOS ligand. *Eur J Immunol,* 30, 1040-1047.

[81] McAdam AJ, Chang TT, Lumelsky AE, Greenfield EA, Boussiotis VA, Duke-Cohan JS, et al. (2000). Mouse inducible costimulatory molecule (ICOS) expression is enhanced by CD28 costimulation and regulates differentiation of CD4+ T cells. *J Immunol,* 165, 5035-5040.

[82] Kopf M, Coyle AJ, Schmitz N, Barner M, Oxenius A, Gallimore A, et al. (2000). Inducible costimulator protein (ICOS) controls T helper cell subset polarization after virus and parasite infection. *J Exp Med*, 192, 53-61.

[83] Liang L, Sha WC. (2002). The right place at the right time: novel B7 family members regulate effector T cell responses. *Curr Opin Immunol*, 14, 384-390.

[84] Khayyamian S, Hutloff A, Buchner K, Grafe M, Henn V, Kroczek RA, et al. (2002). ICOS-ligand, expressed on human endothelial cells, costimulates Th1 and Th2 cytokine secretion by memory CD4+ T cells. *Proc Natl Acad Sci U S A*, 99, 6198-6203.

[85] Wallin JJ, Liang L, Bakardjiev A, Sha WC. (2001). Enhancement of CD8+ T cell responses by ICOS/B7h costimulation. *J Immunol*, 167, 132-139.

[86] Liu X, Bai XF, Wen J, Gao JX, Liu J, Lu P, et al. (2001). B7H costimulates clonal expansion of, and cognate destruction of tumor cells by, CD8(+) T lymphocytes in vivo. *J Exp Med*, 194, 1339-1348.

[87] Dong C, Juedes AE, Temann UA, Shresta S, Allison JP, Ruddle NH, et al. (2001). ICOS co-stimulatory receptor is essential for T-cell activation and function. *Nature*, 409, 97-101.

[88] Guo L, Li XK, Funeshima N, Fujino M, Nagata Y, Kimura H, et al. (2002). Prolonged survival in rat liver transplantation with mouse monoclonal antibody against an inducible costimulator (ICOS). *Transplantation*, 73, 1027-1032.

[89] Coyle AJ, Gutierrez-Ramos JC. (2001). The expanding B7 superfamily: increasing complexity in costimulatory signals regulating T cell function. *Nat Immunol*, 2, 203-209.

[90] Gonzalo JA, Tian J, Delaney T, Corcoran J, Rottman JB, Lora J, et al. (2001). ICOS is critical for T helper cell-mediated lung mucosal inflammatory responses. *Nat Immunol*, 2, 597-604.

[91] Rottman JB, Smith T, Tonra JR, Ganley K, Bloom T, Silva R, et al. (2001). The costimulatory molecule ICOS plays an important role in the immunopathogenesis of EAE. *Nat Immunol,* 2, 605-611.

[92] Tafuri A, Shahinian A, Bladt F, Yoshinaga SK, Jordana M, Wakeham A, et al. (2001). ICOS is essential for effective T-helper-cell responses. *Nature*, 409, 105-109.

[93] McAdam AJ, Greenwald RJ, Levin MA, Chernova T, Malenkovich N, Ling V, et al. (2001). ICOS is critical for CD40-mediated antibody class switching. *Nature*, 409, 102-105.

[94] Ogawa S, Nagamatsu G, Watanabe M, Watanabe S, Hayashi T, Horita S, et al. (2001). Opposing effects of anti-activation-inducible lymphocyte-immunomodulatory molecule/inducible costimulator antibody on the development of acute versus chronic graft-versus-host disease. *J Immunol*, 167, 5741-5748.

[95] Okamoto N, Nukada Y, Tezuka K, Ohashi K, Mizuno K, Tsuji T. (2004). AILIM/ICOS signaling induces T-cell migration/polarization of memory/effector T-cells. *Int Immunol*, 16, 1515-1522.

[96] Harada H, Salama AD, Sho M, Izawa A, Sandner SE, Ito T, et al. (2003). The role of the ICOS-B7h T cell costimulatory pathway in transplantation immunity. *J Clin Invest*, 112, 234-243.

[97] Kosuge H, Suzuki J, Gotoh R, Koga N, Ito H, Isobe M, et al. (2003). Induction of immunologic tolerance to cardiac allograft by simultaneous blockade of inducible co-stimulator and cytotoxic T-lymphocyte antigen 4 pathway. *Transplantation*, 75, 1374-1379.

[98] Ozkaynak E, Gao W, Shemmeri N, Wang C, Gutierrez-Ramos JC, Amaral J, et al. (2001). Importance of ICOS-B7RP-1 costimulation in acute and chronic allograft rejection. *Nat Immunol*, 2, 591-596.

[99] Sporici RA, Beswick RL, von Allmen C, Rumbley CA, Hayden-Ledbetter M, Ledbetter JA, et al. (2001). ICOS ligand costimulation is required for T-cell encephalitogenicity. *Clin Immunol*, 100, 277-288.

[100] Guo L, Fujino M, Kimura H, Funeshima N, Kitazawa Y, Harihara Y, et al. (2004). AdCTLA-4Ig combined with donor splenocytes, bone marrow cells and anti-ICOS antibody treatment induce tolerance in a rat heart transplantation model. *Transpl Int,* 17, 15-21.

[101] Guo L, Li XK, Enosawa S, Funeshima N, Suzuki S, Kimura H, et al. (2004). Significant enhancement by anti-ICOS antibody of suboptimal tacrolimus immunosuppression in rat liver transplantation. *Liver Transpl*, 10, 743-747.

[102] Nakamura Y, Yasunami Y, Satoh M, Hirakawa E, Katsuta H, Ono J, et al. (2003). Acceptance of islet allografts in the liver of mice by blockade of an inducible costimulator. *Transplantation*, 75, 1115-1118.

[103] Nanji SA, Hancock WW, Anderson CC, Adams AB, Luo B, Schur CD, et al. (2004). Multiple combination therapies involving blockade of ICOS/B7RP-1 costimulation facilitate long-term islet allograft survival. *Am J Transplant*, 4, 526-536.

[104] Tao X, Constant S, Jorritsma P, Bottomly K. (1997). Strength of TCR signal determines the costimulatory requirements for Th1 and Th2 CD4+ T cell differentiation. *J Immunol*, 159, 5956-5963.

[105] Ishida Y, Agata Y, Shibahara K, Honjo T. (1992). Induced expression of PD-1, a novel member of the immunoglobulin gene superfamily, upon programmed cell death. *Embo J,* 11, 3887-3895.

[106] Nishimura H, Agata Y, Kawasaki A, Sato M, Imamura S, Minato N, et al. (1996). Developmentally regulated expression of the PD-1 protein on the surface of double-negative (CD4-CD8-) thymocytes. *Int Immunol*, 8, 773-780.

[107] Freeman GJ, Long AJ, Iwai Y, Bourque K, Chernova T, Nishimura H, et al. (2000). Engagement of the PD-1 immunoinhibitory receptor by a novel B7 family member leads to negative regulation of lymphocyte activation. *J Exp Med*, 192, 1027-1034.

[108] Dong H, Zhu G, Tamada K, Chen L. (1999). B7-H1, a third member of the B7 family, co-stimulates T-cell proliferation and interleukin-10 secretion. *Nat Med*, 5, 1365-1369.

[109] Latchman Y, Wood CR, Chernova T, Chaudhary D, Borde M, Chernova I, et al. (2001). PD-L2 is a second ligand for PD-1 and inhibits T cell activation. *Nat Immunol*, 2, 261-268.

[110] Tseng SY, Otsuji M, Gorski K, Huang X, Slansky JE, Pai SI, et al. (2001). B7-DC, a new dendritic cell molecule with potent costimulatory properties for T cells. *J Exp Med,* 193, 839-846.

[111] Eppihimer MJ, Gunn J, Freeman GJ, Greenfield EA, Chernova T, Erickson J, et al. (2002). Expression and regulation of the PD-L1 immunoinhibitory molecule on microvascular endothelial cells. *Microcirculation*, 9, 133-145.

[112] Loke P, Allison JP. (2003). PD-L1 and PD-L2 are differentially regulated by Th1 and Th2 cells. *Proc Natl Acad Sci U S A*, 100, 5336-5341.

[113] Ozkaynak E, Wang L, Goodearl A, McDonald K, Qin S, O'Keefe T, et al. (2002). Programmed death-1 targeting can promote allograft survival. *J Immunol*, 169, 6546-6553.

[114] Nishimura H, Nose M, Hiai H, Minato N, Honjo T. (1999). Development of lupus-like autoimmune diseases by disruption of the PD-1 gene encoding an ITIM motif-carrying immunoreceptor. *Immunity*, 11, 141-151.

[115] Nishimura H, Okazaki T, Tanaka Y, Nakatani K, Hara M, Matsumori A, et al. (2001). Autoimmune dilated cardiomyopathy in PD-1 receptor-deficient mice. *Science*, 291, 319-322.

[116] Nishimura H, Honjo T. (2001). PD-1: an inhibitory immunoreceptor involved in peripheral tolerance. *Trends Immunol,* 22, 265-268.

[117] Carter L, Fouser LA, Jussif J, Fitz L, Deng B, Wood CR, et al. (2002). PD-1:PD-L inhibitory pathway affects both CD4(+) and CD8(+) T cells and is overcome by IL-2. *Eur J Immunol*, 32, 634-643.

[118] Dong H, Strome SE, Matteson EL, Moder KG, Flies DB, Zhu G, et al. (2003). Costimulating aberrant T cell responses by B7-H1 autoantibodies in rheumatoid arthritis. *J Clin Invest*, 111, 363-370.

[119] Kanai T, Totsuka T, Uraushihara K, Makita S, Nakamura T, Koganei K, et al. (2003). Blockade of B7-H1 suppresses the development of chronic intestinal inflammation. *J Immunol,* 171, 4156-4163.

[120] Oflazoglu E, Swart DA, Anders-Bartholo P, Jessup HK, Norment AM, Lawrence WA, et al. (2004). Paradoxical role of programmed death-1 ligand 2 in Th2 immune responses in vitro and in a mouse asthma model in vivo. *Eur J Immunol*, 34, 3326-3336

[121] Salama AD, Chitnis T, Imitola J, Ansari MJ, Akiba H, Tushima F, et al. (2003). Critical role of the programmed death-1 (PD-1) pathway in regulation of experimental autoimmune encephalomyelitis. *J Exp Med*, 198, 71-78.

[122] Baecher-Allan C, Brown JA, Freeman GJ, Hafler DA. (2001). CD4+CD25high regulatory cells in human peripheral blood. *J Immunol*, 167, 1245-1253.

[123] Rodig N, Ryan T, Allen JA, Pang H, Grabie N, Chernova T, et al. (2003). Endothelial expression of PD-L1 and PD-L2 down-regulates CD8+ T cell activation and cytolysis. *Eur J Immunol*, 33, 3117-3126.

[124] Gao W, Demirci G, Strom TB, Li XC. (2003). Stimulating PD-1-negative signals concurrent with blocking CD154 co-stimulation induces long-term islet allograft survival. *Transplantation*, 76, 994-999.

[125] Iwai Y, Terawaki S, Ikegawa M, Okazaki T, Honjo T. (2003). PD-1 inhibits antiviral immunity at the effector phase in the liver. *J Exp Med*, 198, 39-50.

[126] Ansari MJ, Salama AD, Chitnis T, Smith RN, Yagita H, Akiba H, et al. (2003). The programmed death-1 (PD-1) pathway regulates autoimmune diabetes in nonobese diabetic (NOD) mice. *J Exp Med*, 198, 63-69.

[127] Lee I, Wang L, Wells AD, Ye Q, Han R, Dorf ME, et al. (2003). Blocking the monocyte chemoattractant protein-1/CCR2 chemokine pathway induces permanent survival of islet allografts through a programmed death-1 ligand-1-dependent mechanism. *J Immunol*, 171, 6929-6935.

[128] Aramaki O, Shirasugi N, Takayama T, Shimazu M, Kitajima M, Ikeda Y, et al. (2004). Programmed death-1-programmed death-L1 interaction is essential for induction of regulatory cells by intratracheal delivery of alloantigen. *Transplantation*, 77, 6-12.

[129] Riley JL, Blair PJ, Musser JT, Abe R, Tezuka K, Tsuji T, et al. (2001). ICOS costimulation requires IL-2 and can be prevented by CTLA-4 engagement. *J Immunol*, 166, 4943-4948.

In: Immune Tolerance Research Developments
Editor: Emile B. Pontell, pp. 51-73
ISBN: 978-1-60456-209-5

Chapter 3

Regulatory T Cells

Antonio La Cava*
Department of Medicine, University of California Los Angeles,
Los Angeles, California 90095-1670

Abstract

$CD4^+$ T cells that co-express high levels of interleukin (IL)-2 α receptor and the transcription factor Foxp3 ($CD4^+CD25^{high}Foxp3^+$ cells) constitute a lymphocyte subpopulation with an important role in the mechanisms of peripheral immune tolerance. The $CD4^+CD25^{high}Foxp3^+$ cells, commonly called regulatory T cells (Tregs), are capable to regulate innate and adaptive immune responses in several animal models of disease and in human diseases via mechanisms of suppression of the proliferation and cytokine production from several different types of immune cell targets. Although Tregs may not require antigen specificity for suppression, the activation of these cells seems to occur preferentially via the engagement of T-cell receptors on these cells with defined antigen specificity. Numerous data have indicated that within the intricate network of interactions among Tregs, innate and adaptive cells and soluble factors, Tregs represent crucial components of immune tolerance, both *in vitro* and *in vivo*. As a consequence of that, the reconstitution of normal numbers and/or function of Treg cells in autoimmune animals with a deficit of these can beneficially affect disease development, progression and outcome, whereas elimination of these cells can be envisioned in cancer immunotherapy. Recently, the use of Treg cells from experimental animal models into clinical applications in humans has been initiated, and promising Treg-based modalities of therapeutic immune intervention are currently under preclinical investigation.

Introduction

The immune system is capable to balance responsiveness to pathogenic insults with a lack of reactivity to self components. This occurs via several mechanisms that include immune tolerance, which helps to avert autoimmunity by preventing and/or shifting

* E-mail address: alacava@mednet.ucla.edu; Department of Medicine, University of California Los Angeles, Los Angeles, California 90095-1670, USA; Tel.: 310 267-4975; Fax: 310 206-8606; (Corresponding author)

potentially deleterious autoreactive immune response towards non-injurious immune responses.

The immune system is classically divided into two effector arms that act complementarily to counteract the challenges coming from the environment (i.e. pathogens) and from the host (i.e. malignant cells). The two arms of the immune system consist of innate and adaptive immune responses, and the two systems work together to fight pathogens or malignant cells, avoiding at the meantime the risk of autoimmunity. In particular, innate immune responses represent a first-line, primordial defense against bacterial or viral pathogens, whereas adaptive immune responses provide a rather more efficient and specific response to microorganisms [1-2].

One hallmark of the innate immune system is the lack of fine specificity in lieu of the recognition of features shared by many pathogens, while the adaptive immune system typically employs cells with fine specificity for different antigens. Because of the broadness of specificities, the adaptive immune system carries an intrinsic risk for the generation of self-reactive cells potentially capable to trigger autoimmune responses [3-4]. To limit this risk, several mechanisms are in place to control self-reactive lymphocytes. These mechanisms include the deletion of potentially pathogenic clones, hyporesponsiveness to antigenic stimulation, immune ignorance for the antigen, and the suppressive capacity of regulatory cells – which are subsets of lymphocytes with a critical role in the induction and maintenance of immune tolerance.

The immunoregulatory/suppressor cells that modulate immune tolerance include natural killer (NK) and NK T (NKT) cells, $CD8^+CD28^-$ T cells, $CD8^+CD122^+$ T cells, $CD8^+CD25^+$ T cells, Qa-1 restricted $CD8^+$ T cells, dendritic cells (DC), B cells, $\gamma\delta$ T cells, and several subsets of $CD4^+$ T cells (see below) [2, 5-11].

The mechanisms of action of each of these immunoregulatory cell populations may be peculiar of each subset or be among subsets, i.e. NKT cells can secrete transforming growth factor (TGF)-β and interleukin (IL)-10 cytokines like Tr1 cells (see below) and interferon (IFN)-γ, a cytokine which can also be secreted by certain suppressor $CD8^+$ T cells [12].

Types of Regulatory T Cells

Within the population of regulatory $CD4^+$ T cells (Treg cells or Tregs), three major subsets have been described: T-regulatory 1 (Tr1) cells [13-15], Th3 cells [16], and $CD4^+CD25^+$ T cells [17-18].

Tr1 cells are IL-10 producing $CD4^+$ regulatory T cells induced from $CD4^+$ T cells by repetitive antigenic stimulation in the presence of IL-10 [13] or immature DC [19]. Tr1 cells produce high levels of immunosuppressive IL-10 and can be generated by chronic activation in the presence of IL-10 both in the human and murine system [13, 20].

Th3 regulatory T cells are TGF-β-producing $CD4^+$ T cells that suppress $CD4^+$ T cells in an antigen-nonspecific manner [16]. These cells produce not only TGF-β but also varying amount of IL-4 and IL-10 [21], and can be induced *in vitro* by exposure of $CD4^+CD25^-$ T cells to TGF-β. Also, the *in vivo* induction of TGF-β producing Th3 immunoregulatory cells have been reported after oral or intravenous antigen administration [22]. The suppressive effect of *ex vivo*-induced Th3 cells appears mediated by suppressive cytokines and is thus, at least in part, cell-contact-independent [22-23].

Finally, the possibly most widely studied subset of regulatory CD4$^+$ T cells is represented by the CD4$^+$CD25$^+$ T cells, which constitute about 5-10% of peripheral CD4$^+$ T cells in normal mice (less in humans). These cells classically express IL-2 receptor (the CD25 marker, which has been widely used for their identification and isolation). Several other markers have been described to characterize these T cells, including glucocorticoid-induced tumor necrosis factor receptor (GITR), cytotoxic T lymphocyte-associated antigen-4 (CTLA-4, CD152), CD62L^{high}, CD45RB^{low}, CD103, neuropilin-1, membrane-bound TGF- (in form of latency-associated protein, LAP), CD69, CD122, CD5, OX-40L, lymphocyte activation gene 3 (LAG-3) and, last but not least, the intracellular forkhead/winged helix transcription factor Foxp3 [24-28], which is presently considered the most reliable marker to monitor functional Tregs [29].

Another recent approach to discriminate between Tregs and conventional (activated) CD4$^+$ T cells that also express CD25 (a marker of activation) is the differential surface expression of CD127, the α chain of the IL-7 receptor, as Tregs are CD127^{low} while activated conventional T cells are CD127^{high} [30-31]. Despite the wealth of markers on Tregs (Figure 1), no marker can be considered unique for Tregs, and there is substantial overlap in the expressions of most of these molecules on the Tregs with that found on activated effector CD4 T cells.

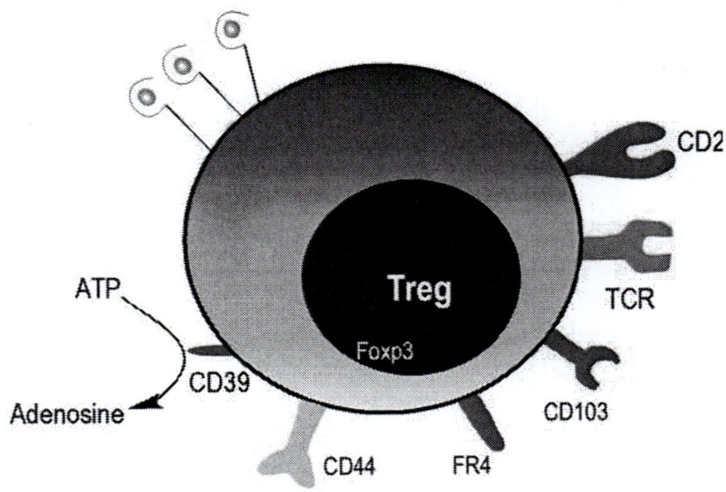

Figure 1. Tregs markers.

Natural Tregs and Adaptive Tregs

CD4$^+$ regulatory T cells are classically divided into two major groups: naturally occurring ("natural") and adaptive ("induced") Tregs.

Natural Tregs

Natural Tregs constitutively express CD4, CD25, and Foxp3, and are potent suppressors of proliferation and cytokine production of target cells both *in vitro* and *in vivo*. Because of their role in the maintenance of self-tolerance and in the prevention of organ-specific autoimmunity, these cells contribute to avert autoimmune disease in several animal model systems, and possibly in humans [17-18].

Natural Tregs arise in the thymus and seed the periphery during day 3 of neonatal life [28, 32-33], suppress the proliferation of activated $CD4^+$ or $CD8^+$ effector T cells by cell contact-dependent and cytokine-independent mechanisms *in vitro* [34-36], and can promote infectious tolerance - a phenomenon by which they can induce conventional $CD4^+$ T cells to also become suppressor cells [37]. This potential therapeutic capacity to amplify immunoregulatory responses of natural Tregs is shared with the adaptive Tregs induced *ex vivo* (i.e. by TGF-β and IL-2), which can also "infectiously" tolerize $CD4^+CD25^-$ cells to become suppressor cells [38].

The number of natural Tregs circulating in peripheral blood in mice comprises 5–10% of the $CD4^+$ cells, while in humans these cells represent only a fraction of $CD25^+$ cells – the ones with brightest staining for this marker ($CD25^{high}$), accounting for about 1% to 2% of total $CD4^+$ T cells [39].

Although natural Tregs are anergic *in vitro*, they can be expanded *ex vivo* with anti-CD3 and IL-2 [40]. Some authors have reported that natural Tregs can proliferate when cultured with high ratios of antigen-loaded DC, and these expanded Tregs retain functional suppressive activity *in vitro* [41]. Another mean to expand natural Tregs and increase their survival is the combination of anti-CD3 and anti-CD28 [42].

Natural Tregs typically mediate their immunoregulatory function through cell-to-cell contact mechanisms that include cytotoxic effector functions involving the synthesis of perforin, CD18, and granzyme A, in a Fas-independent manner [43]. Targets of their cytotoxic effects include $CD4^+CD25^-$ T cells, $CD8^+$ T cells, monocytes, antigen-presenting B cells, and DC [43-44]. A role of LAG-3 in the cell–cell mediated suppression of natural Tregs has also been shown by addition of anti-LAG-3 antibody, which results in the inhibition of the suppressive function of these cells both *in vitro* and *in vivo*, and by the transduction of LAG-3 into $CD4^+CD25^-$ T cells to convey suppressive function [45]. In addition to a somehow controversial role of membrane-bound TGF-β in their mechanisms of suppression [46-47], natural Tregs seem to also mediate suppression of conventional T cells via the ligation of B7 molecules on target T cells, since target cells deficient in B7 molecules (CD80 and, to a lesser degree, CD86) are resistant to Treg suppression [48]. Finally, it is generally thought that natural Tregs cells are enriched in cells that respond to autoantigens [49-50], and that these cells are continuously activated by tissue self-antigens, at least following adoptive transfer [51].

Adaptive Tregs

Adaptive Tregs are generated in the periphery or in *ex vivo* cultures. For example, $CD4^+CD25^+Foxp3^+$ Tregs can be induced *in vitro* from $CD4^+CD25^-$ T cells using TGF-β [38, 52]. However, adoptively transferred polyclonal $CD4^+CD25^-Foxp3^-$ T cells can also differentiate into $CD4^+CD25^+Foxp3^+$ T cells in recipient mice following homeostatic proliferation [53].

The adaptive $CD4^+CD25^+$ T cells have very similar phenotype and function as natural $CD4^+CD25^+$ T cells, e.g. both types of Tregs can suppress immunological responses in multiple ways, possibly including downregulation of antigen presenting cell function and/or induction of other regulatory cells [54]. On the other hand, significant differences may also be present. For example, suppression by natural Tregs requires a direct cell–cell interaction, without the need of soluble factors (and supernatants from these activated Tregs do not have detectable suppressive properties) [48]. Adaptive Tregs may instead require soluble factors (e.g. TGF-β) for optimal action, maintenance, and suppressive capacity [38].

In general, less is known on the modalities of suppression exerted by adaptive Tregs as compared to natural Tregs, and the properties of the different types of adaptive Tregs may depend significantly on the conditions of culture. For example, $CD4^+$ cells can become IL-10-producing Tr1 cells when repeatedly stimulated with IL-10 or with immature DC [13], vitamin D3 and dexamethasone [55]. Those Tr1 cells have strong suppressive effects both *in vitro* and *in vivo*, but there is no evidence to suggest that Tr1 cells can educate other T cells to become suppressor cells.

Characteristics of Tregs

Naïve murine $CD4^+$ T helper cells can differentiate towards T helper (Th)1, Th2, Th17, and regulatory cells (Tregs) both *in vitro* and *in vivo*, depending on the type of stimulation, antigen concentration, co-stimulation, and cytokine milieu where the immune response takes place [56-57]. In general, the presence of interleukin (IL)-12 skews towards Th1; IL-4 towards Th2; TGF–β (+/- IL-2) towards Tregs; and IL-6 and TGF-β towards Th17. The committed cells typically express specific transcription factors: T-bet for Th1, GATA-3 for Th2, Foxp3 for Tregs, and RORγt for Th17 cells [32, 58-62]. Of note, recent studies have suggested that a skewing of murine Th cells towards Tregs and Th17 phenotypes could be mutually exclusive [63].

Table 1. Main characteristics of Treg cell subsets

Treg cell subset	Origin	Mechanisms of action
Natural Tregs	Thymus	Cell-contact dependent, cytokine independent
Adaptive Tregs		
Tr1	*Ex vivo* (with mitogens and IL-10 or immature DC)	Soluble factors (i.e. IL-10)
Th3	*Ex vivo* (with mitogens and IL-2 + TGF-β)	Soluble factors (i.e. TGF-β)
Tregs-like	*Ex vivo* (naïve $CD4^+$ stimulated with alloAg + TGF-β)	Cell-contact dependent, cytokine independent

How Tregs influence immune tolerance was originally seen in experiments in which the transfer of $CD25^+$-depleted $CD4^+$ T cells into neonatally thymectomized mice - a procedure that leads to the development of autoimmunity in multiple organs - results in enrichment of "effector" $CD4^+CD25^-$ T cells causing autoimmunity, and adoptive transfer of $CD4^+CD25^+$ Tregs prevents the development of autoimmune manifestations [64].

In general, while the suppressive capacity of regulatory cells may be deleterious in inhibiting the effector mechanisms of tumor immunosurveillance (because Tregs would inhibit the generation, activation, proliferation, and effector function of tumor-infiltrating T-cells), the activity of Tregs on modulation of activation and peripheral expansion of autoreactive lymphocytes may be essential in the prevention of autoimmunity, both in mice and in humans [65-66]. This is best exemplified by the observation that the genetic deficiency of $Foxp3^+$ cells in scurfy mice [32] or in humans affected by the IPEX syndrome (an X-linked syndrome characterized by immune dysregulation, polyendocrinopathy, enteropathy) [67] causes lethal lymphoproliferative disease.

Additionally, in animal models of organ-specific autoimmunity, a deficiency of Tregs associates with development of organ damage [68-71], and a restoration of the number and/or function of Tregs lead to protection from autoimmunity [69-75]. In systemic autoimmunity, Treg-depleted animals typically develop multi-organ autoimmune disease [76] associated with the presence of anti-nuclear autoantibodies (ANA) and glomerulonephritis, two key features of lupus [64], while supplementation of syngeneic Tregs or adoptive transfer of *in vitro* expanded Tregs abrogates in mice the development of lupus-like disease manifestations [77].

Many studies show that IL-2 is important for the development, peripheral survival, and suppressive function of the Tregs. Mice deficient for IL-2, IL-2R, or IL-2Rβ have a reduced numbers of natural Tregs and die from a lymphoproliferative autoimmune syndrome [78], and an intact IL-2/IL-2R pathway is required for thymic generation of Tregs [79-80]. However, the presence of the thymus may not be an absolute requirement for the generation of Tregs, as these cells can be generated from peripheral expansion and/or from $CD4^+CD25^-$ T cells [81-82].

It is believed that IL-2 production of IL-2 at sites of inflammation can contribute to driving Treg cell-mediated suppression [83], and peripheral survival and expansion of the Tregs may depend on the presence of IL-2 [84]. Incidentally, IL-2 signaling may not be necessarily required for the induction of Foxp3 expression [85], and $IL\text{-}2^{-/-}$ and $IL\text{-}2R^{-/-}$ Tregs can suppress T-cell proliferation *in vitro* [86]. Thus, IL-2 signaling might be required for sustaining *in vivo* the homeostasis of the natural Tregs [84], possibly together with other signals required to survive in the periphery, i.e. the encounter with self peptides presented by MHC II molecules [87], cytokines, and co-stimulatory molecules [88-92].

Mechanisms of Action of Tregs

In vitro Suppression

Tregs need to be activated via the T-cell receptor (TCR) to suppress target cells [93]. Tregs are anergic *in vitro,* and their hyporesponsiveness can be overcome by stimulation with anti-CD3 and IL-2. With no IL-2 added to the system, $CD4^+CD25^+$ T cells suppress the proliferation of $CD4^+CD25^-$ T cells in a cell-contact-dependent, cytokine-independent mechanism, as shown in experiments using Tregs derived from TGF-β -deficient and IL-10-deficient mice, in which the suppressor function of Tregs is retained [91, 94].

Cell contact appears essential, whereas the presence of antigen presenting cells (APC) may not be necessary for Treg suppressor function. CD80 and CD86 ligands on T cells might bind to CTLA-4 on Tregs during suppression, and this might be a reason why cell contact is necessary. Among the molecules involved, the interaction of GITR and GITR-ligand (GITR-L), expressed on effector T cells and APC, respectively, appears to play a relevant role in the susceptibility of the target cells to suppression by the Tregs [95]. Also, cell surface-bound TGF-β might also plays a role in the suppressor function of the Tregs [96].

Regarding the cells target of suppression, there is evidence that some of the effects of the Tregs on target T effector cells include an arrest in cell cycle progression caused by uncoupling of IL-2 signaling [97-98]. Moreover, the activation of Tregs by anti-CD3 and anti-CD46 results in the expression of granzyme A, which facilitates the killing of targets by a perforin-dependent Fas-Fas ligand-independent mechanism [99]. It has also been reported that a granzyme B-dependent perforin-independent mechanism could be involved in the contact-mediated suppression of the Tregs [100].

In vivo Suppression

Although Tregs are anergic *in vitro*, they do proliferate *in vivo* in response to antigenic stimulation [101-103].

These differences are reflected by different Treg activity *in vitro* and *in vivo*. While soluble factors are not involved in the mechanisms of Treg suppression *in vitro*, *in vivo* the Tregs may need IL-10 and TGF-β in their suppression of target cells [104-105].

Also, although Tregs can suppress target cells by inhibiting the transcription of IL-2 in the responder population [91], *in vivo* studies in IL-2 receptor-deficient mice have shown an ability of Tregs to suppress autoimmune responses independently on IL-2 involvement [86]. This is of interest because Tregs require IL-2 for their differentiation, survival, and suppressive capacity [106].

Overall, the data available indicate that *in vitro* suppression of the Tregs may not reflect the *in vivo* situation because additional factors such as *in vivo* migration and homing of the Tregs might significantly influence the activity of these cells, particularly at the sites of inflammation. In that sense, one unanswered question about Treg-mediated suppression regards the location where the induction of tolerance occurs *in vivo*. The accumulation of Tregs in tissues might be beneficial in limiting the activity of target cells by down-modulating inflammation at sites of organ damage, and studies have suggested that differential expression of CD62L and CD27 on human $CD4^+CD25^{high}$ Tregs could distinguish Treg subsets with migratory properties, i.e. $CD27^-CD62L^-$ Tregs could be destined to periphery, $CD62L^+CD27^+$ Tregs would home to lymph nodes [107-109], and Tregs highly express CCR6 and CD45RO would accumulate in tissue [110].

Candidate Molecules of Treg-Mediated Suppression

The molecules that have most frequently been linked to Treg-mediated suppression of target cell proliferation and cytokine production include Foxp3, GITR, and CTLA-4. However, not much is known on the mechanisms by which how each of these molecules may influence suppression, although it is clear that abrogation of the activity of any of these molecules reduces significantly the suppressive capacity of the Tregs. For example, it is generally believed that CTLA-4 on Tregs might act to transduce a costimulatory activating signal along with TCR signaling for the Tregs. This is because after binding of CD80 and CD86 on activated T cells to CTLA-4 on the Tregs, suppression of effector cells ensues [111], and antibody-mediated inhibition of CTLA-4 abrogates the protective effects of Tregs in murine inflammatory bowel disease (IBD) [112].

On the other hand, other molecules can be important in counteracting the suppressive activity of Tregs, as shown by ligation of Toll-like receptor (TLR)-2, -4, -8 and -9 resulting in the abrogation of Treg-mediated suppression [113].

Toll-like receptors (TLR) recognize pathogen-associated molecular patterns (PAMP) common to different pathogens. Upon activation, TLR can stimulate adaptive immune responses through the activation of DC and the upregulation of costimulatory molecules and inflammatory cytokines including IL-6, TNF-α and IL-12 [2, 114].

The engagement of TLR-4 or TLR-9 on murine splenic DC can abrogate the suppressive activity of Tregs *in vitro*, possibly via the induction of a resistance of effector $CD4^+CD25^-$ T cells to Treg-mediated suppression - a phenomenon that is dependent in part of DC-derived IL-6 [115].

Recent studies have shown that TLR-9 deficiency on the MRL background leads to exacerbated lupus, apparently as a result of increased T-cell activation that associates with impaired suppressive capacity *in vitro* of the Tregs [116-117].

Antigen Specificity of Tregs

The issue of antigenic specificity of the Tregs remains unsolved, yet there is evidence suggesting that these cells can express TCR with relatively high affinity for self antigens. Although initial studies of the repertoires of Tregs indicated that these lymphocytes were polyclonal like conventional T cells, subsequent studies on TCR transgenic mice revealed that conventional T cells and Tregs are selected with different affinity/avidity for the TCR [118], and that the TCR repertoire of conventional T cells and Tregs are both diverse and partly overlapping [119].

In vitro, Treg-mediated suppression of effector cells is typically antigen-nonspecific, and Tregs from mice that lack H/K-ATPase can still efficiently prevent autoimmune gastritis induced by H/K-ATPase-specific T cell effectors [120]. Also, in the absence of target antigens, e.g. in athyroid rats or ovariectomized mice, the antigen-reactive Tregs are missing from the repertoire and thus cannot protect new hosts against thyroiditis or oophoritis, although they can still prevent other autoimmune diseases [121-122].

Apparently, however, Tregs activated by antigen act as better, potent suppressor cells. For example, several studies have suggested that Tregs are activated through their TCR (whose specificity can be both to self and foreign antigens) [123] and that co-cultures of Tregs with $CD4^{+}CD25^{-}$ effector T cells with different TCR specificities do not show *in vitro* suppression [124]. Moreover, antigen-specific Tregs generated *in vitro* can suppress autoimmune diabetes [125], and evidence suggests that immune regulation by Tregs can be antigen-specific both *in vivo* [126-128], and *in vitro* [129-133].

Despite that, experimental prevention and/or immunotherapeutic treatment of autoimmunity has mostly been done using polyclonal populations of Tregs, although the therapeutic benefit of antigen-specific regulatory T cells in autoimmunity is also under current evaluation in preclinical studies.

Tregs in Transplantation

The findings that the depletion of $CD4^{+}CD25^{+}$ T cells from normal mice enhances graft rejection and that an increase of the number of Tregs prolongs graft survival strongly suggest that Tregs are involved in transplantation tolerance [134]. The fact that the maintenance of allografts is associated with regulatory T-cell function is also indicated by adoptive transfer studies that show the capacity of Tregs from mice with long-term accepted allografts to regulate rejection of skin allografts in secondary syngeneic hosts [135].

Importantly, several studies have suggested that Tregs not only play a role in solid organ transplantation but may also inhibit graft versus host disease (GVHD) after stem cell transplantation [136-139].

Tregs in Cancer

Although on the one hand Tregs are beneficial in controlling autoimmune responses, on the other hand Tregs may favor the development and growth of tumors.

In murine models of cancer, there is indeed evidence that Tregs hinder anti-tumor immunity [140-141]. For example, depletion of $CD25^{+}$ T cells results in the rejection of a mouse colon tumor and the establishment of long-term anti-tumor immunity [142]. Furthermore, the frequency of Tregs is increased in the peripheral blood of cancer-bearing hosts and/or among the tumor-infiltrating lymphocytes (TIL) and tumor-draining lymph nodes. In haematological malignancies, Tregs are increased in B-cell non-Hodgkin's lymphomas, and intratumoural Tregs are functional in inhibiting effector T-cell proliferation and cytokine production [143].

A study on patients with Hodgkin's lymphoma suggests that Tregs with mixed $CD4^{+}CD25^{+}$ and Tr1 characteristics might be enriched win lymph node-infiltrating T cells [144].

In chronic lymphocytic leukaemia, an increased number of functional Tregs has been correlated with advanced stages of disease, and the chemotherapy-induced induction of Tregs apoptosis sorts beneficial effects on the disease course [145].

In solid tumors, functionally suppressive Tregs are present at high frequency in the peripheral blood and/or TIL of patients with gastric and oesophageal cancer [146] and with squamous cell carcinoma of the head and neck [147].

Increased numbers of Tregs are also found in early-stage non-small cell lung cancer, in late-stage ovarian cancer [148-149] and in lymph nodes in metastatic melanoma [150].

Tregs in Autoimmunity

Tregs in Organ-Specific Autoimmunity

The dysregulation of immune tolerance is a crucial event in the development and progression of pathogenic autoimmunity, and in mice with autoimmune background the numbers of $CD4^+CD25^+$ T cells are usually reduced as compared to the number of Tregs in non-autoimmune mice.

Tregs have been convincingly shown to play a role in human autoimmune diseases such as multiple sclerosis, myasthenia gravis, type 1 diabetes, Kawasaki disease, autoimmune polyglandular syndrome type II, ALPS, rheumatoid arthritis and SLE [151-153]. The importance of the interplay between Tregs and DC in autoimmunity has been reviewed elsewhere [154].

Tregs in Multiple Sclerosis

Experimental autoimmune encephalomyelitis (EAE) is a disease model for human multiple sclerosis and is mediated by encephalitogenic $CD4^+$ T cells. Mice that harbor myelin basic protein (MBP)-specific $CD4^+$ T cells have high incidence of disease due to the failure of Tregs to control pathogenic T cells [155].

Tregs can inhibit *in vitro* the proliferation and cytokine production by myelin oligodendrocyte glycoprotein (MOG)-specific Th1 cells and can confer *in vivo* protection against EAE [156].

In humans, a functional dysfunction and a reduced number of precursor Tregs has been observed in patients with relapsing-remitting MS [157-159].

Tregs in Type-1 Diabetes

The progression of benign to aggressive insulitis in type-1 diabetes-prone female nonobese diabetic (NOD) mice is associated with a temporal peripheral decrease of $FoxP3^+$ Tregs in pancreatic lymph nodes and pancreatic islets [160-161]. Notably, the adoptive transfer of Treg-depleted splenocytes in rodents exacerbates the disease [162], whereas the transfer of Tregs from diabetes-resistant non-lymphopenic animals [163] or *in vitro* expanded Tregs suppress the disease [164].

Since Tregs isolated from pancreatic lymph nodes - but not those from peripheral lymph nodes - delay the progression of diabetes [165], it has been envisioned the use of antigen-specific Tregs for the prevention and/or reversal of experimental diabetes, with encouraging results [166].

In humans, the role of Tregs in patients with type-1 diabetes in the disease pathogenesis is suggested by the functional deficit of these cells and their impaired suppressive capacity [167].

Tregs in Inflammatory Bowel Disease

The development of experimental colitis induced by transfer of naïve $CD4^{+}CD45RB^{high}$ T cells into syngeneic immunodeficient mice [168-169] is prevented by co-transfer of regulatory $CD4^{+}CD45RB^{low}$ T-cells [170].

In humans, the numbers of peripheral Tregs in IBD patients correlate with changes in disease activity, being increased during disease remission and decreased during active disease [171].

Tregs in Experimental Autoimmune Thyroiditis

Several studies suggest that Tregs might effectively modulate experimental autoimmune thyroiditis, a mouse model for Hashimoto's thyroiditis [172-174]. This is relevant because patients with autoimmune thyroiditis seem to suffer from a reduced Treg suppressive activity.

Tregs in Systemic Autoimmunity

Tregs in Systemic Lupus Erythematosus

Studies in murine models of SLE have suggested that a deficiency of Tregs can contribute to loss of self-tolerance and the development of SLE in genetically susceptible mice [175], and/or that lupus-prone mouse have a reduced sensitivity of $CD4^{+}CD25^{-}$ effector T cells to the suppression by Tregs [176]. In other words, in murine lupus, a contribution to the dysfunction of the immune homeostasis observed in the disease could be linked to the abnormal number/function of the Tregs and/or a reduced resistance to their suppressive capacity by the effector target cells.

In any case, the protective role of Tregs in SLE is indicated by *in vivo* studies showing that the adoptive transfer of purified, *ex vivo* expanded Tregs slow the rate of renal disease progression and significantly decrease the mortality of transferred mice [77].

In human SLE, the numbers of natural Tregs are decreased during active flares of SLE [177-178] and during active SLE in pediatric patients [179]. Interestingly, the defects of Tregs in human SLE may be possibly reversible, as SLE Tregs behave as fully functional suppressor cells following *in vitro* activation [180].

Tregs in Rheumatic Autoimmune Diseases

Functional Tregs are enriched in the synovial fluid of patients with rheumatoid arthritis [181]. Although increased numbers of Tregs can be detected in the synovial fluid of patients with active rheumatic disease, Tregs of rheumatoid arthritis patients have a decreased *in vitro* activity in suppressing the production of IFN-γ and TNF-α by target $CD25^-$ T cells [182].

Interestingly, in patients with relatively benign oligoarticular juvenile idiopathic arthritis, a higher frequency of Tregs is observed in comparison with with patients with oligoarticular juvenile arthritis, a disease with a less favorable prognosis [183].

Conclusion

The past few years have seen a significant advance in the understanding of how Tregs can influence immune responses in animal models of disease and in humans.

Although Tregs represent an ideal target of immunomodulation in autoimmunity by virtue of an ability to re-establishing immune tolerance to self-antigens both in new-onset and established disease, the immunosuppressive properties of the Tregs can be detrimental during an immune response to tumors, pathogens, and in vaccination. As discussed before, the enhancement of Tregs activity (in autoimmunity) or abrogation (in cancer) of their suppressive capacity should focus selectively on these cells (i.e. without stimulating effector T cells and DC), to avoid undesirable side effects. This consideration may reveal particularly problematic because of the unreliable nature of CD25 as an exclusive marker for the Tregs, and because of the technically challenging intracellular expression of Foxp3 for the monitoring of $Foxp3^+$ Tregs significantly. These aspects significantly complicate the design of studies specifically targeting this immune cell population *in vivo*. Furthermore, caution should be used in drawing conclusions from animal studies on the modulation of Tregs in human disease because of the different characteristics between human and rodent Tregs. Finally, a better understanding of the cross-talk among Tregs, DC, effector cells, and cytokine milieu where the immune response takes place seems imperative before embarking into Treg-based immunotherapy of human diseases.

Acknowledgments

A.L.C. is supported by the National Institutes of Health grants AR53239 and AI63515.

References

[1] Janeway CA Jr, Medzhitov R. Innate immune recognition. *Annu Rev Immunol* 2002; 20:197-216

[2] La Cava A, Shi FD. Natural and adaptive immune cell-based therapies in autoimmunity. *Curr Med Chem* 2006; 13:1557-66

[3] Nossal GJ. Negative selection of lymphocytes. *Cell* 1994; 76:229–39

[4] von Boehmer H. Positive selection of lymphocytes. *Cell* 1994; 76:219–28

[5] Ghiringhelli F, Menard C, Terme M, *et al.* $CD4^+CD25^+$ regulatory T cells inhibit natural killer cell functions in a transforming growth factor-β-dependent manner. *J Exp Med* 2005; 202:1075–85

[6] Cortesini R, LeMaoult J, Ciubotariu R, Cortesini N, Suciu-Foca N . $CD8^+CD28^-$ T suppressor cells and the induction of antigen-specific, antigen-presenting cell-mediated suppression of Th reactivity. *Immunol Rev* 2001; 182:201–6

[7] Rifa'i M, Kawamoto Y, Nakashima I, Suzuki H. Essential roles of $CD8^+CD122^+$ regulatory T cells in the maintenance of T cell homeostasis. *J Exp Med* 2004; 200:1123–34

[8] Lu L, Werneck MB, Cantor H. The immunoregulatory effects of Qa-1. *Immunol Rev* 2006; 212:51–9

[9] Hanninen A, Harrison LC. γδ T cells as mediators of mucosal tolerance: the autoimmune diabetes model. *Immunol Rev* 2000; 173:109–19

[10] Bacchetta R, Gregori S, Roncarolo MG. $CD4^+$ regulatory T cells: mechanisms of induction and effector function. *Autoimmun Rev* 2005; 4:491-6

[11] Jiang S, Lechler RI, He XS, Huang JF. Regulatory T cells and transplantation tolerance. *Hum Immunol* 2006; 67:765-76

[12] Filaci G, Suciu-Foca N. $CD8^+$ T suppressors are back in the game: are they players in autoimmunity ? *Autoimmun Rev* 2002; 1:279-83

[13] Groux H, O'Garra A, Bigler M, *et al.* A $CD4^+$ T-cell subset inhibits antigen-specific T-cell responses and prevents colitis. *Nature* 1997; 389:737-42

[14] Cong Y, Weaver CT, Lazenby A, Elson CO. Bacterial-reactive T regulatory cells inhibit pathogenic immune responses to the enteric flora. *J Immunol* 2002; 169:6112-9

[15] Veldman C, Hohne A, Dieckmann D, Schuler G, Hertl MJ. Type I regulatory T cells specific for desmoglein 3 are more frequently detected in healthy individuals than in patients with pemphigus vulgaris. *Immunol* 2004 172:6468-75

[16] Weiner HL. Induction and mechanism of action of transforming growth factor-β-secreting Th3 regulatory cells. *Immunol Rev* 2001; 182:207-14

[17] Sakaguchi S. Naturally arising $CD4^+$ regulatory T cells for immunologic self-tolerance and negative control of immune responses. *Annu Rev Immunol* 2004; 22:531-62

[18] Shevach EM. $CD4^+CD25^+$ suppressor T cells: more questions than answers. *Nat Rev Immunol* 2002; 2:389-400

[19] Levings MK, Roncarolo MG. T-regulatory 1 cells: a novel subset of CD4 T cells with immunoregulatory properties. *J Allergy Clin Immunol* 2000; 106:S109-12

[20] Dieckmann D, Bruett CH, Ploettner H, Lutz MB, Schuler G. Human $CD4^+CD25^+$ regulatory, contact-dependent T-cells induce interleukin-10-producing, contact-independent type 1-like regulatory T-cells. *J Exp Med* 2002; 196:247–53

[21] Chen Y, Inobe J, Kuchroo VK, Baron JL, Janeway Jr CA, Weiner HL. Oral tolerance in myelin basic protein T-cell receptor transgenic mice: suppression of autoimmune encephalomyelitis and dose-dependent induction of regulatory cells. *Proc Natl Acad Sci* USA 1996; 93:388-91

[22] Thorstenson KM, Khoruts A. Generation of anergic and potentially immunoregulatory $CD25^+CD4^+$ T-cells in vivo after induction of peripheral tolerance with intravenous or oral antigen. *J Immunol* 2001; 167:188–95

[23] Zheng SG, Gray JD, Ohtsuka K, Yamagiwa S, Horwitz DA. Generation *ex vivo* of TGF-β-producing regulatory T cells from $CD4^+CD25^-$ precursors. *J Immunol* 2002; 169:4183-9

[24] Yi H, Zhen Y, Jiang L, Zheng J, Zhao Y. The phenotypic characterization of naturally occurring regulatory $CD4^+CD25^+$ T cells. *Cell Mol Immunol* 2006; 3:189-95

[25] Piccirillo CA, Shevach EM. Naturally-occurring $CD4^+CD25^+$ immunoregulatory T cells: central players in the arena of peripheral tolerance. *Semin Immunol* 2004; 16:81-8

[26] Wing K, Suri-Payer E, Rudin A. $CD4^+CD25^+$ regulatory T cells from mouse to man. *Scand J Immunol* 2005; 62:1-15

[27] Miyara M, Sakaguchi S. Natural regulatory T cells: mechanisms of suppression. *Trends Mol Med* 2007; 13:108-16

[28] Hori S, Nomura T, Sakaguchi S. Control of regulatory T cell development by the transcription factor Foxp3. *Science* 2003; 299:1057-61

[29] Yagi H, Nomura T, Nakamura K, *et al*. Crucial role of FOXP3 in the development and function of human $CD25^+CD4^+$ regulatory T cells. *Int Immunol* 2004; 16:1643-56

[30] Banham AH. Cell-surface IL-7 receptor expression facilitates the purification of $FOXP3^+$ regulatory T cells. *Trends Immunol* 2006; 27:541-4

[31] Seddiki N, Santner-Nanan B, Martinson J, *et al*. Expression of interleukin (IL)-2 and IL-7 receptors discriminates between human regulatory and activated T cells. *J Exp Med* 2006; 203:1693-700

[32] Fontenot JD, Gavin MA, Rudensky AY. Foxp3 programs the development and function of $CD4^+CD25^+$ regulatory T cells. *Nat Immunol* 2003; 4:330-6

[33] Khattri R, Cox T, Yasayko SA, Ramsdell F. An essential role for scurfin in $CD4^+CD25^+$ T regulatory cells. *Nat Immunol* 2003; 4:337-42

[34] von Boehmer H. Mechanisms of suppression by suppressor T cells. *Nat Immunol* 2005; 6:338-44

[35] Thornton AM, Shevach EM. $CD4^+CD25^+$ immunoregulatory T cells suppress polyclonal T cell activation in vitro by inhibiting interleukin 2 production. *J Exp Med* 1998; 188:287-96

[36] Thornton, AM, Shevach EM. Suppressor effector function of $CD4^+CD25^+$ immunoregulatory T cells is antigen nonspecific. *J Immunol* 2000; 164:183-90

[37] Cobbold SP, Graca L, Lin CY, Adams E, Waldmann H. Regulatory T cells in the induction and maintenance of peripheral transplantation tolerance. *Transpl Int* 2003; 16:66–75

[38] Zheng SG, Wang JH, Gray JG, Soucier H, Horwitz, DA. Natural and induced $CD4^+CD25^+$ cells educate $CD4^+CD25^-$ cells to develop suppressive activity: role of IL-2, TGF-β and IL-10. *J Immunol* 2004; 172:5213-21

[39] Baecher-Allan C, Brown JA, Freeman GJ, Hafler DA. $CD4^+CD25^{high}$ regulatory cells in human peripheral blood. *J Immunol* 2001; 167:1245–53

[40] Taylor PA, Lees CJ, Blazar BR. The infusion of *ex vivo* activated and expanded $CD4^+CD25^+$ immune regulatory cells inhibits graft-versus-host disease lethality. *Blood* 2002; 99:3493–9

[41] Yamazaki S, Iyoda T, Tarbell K, *et al.* Direct expansion of functional $CD25^+CD4^+$ regulatory T cells by antigen-processing dendritic cells. *J Exp Med* 2003; 198:235–47

[42] Tang Q, Henriksen KJ, Boden EK, *et al.*, CD28 controls peripheral homeostasis of $CD4^+CD25^+$ regulatory T cells. *J Immunol* 2003; 171:3348–52

[43] Grossman WJ, Verbsky JW, Barchet W, Colonna M, Atkinson JP, Ley TJ. Human T regulatory cells can use the perforin pathway to cause autologous target cell death. *Immunity* 2004; 21:589–601

[44] Lim HW, Hillsamer P, Banham AH, Kim CH. Direct suppression of B cells by $CD4^+CD25^+$ regulatory T cells. *J Immunol* 2005; 175:4180-3

[45] Huang CT, Workman CJ, Flies D, *et al.* Role of LAG-3 in regulatory T cells. *Immunity* 2004; 21:503–13

[46] Nakamura K, Kitani A, Strober S. Cell-contact-dependent immunosuppression by $CD4^+CD25^+$ regulatory T cells is mediated by cell surface-bound transforming growth factor β. *J Exp Med* 2001; 194:629-44

[47] Piccirillo CA, Letterio JJ, Thornton AM, *et al.* $CD4^+CD25^+$ regulatory T cells can mediate suppressor function in the absence of transforming growth factor β1 production and responsiveness. *J Exp Med* 2002; 196:237-46

[48] Fehervari Z, Sakaguchi S. $CD4^+$ Tregs and immune control. *J Clin Invest* 2004; 114:1209–17

[49] Jordan MS, Boesteanu A, Reed AJ, *et al.*, Thymic selection of $CD4^+CD25^+$ regulatory T cells induced by an agonist self-peptide. *Nat Immunol* 2001; 2:301–6

[50] Bensinger SJ, Bandeira A, Jordan MS, Caton AJ, Laufer TM. Major histocompatibility complex class II-positive cortical epithelium mediates the selection of $CD4^+25^+$ immunoregulatory T cells. *J Exp Med* 2001; 194:427–38

[51] Fisson S, Darrasse-Jeze G, Litvinova E, *et al.*, Continuous activation of autoreactive $CD4^+CD25^+$ regulatory T cells in the steady state. *J Exp Med* 2003; 198:737-46

[52] Chen W, Jin W, Hardegen N, Lei KJ, Li L, Marinos N, McGrady G, Wahl SM. Conversion of peripheral $CD4^+CD25^-$ naïve T cells to $CD4^+CD25^+$ regulatory T cells by TGF-β induction of transcription factor Foxp3. *J Exp Med* 2003; 198:1875-86

[53] Curotto de Lafaille MA, Lino AC, Kutchukhidze N, Lafaille JJ. $CD25^-$ T cells generate $CD25^+Foxp3^+$ regulatory T cells by peripheral expansion. *J Immunol* 2004; 173:7259-68

[54] Lan RY, Ansari AA, Lian ZX, Gershwin ME. Regulatory T cells: development, function and role in autoimmunity. *Autoimmun Rev* 2005; 4:351-63

[55] Barrat FJ, Cua DJ, Boonstra A, *et al.*, *In vitro* generation of interleukin 10-producing regulatory $CD4^+$ T cells is induced by immunosuppressive drugs and inhibited by T helper type 1 (Th1)- and Th2-inducing cytokines. *J Exp M*ed 2002; 195:603–16

[56] Constant SL, Bottomly K. Induction of Th1 and Th2 $CD4^+$ T cell responses: the alternative approaches. *Annu Rev Immunol* 1997; 15:297–322

[57] von Boehmer H. Mechanisms of suppression by suppressor T cells. *Nat Immunol* 2005; 6:338–344

[58] Gately MK, Renzetti LM, Magram J *et al.* The interleukin-12/interleukin-12-receptor system: role in normal and pathologic immune responses. *Annu Rev Immunol* 1998; 16:495–521

[59] Nelms K, Keegan AD, Zamorano J, Ryan JJ, Paul WE. The IL-4 receptor: signaling mechanisms and biologic functions. *Annu Rev Immunol* 1999; 17:701–38

[60] Szabo SJ, Kim ST, Costa GL, Zhang X, Fathman CG, Glimcher LH. A novel transcription factor, T-bet, directs Th1 lineage commitment. *Cell* 2000; 100:655–69

[61] Zheng W, Flavell RA. The transcription factor GATA-3 is necessary and sufficient for Th2 cytokine gene expression in CD4 T cells. *Cell* 1997; 89:587–96

[62] Ivanov II, McKenzie BS, Zhou L, *et al.* The orphan nuclear receptor RORγt directs the differentiation program of proinflammatory IL-17$^+$ T helper cells. *Cell* 2006; 126: 1121–33

[63] Bettelli E, Carrier Y, Gao W, *et al.* Reciprocal developmental pathways for the generation of pathogenic effector TH17 and regulatory T cells. *Nature* 2006; 441:235-8

[64] Sakaguchi S, Sakaguchi N, Asano M, Itoh M, Toda M. Immunologic self-tolerance maintained by activated T cells expressing IL-2 receptor α-chains (CD25). Breakdown of a single mechanism of self-tolerance causes various autoimmune diseases. *J Immunol* 1995; 155:1151-64

[65] Itoh M, Takahashi T, Sakaguchi M, *et al.* Thymus and autoimmunity: production of CD25$^+$CD4$^+$ naturally anergic and suppressive T cells as a function of the thymus in maintaining immunologic self-tolerance. *J Immunol* 1999; 162:5317-26

[66] Bluestone JA, Abbas AK. Natural versus adaptive regulatory T cells. *Nature* 2003; 3:253-7

[67] Bennett CL, Christie J, Ramsdell F, *et al.* The immune dysregulation, polyendocrinopathy, enteropathy, X-linked syndrome (IPEX) is caused by mutations of FoxP3. *Nat Genet* 2001; 27:20-1

[68] Lepault F, Gagnerault MC. Characterization of peripheral regulatory CD4$^+$ T cells that prevent diabetes onset in nonobese diabetic mice. *J Immunol* 2000; 164:240-7

[69] Wu A, Hua S, Munson S, McDevitt H. Tumor necrosis factor-α regulation of CD4$^+$CD25$^+$ T cell levels in NOD mice. *Proc Natl Acad Sci* USA 2002; 99:12287-92

[70] Kohm AP, Carpentier PA, Anger HA, Miller SD. CD4$^+$CD25$^+$ regulatory T cells suppress antigen-specific autoreactive immune responses and central nervous system inflammation during active experimental autoimmune encephalomyelitis. *J Immunol* 2002; 169:4712-6

[71] Bach JF, Chatenoud L. Tolerance to islet autoantigens and type 1 diabetes. *Annu Rev Immunol* 2001; 19:131-61

[72] Taylor PA, Lees CJ, Blazar BR. The infusion of *ex vivo* activated and expanded CD4$^+$CD25$^+$ immune regulatory cells inhibit graft-versus-host disease lethality. *Blood* 2002; 99:3493-9

[73] Szanya V, Ermann J, Taylor C, Holness C, Fathman CG. The subpopulation of CD4$^+$CD25$^+$ splenocytes that delays adoptive transfer of diabetes expresses L-selectin and high levels of CCR7. *J Immunol* 2002; 169:2461-5

[74] Hoffmann P, Ermann J, Edinger M, Fathman CG, Strober S. Donor-type CD4$^+$CD25$^+$ regulatory T cells suppress lethal acute graft-versus-host disease after allogeneic bone marrow transplantation. *J Exp Med* 2002; 196:389-99

[75] Mekala DJ, Geiger TL. Immunotherapy of autoimmune encephalomyelitis with redirected CD4$^+$CD25$^+$ T lymphocytes. *Blood* 2005; 105:2090-2

[76] Sakaguchi S, Takahashi T, Nishizuka Y. Study on cellular events in post-thymectomy autoimmune oophoritis in mice: II. Requirement of Lyt-1 cells in normal female mice for the prevention of oophoritis. *J Exp Med* 1982; 156:1577-86

[77] Scalapino KJ, Tang Q, Bluestone JA, Bonyhadi ML, Daikh DI. Suppression of disease in New Zealand Black/New Zealand White lupus-prone mice by adoptive transfer of *ex vivo* expanded regulatory T cells. *J Immunol* 2006; 177:1451-9

[78] Nelson BH. IL-2, regulatory T cells, and tolerance. *J Immunol* 2004; 172:3983-8

[79] Scheffold A, Huhn J, Hofer T. Regulation of $CD4^+CD25^+$ regulatory T cell activity: it takes (IL-)2 to tango. *Eur J Immunol* 2005: 35:1336-41

[80] Malek TR, Yu A, Vincek V, Scibelli P, Kong L. CD4 regulatory T cells prevent lethal autoimmunity in IL-2Rβ-deficient mice. Implications for the non-redundant function of IL-2. *Immunity* 2002; 17:167-78

[81] Apostolou I, Sarukhan A, Klein L, von Boehmer H. Origin of regulatory T cells with known specificity for antigen. *Nat Immunol* 2002; 3:756–63

[82] Karim M, Kingsley CI, Bushell AR, Sawitzki BS, Wood KJ. Alloantigen-induced $CD25^+CD4^+$ regulatory T cells can develop in vivo from $CD25^-CD4^+$ precursors in a thymus-independent process. *J Immunol* 2004; 172:923-8

[83] Malek TR. The main function of IL-2 is to promote the development of T regulatory cells. *J Leukoc Biol* 2003; 74:961-5

[84] Fontenot JD. Rasmussen JP. Gavin MA, Rudensky AY. A function for interleukin 2 in Foxp3-expressing regulatory T cells. *Nat Immunol* 2005; 6:1142-51

[85] D'Cruz LM, Klein L. Development and function of agonist-induced $CD25^+Foxp3^+$ regulatory T cells in the absence of interleukin 2 signaling. *Nat Immunol* 2005; 6:1152-9

[86] Fontenot JD, Rudensky AY. A well adapted regulatory contrivance: regulatory T cell development and the forkhead family transcription factor Foxp3. *Nat Immunol* 2005; 6:331-7

[87] Bensinger SJ, Bandeira A, Jordan MS, Caton AJ, Laufer TM. Major histocompatibility complex class II-positive cortical epithelium mediates the selection of $CD4^+25^+$ immunoregulatory T cells. *J Exp Med* 2001; 194:427-48

[88] Papiernik M, de Moraes ML, Pontoux C, Vasseur F, Penit C. Regulatory CD4 T cells: expression of IL-2Rα chain, resistance to clonal deletion and IL-2 dependency. *Int Immunol* 1998; 10:371-8

[89] Takahashi T, Tagami T, Yamazaki S, *et al.* Immunologic self-tolerance maintained by $CD25^+CD4^+$ regulatory T cells constitutively expressing cytotoxic T lymphocyte-associated antigen 4. *J Exp Med* 2000; 192:303–10.

[90] Salomon B, Lenschow DJ, Rhee L, *et al.* B7/CD28 costimulation is essential for the homeostasis of the $CD4^+CD25^+$ immunoregulatory T cells that control autoimmune diabetes. *Immunity* 2000; 12:431–40

[91] Belkaid Y, Piccirillo CA, Mendez S, Shevach EM, Sacks DL. $CD4^+CD25^+$ regulatory T cells control *Leishmania major* persistence and immunity. *Nature* 2002; 420:502–7

[92] Malek TR, Porter BO, Codias EK, Scibelli P, Yu A. Normal lymphoid homeostasis and lack of lethal autoimmunity in mice containing mature T cells with severely impaired IL-2 receptors. *J Immunol* 2000; 164:2905–14

[93] Shevach EM. Regulatory T cells in autoimmunity. *Annu Rev Immunol* 2000; 18:423-49

[94] Ichihara F, Kono K, Takahashi A, Kawaida H, Sugai H, Fujii H. Increased populations of regulatory T cells in peripheral blood and tumor-infiltrating lymphocytes in patients with gastric and esophageal cancers. *Clin Cancer Res* 2003; 9:4404-8

[95] Stephens GL, McHugh RS, Whitters MJ, *et al.* Engagement of glucocorticoid-induced TNFR family-related receptor on effector T cells by its ligand mediates resistance to suppression by $CD4^+CD25^+$ T cells. *J Immunol* 2004; 173:5008–20

[96] Chen W, Wahl SM. TGF-β: the missing link in CD4$^+$CD25$^+$ regulatory T cell-mediated immunosuppression. *Cytokine Growth Factor Rev* 2003; 14:85-9

[97] Duthoit CT, Mekala DJ, Alli RS, Geiger TL. Uncoupling of IL-2 signaling from cell cycle progression in naïve CD4$^+$ T cells by regulatory CD4$^+$CD25$^+$ T lymphocytes. *J Immunol* 2005; 174:155–63

[98] Duthoit CT, Nguyen P, Geiger TL. Antigen nonspecific suppression of T cell responses by activated stimulation-refractory CD4$^+$ T cells. *J Immunol* 2004; 172:2238–46

[99] Grossman WJ, Verbsky JW, Barchet W, Colonna M, Atkinson JP, Ley TJ. Human T regulatory cells can use the perforin pathway to cause autologous target cell death. *Immunity* 2004; 21:589–601

[100] Gondek DC, Lu LF, Quezada SA, Sakaguchi S, Noelle RJ. Contact-mediated suppression by CD4$^+$CD25$^+$ regulatory cells involves a granzyme B-dependent, perforin-independent mechanism. *J Immunol* 2005; 174:1783–6

[101] Gavin MA, Clarke SR, Negrou E, Gallegos A, Rudensky A. Homeostasis and anergy of CD4$^+$CD25$^+$ suppressor T cells *in vivo*. *Nat Immunol* 2002; 3:33–41

[102] Fisson S, rrasse-Jeze G, Litvinova E, *et al.* Continuous activation of autoreactive CD4$^+$CD25$^+$ regulatory T cells in the steady state. *J Exp Med* 2003; 198:737–46

[103] Walker LS, Chodos A, Eggena M, Dooms H, Abbas AK. Antigen-dependent proliferation of CD4$^+$CD25$^+$ regulatory T cells *in vivo*. *J Exp Med* 2003; 198:249–58

[104] Dieckmann D, Bruett CH, Ploettner H, Lutz MB, Schuler G. Human CD4$^+$CD25$^+$ regulatory, contact-dependent T cells induce interleukin 10-producing, contact-independent type 1-like regulatory T cells. *J Exp Med* 2002; 196:247–53

[105] Longhi MS, Hussain MJ, Mitry RR *et al.* Functional study of CD4$^+$CD25$^+$ regulatory T cells in health and autoimmune hepatitis. *J Immunol* 2006; 176:4484–91

[106] Thornton AM, Donovan EE, Piccirillo CA, Shevach EM. IL-2 is critically required for the *in vitro* activation of CD4$^+$CD25$^+$ T cell suppressor function. *J Immunol* 2004; 172:6519–23

[107] Ermann J, Hoffmann P, Edinger M, *et al.* Only the CD62L$^+$ subpopulation of CD4$^+$CD25$^+$ regulatory T cells protects from lethal acute GVHD. *Blood* 2005; 105:2220-6

[108] Ruprecht CR, Gattorno M, Ferlito F, *et al.* Coexpression of CD25 and CD27 identifies FoxP3$^+$ regulatory T cells in inflamed synovia. *J Exp Med* 2005; 201:1793-803

[109] Koenen HJ, Fasse E, Joosten I. CD27/CFSE-based ex vivo selection of highly suppressive alloantigen-specific human regulatory T cells. *J Immunol* 2005; 174:7573-83

[110] Kleinewietfeld M, Puentes F, Borsellino G, Battistini L, Rotzschke O, Falk K. CCR6 expression defines regulatory effector/memory-like cells within the CD25$^+$CD4$^+$ T-cell subset. *Blood* 2005; 105:2877-86

[111] Paust S, Lu L, McCarty N, Cantor H. Engagement of B7 on effector T cells by regulatory T cells prevents autoimmune disease. *Proc Natl Acad Sci* USA 2004; 101:10398–403

[112] Read S, Malmstrom V, Powrie F. Cytotoxic T lymphocyte-associated antigen 4 plays an essential role in the function of CD25$^+$CD4$^+$ regulatory cells that control intestinal inflammation. *J Exp Med* 2000; 192:295–302

[113] Mudd PA, Teague BN, Farris AD. Regulatory T cells and systemic lupus erythematosus. Scand *J Immunol* 2006; 64:211-8

[114] Medzhitov R, Preston-Hurlburt P, Janeway CA Jr. A human homologue of the *Drosophila* Toll protein signals activation of adaptive immunity. *Nature* 1997; 388:394-7

[115] Pasare C, Medzhitov R. Toll pathway-dependent blockade of $CD4^{+}CD25^{+}$ T cell-mediated suppression by dendritic cells. *Science* 2003; 299:1033-6

[116] Wu X, Peng SL. Toll-like receptor 9 signaling protects against murine lupus. *Arthritis Rheum* 2006; 54:336-42

[117] Christensen SR, Kashgarian M, Alexopoulou L, Flavell RA, Akira S, Shlomchik MJ. Toll-like receptor 9 controls anti-DNA autoantibody production in murine lupus. *J Exp Med* 2005; 202:321-31

[118] Picca CC, Caton AJ. The role of self-peptides in the development of $CD4^{+}CD25^{+}$ regulatory T cells. *Curr Opin Immunol* 2005; 17:131-6

[119] Hsieh CS, Liang Y, Tyznik AJ, Self SG, Liggitt D, Rudensky AY. Recognition of the peripheral self by naturally arising $CD25^{+}CD4^{+}$ T cell receptors. *Immunity* 2004; 21:267-77

[120] Zwar TD, Read S, van Driel IR, Gleeson PA. $CD4^{+}CD25^{+}$ regulatory T cells inhibit the antigen-dependent expansion of self-reactive T cells *in vivo. J Immunol* 2006; 176:1609-17

[121] Seddon B, Mason D. Peripheral autoantigen induces regulatory T cells that prevent autoimmunity. *J Exp Med* 1999; 189:877-82

[122] Samy ET, Parker LA, Sharp CP, Tung KS. Continuous control of autoimmune disease by antigen-dependent polyclonal $CD4^{+}CD25^{+}$ regulatory T cells in the regional lymph node. *J Exp Med* 2005; 202:771-81

[123] Taams LS, Vukmanovic-Stejic M, Smith J, *et al.* Antigen-specific T cell suppression by human $CD4^{+}CD25^{+}$ regulatory T cells. *Eur J Immunol* 2002; 32:1621–30

[124] Takahashi T, Kuniyasu Y, Toda M, *et al.* Immunologic self-tolerance maintained by $CD25^{+}CD4^{+}$ naturally anergic and suppressive T cells: induction of autoimmune disease by breaking their anergic/suppressive state. *Int Immunol* 1998; 10:1969-80

[125] Tang Q, Henriksen KJ, Bi M, *et al. In vitro*-expanded antigen-specific regulatory T cells suppress autoimmune diabetes. *J Exp Med* 2004; 199:1455–65

[126] Samy ET, Parker LA, Sharp CP, Tung KS. Continuous control of autoimmune disease by antigen-dependent polyclonal $CD4^{+}CD25^{+}$ regulatory T cells in the regional lymph node. *J Exp Med* 2005; 202:771–81

[127] Yu P, Gregg RK, Bell JJ, *et al.* Specific T regulatory cells display broad suppressive functions against experimental allergic encephalomyelitis upon activation with cognate antigen. *J Immunol* 2005; 174 :6772-80

[128] Crispin, JC, Martinez A, Alcocer-Varela J. Quantification of regulatory T cells in patients with systemic lupus erythematosus. *J Autoimmun* 2003; 21:273-6

[129] Tanchot C, Vasseur F, Pontoux C, Garcia C, Sarukhan A. Immune regulation by self-reactive T cells is antigen specific. *J Immunol* 2004; 172:4285-91

[130] Joffre O, Gorsse N, Romagnoli P, Hudrisier D, van Meerwijk JP. Induction of antigen-specific tolerance to bone marrow allografts with $CD4^{+}CD25^{+}$ T lymphocytes. *Blood* 2004; 103:4216–21

[131] Kohm AP, Carpentier PA, Anger HA, Miller SD. $CD4^{+}CD25^{+}$ regulatory T cells suppress antigen-specific autoreactive immune responses and central nervous system

inflammation during active experimental autoimmune encephalomyelitis. *J Immunol* 2002; 169:4712-6

[132] La Cava A, Ebling FM, Hahn BH. Ig-reactive $CD4^+CD25^+$ T cells from tolerized (New Zealand Black x New Zealand White)F_1 mice suppress *in vitro* production of antibodies to DNA. *J Immunol* 2004; 173:3542-8

[133] Wang HY, Lee DA, Peng G, *et al.* Tumor-specific human $CD4^+$ regulatory T cells and their ligands: implications for immunotherapy. *Immunity* 2004; 20:107-18

[134] Sakaguchi S, Sakaguchi N, Shimizu J, *et al.* Immunologic tolerance maintained by $CD4^+CD25^+$ regulatory T-cells: their common role in controlling autoimmunity, tumor immunity and transplantation tolerance. *Immunol Rev* 2001; 182:18–32

[135] Suri-Payer E, Amar AZ, Thornton AM, Shevach EM. $CD4^+CD25^+$ T-cells inhibit both the induction and effector function of autoreactive T-cells and represent a unique lineage of immunoregulatory cells. *J Immunol* 1998; 160:1212–8

[136] Cohen JL, Trenado A, Vasey D, Klatzmann D, Salomon BL. $CD4^+CD25^+$ immunoregulatory T-cells: new therapeutics for graft-vs.-host disease. *J Exp Med* 2002; 196:401-6

[137] Hoffmann P, Ermann J, Edinger M, Fathman CG, Strober S. Donor-type $CD4^+CD25^+$ regulatory T-cells suppress lethal acute graft-versus-host disease after allogenic bone marrow transplantation. *J Exp Med* 2002; 196:389-99

[138] Taylor PA, Noelle RJ, Blazar BR. $CD4^+CD25^+$ immune regulatory cells are required for induction of tolerance to alloantigen via costimulatory blockade. *J Exp Med* 2001; 193:1311-8

[139] Edinger M, Hoffmann P, Ermann J, *et al.* $CD4^+CD25^+$ regulatory T-cells preserve graft-versus-tumor activity while inhibiting graft-versus-host disease after bone marrow transplantation. *Nature Med* 2003; 9:1144–50

[140] Beyer M, Schultze JL. Regulatory T cells in cancer. *Blood* 2006; 108:804-11

[141] Baecher-Allan C, Anderson DE. Regulatory cells and human cancer. *Semin Cancer Biol* 2006; 16:98-105

[142] Golgher D, Jones E, Powrie F, Elliott T, Gallimore A. Depletion of $CD25^+$ regulatory cells uncovers immune responses to shared murine tumor rejection antigens. *Eur J Immunol* 2002; 32:3267-75

[143] Yang ZZ, Novak AJ, Stenson MJ, Witzig TE, Ansell SM. Intratumoral $CD4^+CD25^+$ regulatory T-cell-mediated suppression of infiltrating $CD4^+$ T cells in B-cell non-Hodgkin lymphoma. *Blood* 2006; 107:3639-46

[144] Marshall NA, Christie LE, Munro LR, *et al.* Immunosuppressive regulatory T cells are abundant in the reactive lymphocytes of Hodgkin lymphoma. *Blood* 2004; 103:1755-62

[145] Beyer M, Kochanek M, Darabi K, *et al.* Reduced frequencies and suppressive function of $CD4^+CD25^{hi}$ regulatory T cells in patients with chronic lymphocytic leukemia after therapy with fludarabine. *Blood* 2005; 106:2018-25

[146] Ichihara F, Kono K, Takahashi A, Kawaida H, Sugai H, Fujii H. Increased populations of regulatory T cells in peripheral blood and tumor-infiltrating lymphocytes in patients with gastric and esophageal cancers. *Clin Cancer Res* 2003; 9:4404-8

[147] Schaefer C, Kim GG, Albers A, Hoermann K, Myers EN, Whiteside TL. Characteristics of $CD4^+CD25^+$ regulatory T cells in the peripheral circulation of patients with head and neck cancer. *Br J Cancer* 2005; 92:913-20

[148] Woo EY, Chu CS, Goletz TJ, *et al.* Regulatory $CD4^+CD25^+$ T cells in tumors from patients with early-stage non-small cell lung cancer and late-stage ovarian cancer. *Cancer Res* 2001; 61:4766-72

[149] Woo EY, Yeh H, Chu CS, *et al.* Regulatory T cells from lung cancer patients directly inhibit autologous T cell proliferation. *J Immunol* 2002; 168:4272-6

[150] Viguier M, Lemaitre F, Verola O, *et al.* Foxp3 expressing $CD4^+CD25^{high}$ regulatory T cells are overrepresented in human metastatic melanoma lymph nodes and inhibit the function of infiltrating T cells. *J Immunol* 2004; 173:1444-53

[151] Lan RY, Ansari AA, Lian ZX, Gershwin ME. Regulatory T cells: development, function and role in autoimmunity. *Autoimmun Rev* 2005; 4:351–63

[152] Lawson CA, Brown AK, Bejarano V, *et al.* Early rheumatoid arthritis is associated with a deficit in the $CD4^+CD25^{high}$ regulatory T cell population in peripheral blood. *Rheumatology* 2006; 45:1210-7

[153] Zhang X, Reddy J, Ochi H, Frenkel D, Kuchroo VK, Weiner HL. Recovery from experimental allergic encephalomyelitis is TGF-β dependent and associated with increases in $CD4^+LAP^+$ and $CD4^+CD25^+$ T cells. *Int Immunol* 2006; 18:495–503

[154] Tang Q, Bluestone JA. Regulatory T-cell physiology and application to treat autoimmunity. *Immunol Rev* 2006; 212:217-37

[155] Paust S, Cantor H. Regulatory T cells and autoimmune disease. *Immunol Rev* 2005; 204:195-207

[156] Kohm AP, Carpentier PA, Anger HA, Miller SD. $CD4^+CD25^+$ regulatory T cells suppress antigen-specific autoreactive immune responses and central nervous system inflammation during active experimental autoimmune encephalomyelitis. *J Immunol* 2002; 169:4712-6

[157] Viglietta V, Baecher-Allan C, Weiner HL, Hafler DA. Loss of functional suppression by $CD4^+CD25^+$ regulatory T cells in patients with multiple sclerosis. *J Exp Med* 2004; 199:971–9

[158] Fahlén L, Read S, Gorelik L, *et al.* T cells that cannot respond to TGF-β escape control by $CD4^+CD25^+$ regulatory T cells. *J Exp Med* 2005; 201:737-46

[159] Matarese G, Carrieri PB, La Cava A, *et al.* Leptin increase in multiple sclerosis associates with reduced number of $CD4^+CD25^+$ regulatory T cells. *Proc Natl Acad Sci* USA 2005; 102:5150-5

[160] Pop SM, Wong CP, Culton DA, Clarke SH, Tisch R. Single cell analysis shows decreasing FoxP3 and TGFβ1 coexpressing $CD4^+CD25^+$ regulatory T cells during autoimmune diabetes. *J Exp Med* 2005; 201:1333-46

[161] You S, Thieblemont N, Alyanakian MA, Bach JF, Chatenoud L. Transforming growth factor-β and T-cell-mediated immunoregulation in the control of autoimmune diabetes. *Immunol Rev* 2006; 212:185-202

[162] Gregori S, Giarratana N, Smiroldo S, Adorini L. Dynamics of pathogenic and suppressor T cells in autoimmune diabetes development. *J Immunol* 2003; 171:4040–7

[163] Poussier P, Ning T, Murphy T, Dabrowski D, Ramanathan S. Impaired post-thymic development of regulatory $CD4^+25^+$ T cells contributes to diabetes pathogenesis in BB rats. *J Immunol* 2005; 174:4081-9

[164] Tarbell KV, Yamazaki S, Olson K, Toy P, Steinman RM. $CD25^+CD4^+$ T cells, expanded with dendritic cells presenting a single autoantigenic peptide, suppress autoimmune diabetes. *J Exp Med* 2004; 199:1467–77

[165] Green EA, Choi Y, Flavell RA. Pancreatic lymph node-derived $CD4^+CD25^+$ Treg cells: highly potent regulators of diabetes that require TRANCE-RANK signals. *Immunity* 2002; 16:183-91

[166] Bluestone JA, Tang Q. Therapeutic vaccination using $CD4^+CD25^+$ antigen-specific regulatory T cells. *Proc Natl Acad Sci* USA 2004; 101:14622-6

[167] Lindley S, Dayan CM, Bishop A, Roep BO, Peakman M, Tree TI. Defective suppressor function in $CD4^+CD25^+$ T-cells from patients with type 1 diabetes. *Diabetes* 2005; 54:92-9

[168] Powrie F, Mason D. $OX\text{-}22^{high}$ $CD4^+$ T cells induce wasting disease with multiple organ pathology: prevention by the $OX\text{-}22^{low}$ subset. *J Exp Med* 1990; 172:1701-8

[169] Izcue A, Coombes JL, Powrie F. Regulatory T cells suppress systemic and mucosal immune activation to control intestinal inflammation. *Immunol Rev* 2006: 212:256-71

[170] Powrie F, Carlino J, Leach MW, Mauze S, Coffman RL. A critical role for transforming growth factor-beta but not interleukin 4 in the suppression of T helper type 1-mediated colitis by $CD45RB^{low}$ $CD4^+$ T cells. *J Exp Med* 1996; 183:2669-74

[171] Maul J, Loddenkemper C, Mundt P, *et al.* Peripheral and intestinal regulatory $CD4^+CD25^{high}$ T cells in inflammatory bowel disease. *Gastroenterology* 2005; 128:1868-78

[172] Vasu C, Dogan RN, Holterman MJ, Prabhakar BS. Selective induction of dendritic cells using granulocyte macrophage-colony stimulating factor, but not *fms*-like tyrosine kinase receptor 3-ligand, activates thyroglobulin-specific $CD4^+CD25^+$ T cells and suppresses experimental autoimmune thyroiditis. *J Immunol* 2003; 170:5511-22

[173] Gangi E, Vasu C, Cheatem D, Prabhakar BS. IL-10-producing $CD4^+CD25^+$ regulatory T cells play a critical role in granulocyte-macrophage colony-stimulating factor-induced suppression of experimental autoimmune thyroiditis. *J Immunol* 2005; 174:7006-13

[174] Verginis P, Li HS, Carayanniotis G. Tolerogenic semimature dendritic cells suppress experimental autoimmune thyroiditis by activation of thyroglobulin-specific $CD4^+CD25^+$ T cells. *J Immunol* 2005; 174:7433-9

[175] Wolf D, Hochegger K, Wolf AM, *et al.* $CD4^+CD25^+$ regulatory T cells inhibit experimental anti-glomerular basement membrane glomerulonephritis in mice. *J Am Soc Nephrol.* 2005; 16:1360-70

[176] Monk CR, Spachidou M, Rovis F, *et al.* MRL/Mp $CD4^+$, $CD25^-$ T cells show reduced sensitivity to suppression by $CD4^+$, $CD25^+$ regulatory T cells in vitro: a novel defect of T cell regulation in systemic lupus erythematosus. *Arthritis Rheum* 2005; 52: 1180-4

[177] Miyara M, Amoura Z, Parizot C, *et al.* Global natural regulatory T cell depletion in active systemic lupus erythematosus. *J Immunol* 2005; 175:8392-400

[178] Mellor-Pita S, Citores MJ, Castejon R, *et al.* Decrease of regulatory T cells in patients with systemic lupus erythematosus. *Ann Rheum Dis* 2006; 65:553-4

[179] Lee JH, Wang LC, Lin YT, Yang YH, Lin DT, Chiang BL. Inverse correlation between CD4 regulatory T-cell population and autoantibody levels in pediatric patients with systemic lupus erythematosus. *Immunology* 2006; 117:280-6

[180] Valencia X, Yarboro C, Illei G, Lipsky P. Deficient $CD4^{+}CD25^{high}$ T regulatory cell function in patients with active systemic lupus erythematosus. *J Immunol* 2007; 178: 2579-88

[181] Cao D, Malmstrom V, Baecher-Allan C, Hafler D, Klareskog L, Trollmo C. Isolation and functional characterization of regulatory $CD25^{bright}CD4^{+}$ T cells from the target organ of patients with rheumatoid arthritis. *Eur J Immunol* 2003; 33:215-23

[182] Ehrenstein MR, Evans JG, Singh A, *et al.* Compromised function of regulatory T-cells in rheumatoid arthritis and reversal by anti-TNF-α therapy. *J Exp Med* 2004; 200:277-285

[183] de Kleer IM, Wedderburn LR, Taams LS, *et al.* $CD4^{+}CD25^{bright}$ regulatory T cells actively regulate inflammation in the joints of patients with the remitting form of juvenile idiopathic arthritis. *J Immunol* 2004; 172:6435-43

In: Immune Tolerance Research Developments
Editor: Emile B. Pontell, pp. 75-91
ISBN: 978-1-60456-209-5

Chapter 4

Plant-Based Pharmaceuticals and Its Application in Oral Tolerance

Shengwu Ma[1,2,3*], Reynald Tremblay[1], Xiaofeng Wang[1] and Anthony M. Jevnikar[2,3]

[1]Department of Biology, University of Western Ontario, London, Ontario, Canada N6A 5B7

[2]Lawson Health Research Institute, London, Ontario, Canada N6A 4G5

[3]Plantigen Inc., 700 Collip Circle, London, Ontario, Canada N6G 4X8;

Abstract

Genetically engineered plants have emerged as an attractive alternative expression platform for the production of therapeutic proteins in order to meet the ever-increasing need for protein-based human therapeutics that would be difficult to achieve by using conventional methods. This rise is due in part to a greater understanding of disease pathogenesis that has led to the development of new therapeutic treatments. One such treatment utilizes the natural phenomena of oral immune tolerance, whereby ingested protein antigens induce a state of immunologic unresponsiveness to subsequent antigen stimulation. Oral tolerance has proven to be very effective in treating experimental autoimmune diseases including type 1 diabetes. Although still preliminary, oral tolerance has shown promising results in humans as well. However, as oral tolerance induction requires repeated administration of large amounts of protein antigens, the clinical application of oral tolerance strategy may be limited by the potentially huge cost of producing the protein. The use of transgenic plant to express and deliver protein antigens may provide a highly effective, low-cost method for inducing oral tolerance to the treatment of human autoimmune diseases as well as allergy and organ transplantation. This review will examine 1) recombinant protein biotechnology in plants; 2) oral tolerance induction in animal models using transgenic plants expressing specific antigenic proteins; and 3) future prospects for plant-based therapies against immune-mediated diseases.

[*] E-mail address: sma@uwo.ca; Tel. 519-858-5088; Fax: 519-858-5142; (Corresponding author)

1. Introduction

Over the last decade, there has been a significant increase in demand for protein therapeutics, including therapeutic and diagnostic antibodies, cytokines, growth factors, growth factor receptors, and many other immunomodulators, largely due to a better understanding of disease pathogenesis and the identification of new molecular targets. It is anticipated that the demand for protein therapeutics will continue to grow at a phenomenal rate. Conventional cell culture-based expression systems, such as *E. coli,* yeast and mammalian cells, cannot meet such an increasing need.

The use of genetically engineered (transgenic) plants as an alternative platform to conventional cell culture-based systems for the production of high-value recombinant proteins has gained much interest [1]. Several efficient plant-based expression systems have emerged in the last 10 years. The main advantage is the anticipated cost savings, reflecting the large amount of biomass that can be produced in a short time with no need for specialized equipment or expensive media. Plants can be contained, grown easily and inexpensively in large quantities, can be harvested and processed with available agronomic infrastructures, and has simple, unlimited scalability. Moreover, being higher eukaryotes, plants also have a crucial advantage over bacteria in being able to perform many of the complex protein processing steps, such as isoprenylation, oligomerization, disulfide bridge formation and proteolytic cleavage found in a mammalian system. This may be particularly important in producing recombinant proteins that have *in vivo* activities identical to their animal counterparts. In addition, plants do not harbor infectious agents such as viruses and prions harmful to humans as these agents cannot replicate in plants. Safety is a primary concern when any therapeutic proteins for human use are prepared from animal tissues or bacterial cells.

Over the last several years, our group has been exploring transgenic plants for the expression of diabetes-associated autoantigens such as glutamic acid decarboxylase (GAD) intended for inducing oral tolerance to prevent autoimmune diabetes [2, 3]. The use of transgenic plants for oral tolerance induction offers unique advantages. One such advantage is that transgenic plant tissues can be used for direct oral delivery of the expressed antigens without extensive purification, a cost-effective approach for oral tolerance. Moreover, augmented immune responses to plant produced vaccines may suggest increased stability for plant expressed recombinant proteins to gastrointestinal degradation [4]. This review aims to provide an update on progress in oral tolerance induction using transgenic plants. We will first discuss the current state of the technology for plant transformation, followed by a discussion on the application of plant-derived antigens in oral tolerance induction. In the final part of the article, we will discuss the future directions in the area of oral tolerance induction using transgenic plants.

2. Technology for Plant Transformation

There are two basic methods for expressing recombinant foreign proteins in plants. One involves the generation of transgenic plants by stable genomic integration of transgene. The other involves the expression of transgenes in transiently transformed plants or tissues. Each approach has its advantages and disadvantages [5]. Compared to stable plant transformation, transient gene expression is rapid and relatively simple to handle, and the experiment is usually completed within a few days. Furthermore, the absence of chromosomal position effects allows for better reproducibility and reliable levels of gene expression in transient assays [6]. Transient gene expression, however, is limited in scale and is neither permanent nor heritable. In contrast, stably transformed plants allow for the permanent and heritable expression of a particular protein, although generating stably transformed plants requires a longer scale-up time.

2.1. Expression in Stably Transformed Plants

The introduction of foreign genes into plant genomes to develop stably transformed plant lines has almost become a routine practice for many crops. The principle transformation technologies currently used in plant biotechnology are *Agrobacterium*- mediated gene transfer and direct gene transfer via particle bombardment (biolistic delivery). *Agrobacterium tumefaciens*, a soil-borne plant pathogen, has been widely used for the transformation of most dicotyledonous plants such as tobacco and pea [7]. The molecular mechanisms of *Agrobacterium*-mediated transformation are now well understood [8]. Agrobacterium-based gene transfer system offers many unique advantages in plant transformation: (1) The naturally evolved unique ability of *Agrobacterium* to transfer part of its tumor-inducing plasmid (T-DNA) into plants makes it a simple and efficient plant transformation vector. (2) A precise integration of a small number of gene copies into the plant genome and a greater degree of stability for the transgene. (3) Reasonably low incidence of transgene silencing. (4) The ability to transfer long stretches of foreign DNA. The disadvantage of *Agrobacterium*-mediated gene transfer is that it has limited host range, resulting in a low efficiency of transformation in certain crops such as wheat, rice and corn [9]. Particle bombardment, on the other hand, delivers DNA-coated microprojectiles into host cell or tissue. DNA diffuses from particles, interacts with genomic DNA and integrates into the host genome randomly. This method relies on physical principles and is therefore not limited by the cell type, species or genotype. For example, both undifferentiated cells (immature embryo, embryogenic callus, or mature seeds) and differentiated cells (leaves, microtubers) are amenable to this method. Almost all major crops have been transformed by this technique [10]. Another major advantage of particle bombardment is that it requires only minimal gene cassettes (the promoter, transgene and polyadenylation site). This clean-DNA technique introduces only the transgene and no vector backbone into host genome, which frequently but not always happens in the *Agrobacterium*-mediated transformation. Particle bombardment is also able to introduce multiple genes simultaneously and is a much quicker and more straightforward method compared to *Agrobacterium*-based transformation. A major drawback of biolistic delivery is the considerable variation seen in stability, integration, and expression of the introduced transgene.

Nuclear genome transformation is by far the most commonly used approach to express foreign proteins in stably transformed plants. However, a major limitation of using nuclear transformed plants as an expression system is the low accumulation levels of recombinant proteins. In general, the expression did not exceed 0.4% of total soluble protein (TSP). In recent years, stable chloroplast genome transformation in higher plants has emerged as an attractive alternative to conventional nuclear transformation for the expression of recombinant proteins [11]. Chloroplasts are found in plant cells and are responsible for photosynthesis. In a typical leaf cell, there are about 100 chloroplasts, each containing about 100 copies of the chloroplast genome. Consequently, about 10,000 copies per cell of the gene of interest can be amplified in transformed chloroplasts, as compared to one or two copies per cell as typically found after nuclear transformation. This, in turn, results in the generation of very high levels of the desired expression product. For example, the accumulation of foreign protein of up to 40% TSP has been achieved in chloroplast-transformed tobacco plants [12, 13]. Moreover, chloroplast transformation provides better environmental containment, as chloroplasts are inherited maternally and cannot be transferred by pollen to conventional crops or other sexually compatible plants in the environment. As transgene integration into the chloroplast genome takes place via homologous recombination which is in contrast to nuclear transformation where random insertions occur, chloroplast transformation also eliminates positional effects that are frequently observed with nuclear transformation and no gene silencing or co-suppression has been observed [14]. So far particle bombardment has been the major and the most convenient method used for chloroplast genome transformation, and chloroplast transformation has been achieved in several major crops, such as tobacco, tomato and potato [15, 16]. It has been demonstrated that chloroplast is able to process certain post-translational modifications such as forming disulfide bond and phosphorylation, but it is not able to perform glycosylation, often required for the biological function of many proteins.

2.2. Expression in Transiently Transformed Plants

Transient expression can be used to test the function of an expression construct before progressing to large-scale production in stably transformed plants, as well as for protein production. Transient gene expression can be achieved via different methods including using plant virus, infiltration of *Agrobacterium* and particle bombardment. Plant virus such as tobacco mosaic virus (TMV) has been used to transiently express genes that had been inserted into its viral genome. This virus-mediated transformation can achieve relative high yield in a short time. Since plant viruses do not integrate into the host genome, there is no stable transformation and the transgene is not passed through the germ line [17, 18]. Agroinfiltation is another major strategy to achieve transient expression, in which *A. tumefaciens* are infiltrated into plant tissue [19]. The T-DNA is transferred to the nucleus in a large number of plant cells resulting in the production of micro- to milligram amounts of recombinant protein within a few days [20]. Biolistic delivery offers a useful alternative delivery system that avoids the need for a pathogen and allows use of simple vectors lacking T-DNA or virus sequences [21]. The drawbacks to this system, as stated above, is the transient expression system is neither stable nor heritable and has limited scalability, limiting its economic value.

3. Overview of Oral Immune Tolerance and Its Potential for Treating Autoimmune Diseases

Oral tolerance refers to the oral administration of protein antigens, which induces a state of systemic non-responsiveness specific for the fed antigen. The phenomenon of orally-induced tolerance was first described by Wells in 1911 [22]. In these early studies, Guinea pigs fed hen proteins or dinitrochlorobenzene (DNB) did not develop responses to subsequent systemic challenges with the same antigen. Later, it was shown that ingestion of a wide range of proteins can lead to attenuated or absent systemic immune responses to those particular antigens [23]. It is now well established that oral tolerance is a important natural physiological property of the immune system, whereby the host can avoid dangerous reactions such as DTH (delayed-type hypersensitivity) to "non-dangerous" antigens and other substances encountered in our diets [23].

A milestone in the area of oral tolerance was the recognition that self-antigens could be administered to treat and prevent autoimmune diseases. Oral tolerance has been shown to suppress several autoimmune diseases in animal models including experimental allergic encephalomyelitis (EAE), uveitis, thyroiditis, myasthenia, arthritis and diabetes in the nonobese diabetic (NOD) mouse [24]. Oral tolerance has also been shown to suppress other inflammatory conditions such as allergy and transplantation. Encouraged by the promising results of animal tests and the safety of the approach, oral tolerance induction has been further tested in human autoimmune diseases, including multiple sclerosis (MS), rheumatoid arthritis (RA), uveitis and diabetes. The results of human trials suggest that there is no systemic toxicity or exacerbation of disease, although clinical improvements have not yet been definitively demonstrated [24]. However, many lessons have been learned from these initial human trials as well as from the successful experiments with animal models. It is now clear from these studies that several factors need to be considered in order to improve the effectiveness of oral tolerance in human disease: (1) the form of antigen (requirement for purified antigen) is important; (2) the dose of antigen (low-dose versus high-dose tolerance) is crucial; (3) frequency of antigen administration affects the efficiency of oral tolerance induction; (4) mucosal adjuvants may need to be used to enhance oral tolerance; and (5) early therapy is an important factor since oral tolerance is mostly effective before or shortly after disease onset.

There are two primary mechanisms for oral tolerance induction, and the determining factor is the dose of antigen administered. Low doses of antigen administration favor the generation of regulatory cell-driven tolerance, whereas high doses of antigen favor clonal anergy or deletion of specific T cells [24, 25]. Low doses of antigen would preferentially induce regulatory T cells (Tregs) that secrete anti-inflammatory T helper 2 (Th2) type cytokines such as IL-4, IL-10 or Th3 type cytokines such as TGF-β. These regulatory T cells, originated in the gut, will migrate to lymphoid organs suppressing immune responses by inhibiting the generation of effector cells and to target organs, suppressing disease by releasing antigen nonspecific cytokines (bystander suppression). These two mechanisms of tolerance are not mutually exclusive and may overlap.

There are still some issues that need to be addressed when considering oral tolerance as a therapy. One is the choice of a suitable target antigen. The primary reason that oral tolerance has been promoted as a potential therapy for autoimmune disorders is it provides a type of antigen-specific immunosuppression avoiding the toxic side effects associated with drug immunosuppression. Furthermore, it has the advantage of oral administration. One potential problem in its use is the difficulty in choosing the correct target antigen. It is not always clear which autoantigens are relevent or what is the early primary autoantigen that triggers the initiation of autoimmune pathogenesis. The other problem is the limiting effect of oral tolerance on treating already sensitized subjects. Several previous studies have shown that it is relatively easy to induce oral tolerance in naïve animals, but becomes increasingly difficult to induce oral tolerance in primed or immune animals [24]. The third problem is the requirement of large doses of antigen for its efficient induction. Clinical application of oral tolerance strategies is limited by the potentially huge cost of producing autoantigens, particularly if repeated regular doses are required to maintain beneficial effects. To make oral tolerance a more efficient and affordable therapeutic regimen, a new expression platform that provides large amounts of functional protein at extremely low cost is needed. Transgenic plant expression systems have the potential to produce not only large amounts of protein economically, but also to be used as a vehicle for direct oral delivery of peptides or proteins to induce oral tolerance.

Oral tolerance can be enhanced by the use of mucosal adjuvants. The most commonly used mucosal adjuvant is the cholera toxin B subunit (CTB) [26, 27]. It has been shown that CTB given simultaneously with a variety of antigens orally can enhance oral tolerance and allows a reduction in the antigen dose and dosing schedule (frequency of antigen feeding) [28, 29]. One mechanism of such enhancement is that CTB bound to antigen, by virtue of its capacity to bind to eukaryotic cell surfaces *via* GM1 ganglioside receptors present on intestinal epithelial cell surfaces, focuses or concentrates antigens in specialized mucosal cells with antigen presentation capacity and thus facilitates the development of immune tolerance. However, responses may be limited, as the immune system will have neutralizing effects on any components of infectious agents that may represent "danger". In addition to CTB, Th2 cytokines have also been examined for possible enhancement of oral tolerance, because of their known roles in differentiating precursor Th0 cells to Th2 lineages [30]. Parenterally administered IL-4, orally administered IL-4 or IL-10 have been shown to enhance oral tolerance [24, 25].

4. Induction of Oral Tolerance to Prevent Autoimmune Diabetes Using Transgenic Plants Expressing β-cell Autoantigens

Insulin-dependent diabetes mellitus, or type 1 diabetes (T1D), is a common chronic autoimmune disease caused by the body's immune system attacking the insulin-producing cells of the pancreas [31]. Treatment options are currently limited to a daily insulin injection, which is not a cure, or islet transplantation that requires daily drug immunosuppression leading to severe side effects such as increased risk of infection. Oral tolerance induction may represent an attractive alternative treatment for T1D because of its unique advantages: high specificity, low toxicity and simplicity. In type 1 diabetes, several islet cell target autoantigens have been identified including GAD, insulin, and tyrosine phosphatase-like IA-2 which play a role in the initiation and maintenance of the pathogenic events that lead to T1D [31]. In non-obese diabetic (NOD) mouse model, which closely resembles human IDDM, overt diabetes is preceded by a period in which there is a characteristic lymphocytic infiltration of pancreatic islets termed insulitis. Intervention can alter disease progression during this period. Results in this mouse model have suggested that there may be a potential for immunological intervention and prevention of T1D in clinical practice.

4.1. Demonstration of Oral Administration of Transgenic Plants Expressing Mouse GAD67 to Prevent Diabetes in NOD Mice

In a first proof-of-concept demonstration, we produced transgenic tobacco and potato plants expressing mouse glutamic acid decarboxylase (GAD67) [3]. The expression of GAD67 in plants was under the control of strong constitutive cauliflower mosaic 35S promoter, with the expression level accounting for 0.4% of total soluble protein (TSP). GAD is an enzyme that catalyzes the decarboxylation of glutamate to γ-aminobutyric acid (GABA) and CO2, but the immunogenicity of GAD is not dependent on its enzymatic activity but rather its primary amino acid sequences which form immunodominant epitopes upon processing in antigen presenting cells *in vivo* [32]. There are two isomers of GAD, GAD65 and 67, in rodents and humans, both of which are implicated in T1D [33, 34]. Rat and human islets express GAD65 predominantly, as opposed to mouse islets expression of GAD67 [35]. As it has been shown that administration of purified GAD67 to young NOD mice specifically prevented development of diabetes [34], the selection of mouse GAD67 for initial expression in plants facilitated the design of animal experiments for testing plant-derived GAD. To demonstrate the effect of plant-derived mouse GAD67 on diabetes prevention, young pre-diabetic female NOD mice were fed transgenic potato tuber or tobacco leaf tissue as dietary supplementation for a period of seven months starting at 5 weeks of age. The amount of GAD delivered was less than 1 mg per mouse daily. Control mice received an equivalent amount of vector-minus insert transformed tobacco or potato tissue. NOD mice develop diabetes spontaneously and at age of 6 to 7 months, typically 75 to 90% of female mice will become diabetic. Ten out of twelve NOD mice fed GAD67 potato tuber (n=6) or GAD67 tobacco leaf tissue (n=6) remained free of disease (p=0.007 from controls). On the contrary, eight out of twelve control plant-fed mice (67%) developed diabetes [3]. These results demonstrate that oral administration of transgenic plants expressing a β-cell autoantigen is able to prevent autoimmune diabetes by inducing oral immune tolerance. To determine the mechanism by which oral administration of GAD67 transgenic plants prevents diabetes, NOD mice at age of 4 weeks were fed either GAD67 or control plants for 4 to 5 weeks followed by immunization with purified *E. coli*-derived GAD67 in IFA (incomplete Freund's adjuvant). Ten days post-immunization mice were sacrificed and spleen cells were isolated and analysed for their capacity to proliferate in response to GAD67. It was found that proliferation of splenic T cells isolated from GAD67 plant-fed mice was markedly reduced, whereas splenic T cells from control plant-fed mice retained their proliferating capacity. Furthermore, cytokine analyses of supernatants derived from T cells of GAD67 plant treated mice showed a reduction in the production of IFN-γ with a concurrent increase in the production of IL-4 compared with control plant fed mice. In addition, there was an increase in the serum anti-GAD IgG1 levels in GAD67 plant fed mice compared with control plant fed mice, consistent with skewing of responses to Th2. Together, these results demonstrate that the protection from diabetes in GAD67 plant fed mice is associated with the induction of Th2 responses.

4.2. Prevention of Diabetes by Oral Administration of Transgenic Plants Expressing Human GAD65 and IL-4.

While the demonstration that oral administration of transgenic plants expressing mouse GAD67 prevented diabetes is an important proof of concept for the use of plants to induce oral tolerance, such mouse GAD67 expressing plants cannot be given to diabetes patients. To apply the plant-based oral tolerance induction strategy to the treatment of human diseases such as diabetes, the use of a human version of GAD for plant expression would be necessary. GAD65 has been implicated as being a key autoantigen in humans as well as in NOD mice [36]. To this end, we produced transgenic tobacco plants expressing human GAD65. Human GAD65 was expressed at lower levels compared to mouse GAD67, accounting for 0.04% of TSP. Oral administration of GAD65 plants alone failed to provide protection against diabetes in NOD mice. Co-administration of a mucosal adjuvant may enhance oral tolerance to GAD65. To test this possibility, we additionally produced transgenic tobacco plants expressing mouse IL-4 at levels of approximately 0.1% TSP. IL-4 is species specific and does not cross-react between human and mouse [37]. IL-4, being a typical Th2 cytokine, is known to strongly induce Th2 responses [30]. Using an *in vitro* cell proliferation assay, we showed that plant-derived mouse IL-4 is biologically active, a requirement for the immunomodulating effect if given *in vivo* [2]. To demonstrate the effect of combined feeding of IL-4 and GAD65 transgenic plants on diabetes prevention, young pre-diabetic female NOD mice were given IL-4+GAD65 transgenic tobacco leaf tissue as dietary supplementation from 5 weeks to 30 weeks of age. The amount of IL-4 delivered daily per mouse was approximately 1 to 2 μg, while the amount of GAD65 delivered was roughly 6 to 8 μg per mouse daily. Control mice were given either IL-4 or GAD65 transgenic tobacco leaf tissue alone. The feeding results showed that only 23% (4/15) of the NOD mice that received IL-4+GAD65 transgenic plant tissue developed diabetes by 30 weeks of age, whereas 83% (15/18) of the NOD mice that received GAD65 transgenic plant tissue and 100% (18/18) of the NOD mice that received IL-4 transgenic plant tissue developed diabetes by the same age ($p=0.0002$) [2]. It appears that human GAD65, when co-administered with IL-4, can suppress development of diabetes in NOD mice at lower doses than that required for GAD65 alone, suggesting the potential usefulness of IL-4 as a mucosal adjuvant in enhancing oral tolerance, especially in cases where only low levels of the target autoantigen are expressed in transgenic plants. The Enzyme-linked immunosorbent spot (ELISPOT) analysis of the frequency of GAD-specific splenic T cells secreting IFN-γ or IL-4 showed that the ratio of IL-4:IFN-γ secreting cells rose in mice fed with IL-4 plus GAD65 plants but unchanged in control plant treated mice, suggesting a shift in the Th1/Th2 balance toward Th2 dominance. Furthermore, the results of adoptive transfer experiments indicated that the protection from diabetes in IL-4+GAD65 plant fed mice is associated with the induction of regulatory GAD-specific T cells. Together, these data suggest that orally administered plant IL-4 remains biologically active in gastrointestinal tract and is synergistic when given with hGAD65 in inducing robust oral immune tolerance.

4.3. Prevention of Diabetes by Oral Administration of Transgenic Plants Expressing a Cholera Toxin B Subunit (CTB)-Human Insulin Fusion Protein

Insulin is another major autoantigen in type 1 diabetes. Injection of NOD mice with insulin or insulin peptides was shown to inhibit both insulitis and the subsequent development of diabetes [38]. Insulin therapy by injection has also been shown to delay IDDM in humans [39]. Arakawa et al. (1998) generated transgenic potato plants synthesizing a fusion protein consisting of CTB and human proinsulin (CTB-INS) to develop a transgenic plant-based strategy for oral tolerance induction to the prevention of autoimmune diabetes using a different β-cell autoantigen plus a mucosal adjuvant. The expression of the CTB-INS fusion protein was driven by the mannopine synthase (*mas*) promoter. Transgenic potato tubers produced 0.1% of total soluble protein as the petameric CTB-insulin fusion, which retained GM1-ganglioside binding affinity and native antigenicity of both CTB and insulin. NOD mice fed transgenic potato tubers containing ug amounts of the CTB-Insulin fusion protein showed a reduction in insulitis, and a delay in the progression of clinical diabetes, while those receiving transgenic potato tissues producing insulin or CTB protein alone were not protected. When serum anti-insulin IgG antibody subclasses were analysed, there was a significant increase in the anti-insulin IgG1 subclass but not in the IgG2a subclass indicative of a bias toward an insulin-specific Th2 response in mice fed transgenic potato tissues synthesizing the CTB-INS fusion protein. These results provide further evidence supporting the oral tolerance approach to treat autoimmune diabetes by using transgenic plants. Moreover, these results indicate a role of plant-derived CTB in enhancing oral tolerance. A possible concern with the use of CTB as a mucosal adjuvant or carrier molecule for conjugated antigens in the induction of oral tolerance is that prolonged feeding of CTB may induce neutralizing mucosal and systemic antibodies specific for CTB and prevent long lasting tolerance induction. In NOD mice fed transgenic potato tubers containing CTB-Insulin fusion protein, serum and mucosal anti-CTB antibodies were detected [40].

5. Prevention of Allergy and other Inflammatory Disorders by Oral Administration of Transgenic Plants Expressing Relevant Antigens

Allergic reactions represent exaggerated or inappropriate adaptive responses to a wide variety of environmental triggers. These allergen hypersensitivity reactions (AH) typically involve the skin, respiratory tract, and gut. AH is a significant health problem; it currently affects >15% of children and adults worldwide and is rising in incidence [41]. AH appears to be a major factor in the pathogenesis of most asthma and rhinitis, especially in children and young adults [42]. Although a number of immune factors participate in AH, interaction of IgE antibody with mast cells that express high-affinity IgE receptors (FcεR1) is central to the most severe and immediate form of hypersensitivity (type I). Allergen-specific IgE attachment predisposes mast cells to activation, because contact with multivalent allergen crosslinks surface-bound IgE and leads to the release of inflammatory autocoids, including histamine [43]. Current therapies such as corticosteroids and bronchodilators are nonspecific and expensive and are associated with adverse side effects [44]. There is an urgent need for more effective and specific therapies, including neutralization of IgE with monoclonal antibodies (omalizumab for example) [45], and targeting of inflammatory cytokines and chemokine receptors [46]. Although these strategies hold promise, they focus primarily on inhibiting effector phases of allergy, whereas prevention of allergy would likely be more effective. One appealing prevention/intervention strategy may be through oral tolerance induction. Recently, a similar transgenic plant-based oral antigen or cytokine approach has been applied for preventing/treating allergy or other inflammatory disorders.

5.1. Inhibition of Allergy-Specific *Th2 Responses* by Oral Administration of Transgenic Rice Expressing *Specific T Cell Epitopes of Allergen*

Takagi *et al* (2005) reported the production of transgenic rice expressing mouse dominant T cell epitope peptides of Cry j I and Cry j II allergens of Japanese cedar (*Cryptomeria japonica*) pollen as a fusion protein with the soybean seed storage protein glycinin, with the long-term goal of their study being the development a plant-based edible vaccine against allergens through induction of oral tolerance [47]. The use of rice seed systems as a carrier has advantages beyond transgenic plant leaf or root expression. Seeds, as a major storage organ, are designed to be natural reservoirs of products required for seedling growth, including substantial amounts of protein. Rice is easy to store and transport, and recombinant proteins expressed in seeds are highly stable at room temperature. The design of expressing these short T cell epitope peptides as a fusion protein with a seed protein was intended to increase the accumulation of target proteins. Achieving high levels of expression of recombinant peptide antigens in transgenic plants is challenging, because small peptides cannot form stable secondary structures and thus are more vulnerable to proteolytic degradation in plant cells. Expression of the fusion protein was under the control of the robust rice seed storage protein glutelin promoter *GluB-1*. Using this strategy, accumulation reached 0.5% of the total seed protein. Daily oral delivery of transgenic rice seeds containing approximately 70 μg of the fusion protein for 4 weeks inhibited the development of allergen-specific serum IgE and IgG antibodies in BALB/c mice; reduced the allergen-specific proliferative responses of $CD4^+$ T cells; decreased the secretion of allergen-specific Th2 cytokines such as IL-4, IL-5, and IL-13; and decreased the level of serum histamine in mice systemically primed with intact cedar pollen antigen. Moreover, they were able to show clinical benefit in a mouse model of upper-airway pollen allergy using orally administered transgenic rice seeds. These results demonstrate the efficacy of T cell epitope peptides expressed in transgenic rice seeds for oral delivery and induction of oral tolerance against pollen allergen-specific responses.

As demonstrated here, the success of rice-based allergy immunotherapy is critically dependent on the inhibition of $CD4^+$ Th2 responses and IgE production, which is a totally opposite response compared with the previous demonstration that oral administration of transgenic plants expressing GAD or insulin prevented the onset of autoimmune diabetes by specific inhibition of $CD4^+$ T helper 1 (Th1) cells [2, 40]. This may be the first example demonstrating that oral administration of edible transgenic plants expressing a peptide allergen can prevent a Th2-type T cell-mediated allergic disease, although oral administration of transgenic plants expressing a candidate whole allergen has been demonstrated to prevent experimental allergic asthma (see Section 5.2).

5.2. Suppression of Experimental Asthma by Oral Administration of Transgenic Lupin Plants Expressing Allergen Sunflower Seed Albumin

Smart et al., (2003) produced transgenic lupin ((*Lupinus angustifolius L.*) plants synthesizing sunflower seed albumin (SSA), a potential allergen in sunflower seed hypersensitivity, to examine whether a food plant-based vaccine strategy can be used to suppress the development of experimental asthma via the induction of oral tolerance [48]. Allergic asthma is characterized by airway hyperresponsiveness (AHR) to a variety of specific and nonspecific stimuli, chronic pulmonary eosinophilia, elevated serum immunoglobulin E (IgE), and excessive airway mucus production [49]. Clinical and experimental investigations have shown that $CD4^+$ T lymphocytes producing an array of type 2 cytokines (IL-4, IL-5, IL-6, IL-9, IL-10, IL-13) that activate inflammatory and resident effector pathways in the lung and predipose to the pathophysiological features of asthma [49]. Murine models of experimental asthma have also supported the importance of the $CD4^+$ Th2-type cells and Th2-type cytokines in the modulation of allergic airways disease. Using a mouse model of allergic airways disease (AAD), the authors showed that oral consumption of seed meal prepared from lupin expressing SSA protein in the seeds promoted a SSA-specific Th1-type antibody response (IgG2a), attenuated the induction of delayed-type hypersensitivity, and suppressed pathological features of asthma (mucus hypersecretion, eosinophilic inflammation, and enhanced bronchial reactivity (airways hyperreactivity). The suppression of experimental asthma by SSA expressing lupin was associated with the production of $CD4^+$ T cell-derived IFN-γ and IL-10. Furthermore, the authors showed that oral administration of SSA expressing lupin seeds induced $CD4^+CD45RB^{low}$ regulatory T cells that can mediate suppression of AAD, and that the specific suppression of experimental asthma was mediated by both $CD4^+CD45RB^{low}$ regulatory T cells and IFN-γ. This study provides additional support for using transgenic plants as a novel therapeutic strategy to treat allergic diseases.

5.3. Treatment of Experimental Colitis by Oral Administration of Transgenic Low-Alkaloid Tobacco Expressing Human Interleukin-10

Inflammatory bowel disease (IBD) is a chronically relapsing intestinal disorder that is characterized by diarrhea and abdominal pain. It is a significant health issue, as more than one million North Americans are currently affected. For reasons that are unclear, the incidence of IBD is increasing [50]. Two major types of IBD are described: ulcerative colitis (UC) and Crohn disease (CD). As the name suggests, ulcerative colitis is limited to the colon (large intestine). Although Crohn disease can involve any part of the gastrointestinal tract from the mouth to the anus, it most commonly affects the small intestine and/or the colon. The mechanisms responsible for development of IBD have not been fully elucidated, although the main cause of disease pathology is attributed to up-regulated inflammatory processes. Both UC and CD are characterized by activation of macrophages and T cells, pro-inflammatory cytokine, chemokine, and adhesion molecule expression; and an inability to adequately down-regulate immune activation. IBD, particularly CD, is characterized by a predominantly Th1 type profile, involving the up-regulation of cytokines such as IL-6, IL-8, IL-1β, and tumor necrosis factor (TNF)-α [51]. Treatment of IBD involves the systemic reduction of inflammation through the administration of corticosteroids or immunosuppressive agents. Unfortunately, in many patients, such therapy is limited in efficacy as it is poorly tolerated with numerous serious side-effects associated with systemic administration [52, 53]. Inhibition of TNF-α with monoclonal antibodies can induce clinical remission in CD and other forms of IBD. However, antibody therapy is expensive, requires systemic administration [54], and is associated with side-effects which may limit its long-term use. Clearly, alternative therapies need to be developed.

Menassa et al., (2007) produced transgenic low-alkaloid tobacco plants expressing human IL-10 to test whether a plant-based oral cytokine strategy can be used as a luminal therapy for IBD [55]. IL-10 has been shown to be a potent anti-inflammatory cytokine through its capacity to inhibit macrophage and T-helper-1 (Th1) T-cell activation, as well as the expression of TNF-α [56, 57]. Human IL-10 expression in tobacco was under the control of an enhanced 35S promoter. Plant-derived recombinant IL-10 is biologically active, non-glycosylated, and resistant to gastric and intestinal fluid digestion. To evaluate the ability of transgenic plants expressing IL-10 to modify pro-inflammatory cytokine expression in the gut, IL-$10^{-/-}$ mice, which spontaneously develop colitis, were fed IL-10 low-alkaloid tobacco delivering up to 9 μg of human IL-10 daily for 4 weeks. Results of the feeding experiment showed that oral administration of IL-10 plants reduced the severity of colitis by down-regulating TNF-α expression directly at the sites of inflammation in IBD-susceptible IL-$10^{-/-}$ mice. Gut histology was significantly improved relative to controls ($P = 0.002$), and was correlated with a decrease in small bowel TNF-α mRNA levels and an increase in IL-2 and IL-1β mRNA levels. These results demonstrate transgenic plants expressing an anti-inflammatory cytokine have the potential for treating gut-associated inflammatory diseases such as IBD.

6. Conclusion and future perspectives

There is growing evidence to support oral tolerance induction as a safe, effective therapeutic modality for the treatment of autoimmune diseases, allergy, and possibly organ transplantation rejections. The use of transgenic plants to express and deliver antigens may offer an attractive strategy for oral tolerance induction. This strategy has several unique advantages. (1) The cost to produce a recombinant protein is low and scale-up for mass production is as simple as growing more plants with minimal capital investment. (2) Plant-derived proteins are safer to use, as they are free of contamination with endotoxins or human pathogens. (3) In the case of oral tolerance application, antigen candidates can be expressed in edible plant organs, allowing them to be administered as unprocessed or partially processed material. This last point is important as downstream purification of proteins is very costly and can eliminate the economic advantage of any production system. The successful demonstration of oral tolerance induction in animal autoimmune diabetes and allergy by using transgenic plants expressing GAD, insulin, allergen or allergen peptides brings us closer to the reality of oral tolerance therapy in humans using a novel transgenic plant-based approach.

As oral tolerance induction is usually less efficient in systematically sensitized hosts than in naïve hosts [58], one of the obvious challenges is to identify those at risk and treat prior to disease onset. Additionally, we will need to enhance the efficacy of oral tolerance in clinical autoimmune disease. A potentially useful approach is to produce single transgenic plants that express multiple antigens such as GAD, insulin and tyrosine phosphorylase IA-2, or a synthetic "multiantigen/multiepitope" protein containing T-cell epitopes from these antigens for use in oral tolerance induction. It is known that there are multiple antigens involved in immune and autoimmune diseases during disease progression, inhibition of immune responses to just one antigen is often ineffective. Another useful approach is to synthesize adjuvanted antigens in which protein adjuvants are linked to antigens such as IL-4-GAD or CTB-insulin.

Oral tolerance has clear benefit in animals, but has not been conclusively shown in humans, in part due to the larger demand for therapeutic proteins that such trials require. One of the limitations of this strategy, namely cost and delivery, may be addressed by plant systems. In general, levels of recombinant proteins produced by transgenic plants range from 0.001 to 1% of total soluble protein [5]. While these levels of recombinant protein production are sufficient for animal trials, they may limit the ability to induce oral tolerance by direct oral administration of transgenic plants to humans. To make transgenic plants an even more efficient tool for oral tolerance induction, increased protein production levels need to be achieved. Recent advances in plant biotechnology, molecular biology, and genomics have opened up a number of avenues of approach for improving the foreign protein accumulation in plants. These approaches include the use of stronger and/or tissue specific promoters, codon optimization, targeting of proteins to the endoplasmic reticulum (ER) or cellular organelles, expression of a foreign protein as a fusion to plant proteins, the use of native signal sequences, and the introduction of foreign genes into plant chloroplasts via chloroplast transformation [59]. These plant-based approaches may indeed hold promise for treating immune-mediated diseases such as autoimmune diseases and allergic diseases via oral tolerance induction.

Acknowledgments

We gratefully acknowledge the support of the National Sciences and Engineering Research Council of Canada for our work on the use of transgenic plants to induce oral tolerance for the treatment of autoimmune diabetes.

References

[1] Goddijn OJM, Pen J. Plants as bioreactors. *Trends in Biotechnology* 1995;13(9): 379-387.

[2] Ma S, Huang Y, Yin Z, Menassa R, Brandle JE, Jevnikar AM. Induction of oral tolerance to prevent diabetes with transgenic plants requires glutamic acid decarboxylase (GAD) and IL-4. *Proc Natl Acad Sci U S A* 2004;101(15):5680-5.

[3] Ma SW, Zhao DL, Yin ZQ, Mukherjee R, Singh B, Qin HY, et al. Transgenic plants expressing autoantigens fed to mice to induce oral immune tolerance. *Nat Med* 1997;3(7):793-6.

[4] Ma SW, Jevnikar AM. Suppression of autoimmune diabetes by the use of transgenic plants expressing autoantigens to induce oral tolerance. In: Erickson L, Yu W, Brandle

JE, Rymerson RT, editors. Molecular Farming of Plants and Animals for Human and Veterinary Medicine. *Amsterdam: Kluwer*; 2002. p. 156-167.

[5] Fischer R, Stoger E, Schillberg S, Christou P, Twyman RM. Plant-based production of biopharmaceuticals. *Curr Opin Plant Biol* 2004;7(2):152-8.

[6] Janssen BJ, Gardner RC. Localized transient expression of GUS in leaf discs following cocultivation with Agrobacterium. *Plant Mol Biol* 1990;14(1):61-72.

[7] Horsch RB, Fry JE, Hoffmann NL, Eichholtz D, Rogers SG, Fraley RT. A simple and general method for transferring genes into plants. *Science* 1985;227:1229-1231.

[8] McCullen CA, Binns AN. Agrobacterium tumefaciens and plant cell interactions and activities required for interkingdom macromolecular transfer. *Annu Rev Cell Dev Biol* 2006;22:101-27.

[9] Gelvin SB. Agrobacterium-mediated plant transformation: the biology behind the "gene-jockeying" tool. *Microbiol Mol Biol Rev* 2003;67(1):16-37, table of contents.

[10] Taylor NJ, Fauquet CM. Microparticle bombardment as a tool in plant science and agricultural biotechnology. *DNA Cell Biol* 2002;21(12):963-77.

[11] Maliga P. Progress towards commercialization of plastid transformation technology. *Trends Biotechnol* 2003;21(1):20-8.

[12] Staub JM, Garcia B, Graves J, Hajdukiewicz PT, Hunter P, Nehra N, et al. High-yield production of a human therapeutic protein in tobacco chloroplasts. *Nat Biotechnol* 2000;18(3):333-8.

[13] De Cosa B, Moar W, Lee SB, Miller M, Daniell H. Overexpression of the Bt cry2Aa2 operon in chloroplasts leads to formation of insecticidal crystals. *Nat Biotechnol* 2001;19(1):71-4.

[14] Heifetz PB. Genetic engineering of the chloroplast. *Biochimie* 2000;82(6-7):655-66.

[15] Bock R. Plastid biotechnology: prospects for herbicide and insect resistance, metabolic engineering and molecular farming. *Curr Opin Biotechnol* 2007;18(2):100-6.

[16] Daniell H. Production of biopharmaceuticals and vaccines in plants via the chloroplast genome. *Biotechnol J* 2006;1(10):1071-9.

[17] Gleba Y, Marillonnet S, Klimyuk V. Engineering viral expression vectors for plants: the 'full virus' and the 'deconstructed virus' strategies. *Curr Opin Plant Biol* 2004;7(2):182-8.

[18] Verch T, Yusibov V, Koprowski H. Expression and assembly of a full-length monoclonal antibody in plants using a plant virus vector. *J Immunol Methods* 1998;220(1-2):69-75.

[19] Kapila J, De Rycke R, Van Montagu M, Angenon G. An *Agrobacterium*-mediated transient gene expression system for intact leaves. *Plant Sciences* 1997;122:101-108.

[20] Schillberg S, Twyman RM, Fischer R. Opportunities for recombinant antigen and antibody expression in transgenic plants--technology assessment. *Vaccine* 2005;23(15):1764-9.

[21] Seki M, Iida A, Morikawa H. Transient expression of the beta-glucuronidase gene in tissues of Arabidopsis thaliana by bombardment-mediated transformation. *Mol Biotechnol* 1999;11(3):251-5.

[22] Wells HG. Studies on the chemistry of anaphylaxix III. Experiments with isolated proteins, especially those of hen's egg. *Journal of Infectious Disease* 1911;9:147-151.

[23] Mowat AM. The regulation of immune response to dietary protein antigens. *Immunology Today* 1987;8:93-98.

[24] Faria AM, Weiner HL. Oral tolerance: therapeutic implications for autoimmune diseases. *Clin Dev Immunol* 2006;13(2-4):143-57.

[25] Weiner HL, Friedman A, Miller A, Khoury SJ, al-Sabbagh A, Santos L, et al. Oral tolerance: immunologic mechanisms and treatment of animal and human organ-specific autoimmune diseases by oral administration of autoantigens. *Annu Rev Immunol* 1994;12:809-37.

[26] Czerkinsky C, Sun JB, Lebens M, Li BL, Rask C, Lindblad M, et al. Cholera toxin B subunit as transmucosal carrier-delivery and immunomodulating system for induction of antiinfectious and antipathological immunity. *Annals of the New York Academy of Sciences* 1996;778:185-193.

[27] Sun JB, Holmgren J, Czerkinsky C. Cholera toxin B subunit: an efficient transmucosal carrier-delivery system for induction of peripheral immunological tolerance. *Proc Natl Acad Sci* U S A 1994;91(23):10795-9.

[28] Bergerot I, Ploix C, Petersen J, Moulin V, Rask C, Fabien N, et al. A cholera toxoid-insulin conjugate as an oral vaccine against spontaneous autoimmune diabetes. *Proc Natl Acad Sci* U S A 1997;94(9):4610-4.

[29] Sun JB, Rask C, Olsson T, Holmgren J, Czerkinsky C. Treatment of experimental autoimmune encephalomyelitis by feeding myelin basic protein conjugated to cholera toxin B subunit. *Proc Natl Acad Sci* U S A 1996;93(14):7196-201.

[30] Mosmann TR, Coffman RL. TH1 and TH2 cells: different patterns of lymphokine secretion lead to different functional properties. *Annu Rev Immunol* 1989;7:145-73.

[31] Atkinson MA, Maclaren NK. The pathogenesis of insulin-dependent diabetes mellitus. *N Engl J Med* 1994;331(21):1428-36.

[32] Baekkeskov S, Aanstoot HJ, Christgau S, Reetz A, Solimena M, Cascalho M, et al. Identification of the 64K autoantigen in insulin-dependent diabetes as the GABA-synthesizing enzyme glutamic acid decarboxylase. *Nature* 1990;347(6289):151-6.

[33] Bu DF, Erlander MG, Hitz BC, Tillakaratne NJ, Kaufman DL, Wagner-McPherson CB, et al. Two human glutamate decarboxylases, 65-kDa GAD and 67-kDa GAD, are each encoded by a single gene. *Proc Natl Acad Sci* U S A 1992;89(6):2115-9.

[34] Elliott JF, Qin HY, Bhatti S, Smith DK, Singh RK, Dillon T, et al. Immunization with the larger isoform of mouse glutamic acid decarboxylase (GAD67) prevents autoimmune diabetes in NOD mice. *Diabetes* 1994;43(12):1494-9.

[35] Kim J, Richter W, Aanstoot HJ, Shi Y, Fu Q, Rajotte R, et al. Differential expression of GAD65 and GAD67 in human, rat, and mouse pancreatic islets. *Diabetes* 1993;42(12):1799-808.

[36] Tisch R, Yang XD, Singer SM, Liblau RS, Fugger L, McDevitt HO. Immune response to glutamic acid decarboxylase correlates with insulitis in non-obese diabetic mice. *Nature* 1993;366(6450):72-5.

[37] Ma S, Huang Y, Davis A, Yin Z, Mi Q, Menassa R, et al. Production of biologically active human interleukin-4 in transgenic tobacco and potato. *Plant Biotechnol J* 2005;3(3):309-18.

[38] Atkinson MA, Maclaren NK, Luchetta R. Insulitis and diabetes in NOD mice reduced by prophylactic insulin therapy. *Diabetes* 1990;39(8):933-7.

[39] Keller RJ, Eisenbarth GS, Jackson RA. Insulin prophylaxis in individuals at high risk of type I diabetes. *Lancet* 1993;341(8850):927-8.

[40] Arakawa T, Yu J, Chong DK, Hough J, Engen PC, Langridge WH. A plant-based cholera toxin B subunit-insulin fusion protein protects against the development of autoimmune diabetes. *Nat Biotechnol* 1998;16(10):934-8.

[41] Arshad SH. Primary prevention of asthma and allergy. *J Allergy Clin Immunol* 2005;116(1):3-14; quiz 15.

[42] Weiss KB, Sullivan SD. The health economics of asthma and rhinitis. I. Assessing the economic impact. *J Allergy Clin Immunol* 2001;107(1):3-8.

[43] Wills-Karp M. Immunologic basis of antigen-induced airway hyperresponsiveness. *Annu Rev Immunol* 1999;17:255-81.

[44] Biedermann T, Rocken M. Thl/Th2 balance in atopy. *Springer Seminars in Immunopathology* 1999;21(3):295-316.

[45] Presta LG, Lahr SJ, Shields RL, Porter JP, Gorman CM, Fendly BM, et al. Humanization of an antibody directed against IgE. *J Immunol* 1993;151(5):2623-32.

[46] Peachell P. Targeting the mast cell in asthma. *Curr Opin Pharmacol* 2005;5(3):251-6.

[47] Takagi H, Hiroi T, Yang L, Tada Y, Yuki Y, Takamura K, et al. A rice-based edible vaccine expressing multiple T cell epitopes induces oral tolerance for inhibition of Th2-mediated IgE responses. *Proc Natl Acad Sci* U S A 2005;102(48):17525-30.

[48] Smart V, Foster PS, Rothenberg ME, Higgins TJ, Hogan SP. A plant-based allergy vaccine suppresses experimental asthma via an IFN-gamma and CD4+CD45RBlow T cell-dependent mechanism. *J Immunol* 2003;171(4):2116-26.

[49] Bochner BS, Undem BJ, Lichtenstein LM. Immunological aspects of allergic asthma. *Annu Rev Immunol* 1994;12:295-335.

[50] Hanauer SB. Inflammatory bowel disease: epidemiology, pathogenesis, and therapeutic opportunities. *Inflamm Bowel Dis* 2006;12 Suppl 1:S3-9.

[51] Balding J, Livingstone WJ, Conroy J, Mynett-Johnson L, Weir DG, Mahmud N, et al. Inflammatory bowel disease: the role of inflammatory cytokine gene polymorphisms. *Mediators Inflamm* 2004;13(3):181-7.

[52] Lapidus A, Bernell O, Hellers G, Lofberg R. Clinical course of colorectal Crohn's disease: a 35-year follow-up study of 507 patients. *Gastroenterology* 1998;114(6):1151-60.

[53] Farrell RJ, Kelleher D. Glucocorticoid resistance in inflammatory bowel disease. *J Endocrinol* 2003;178(3):339-46.

[54] Targan SR, Hanauer SB, van Deventer SJ, Mayer L, Present DH, Braakman T, et al. A short-term study of chimeric monoclonal antibody cA2 to tumor necrosis factor alpha for Crohn's disease. Crohn's Disease cA2 Study Group. *N Engl J Med* 1997; 337 (15): 1029-35.

[55] Menassa R, Du C, Yin ZQ, Ma S, Poussier P, Brandle J, et al. Therapeutic effectiveness of orally administered transgenic low-alkaloid tobacco expressing human interleukin-10 in a mouse model of colitis. *Plant Biotechnol J* 2007;5(1):50-9.

[56] Vieira P, de Waal-Malefyt R, Dang MN, Johnson KE, Kastelein R, Fiorentino DF, et al. Isolation and expression of human cytokine synthesis inhibitory factor cDNA clones: homology to Epstein-Barr virus open reading frame BCRFI. *Proc Natl Acad Sci U S A* 1991;88(4):1172-6.

[57] Schreiber S, Heinig T, Thiele HG, Raedler A. Immunoregulatory role of interleukin 10 in patients with inflammatory bowel disease. *Gastroenterology* 1995;108(5):1434-44.

[58] Zhang ZJ, Davidson L, Eisenbarth G, Weiner HL. Suppression of diabetes in nonobese diabetic mice by oral administration of porcine insulin. *Proc Natl Acad Sci U S A* 1991;88(22):10252-6.

[59] Twyman RM, Stoger E, Schillberg S, Christou P, Fischer R. Molecular farming in plants: host systems and expression technology. *Trends Biotechnol* 2003;21(12):570-8.

In: Immune Tolerance Research Developments
Editor: Emile B. Pontell, pp. 93-115
ISBN: 978-1-60456-209-5

Chapter 5

Immune Tolerance in Transplantation

Phillip Ruiz, Jennifer Barker and Andreas Tzakis
University of Miami School of Medicine, FL USA

Abstract

The advent and successful evolution of human solid organ transplantation over the past 50 years has been a remarkable achievement that has provided thousands of patients with certain types of end stage organ disease an improved life with notably reduced morbidity and mortality. In order to achieve this success there has been the need for significant immunosuppression of the host to prevent recipient alloimmune responses from rejecting the genetically disparate donor organ. Unfortunately, the application of immunosuppression comes at a price and carries with it the potential for numerous life threatening and debilitating side effects. Since donor allograft tolerance has been extensively characterized and accomplished in animal models, transplant physicians have always attempted to achieve immunological tolerance in human transplant recipients in order to attain a state of specific nonreactivity to the donor transplant with little or no immunosuppression but without sacrificing graft function. To date, the realization of true immunological tolerance in human transplantation remains elusive; however, there have been many examples where a state of "operational" tolerance has been achieved. This chapter will describe these clinical occurrences and based upon animal models, an overview of some postulated mechanisms in immune tolerance.

I. Introduction: Definition of Immunological Tolerance

In order to maintain proper homeostasis in the face of exogenous microorganisms and endogenously generated pathological processes with novel antigenic epitopes, a host must have a properly functioning adaptive immune system capable of selectively mounting immune responses to non-self molecules while remaining unresponsive to molecules produced by the host. This state of selective and non-injurious immunity that ignores host structures in a healthy individual is designated as *immune tolerance*. It is the amalgamation of a variety of complex changes that occur among and between different cell lineages of the immune system. As with many aspects of the immune system, there are often overlapping and recapitulating effects of the various components of the immune system so that depending on the particular deficiency there may not be a notable change in the overall immune response or tolerance status. Malleability and induction of alternative cellular pathways may compensate for one or more given defects. However, a more central or critical flaw in the immune networks supporting the maintenance of immune tolerance, such as the steps involved in blocking autoreactive cells from maturation, can result in the generation of systemic autoimmunity or dysfunctional response to neoantigens. While immune tolerance occurs normally in the healthy immunocompetent host, there are also several experimental animal models that have demonstrated how an *alteration* of the immune pathways can make the host artificially tolerant to foreign antigens. The most notable example of beneficial *actively acquired* immune tolerance and the core topic of this chapter is an attempt to induce tolerance in the host response to allogeneic or xenogeneic organ transplants while maintaining normal immunity to other pathogens. This highly desirable state of *transplantation tolerance*, is as of yet, not easily attainable in humans and remains the "holy grail" of transplant physicians.

The modern-day notion of inducing tolerance to foreign grafts was originally conceived in 1945 with the observation by Owen [1] that Freemartin cattle sharing the same placenta exhibited hematopoietic chimerism and accepted allogeneic skin grafts from their twins later in life without the need for immunosuppression. This observation was the basis of ground breaking experiments by Billingham, Brent, and Medawar who attempted in 1953 [2] to *induce* tolerance artificially in experimental animals. These investigators inoculated tissues from allogeneic adult donors into fetal mice which led to hematopoietic chimerism; in adulthood, the inoculated mice showed specific acceptance (i.e., tolerance) to donor strain graft challenge (unrelated third party grafts were rejected) and this provided the first direct experimental evidence that artificial tolerance was attainable. Since then, the field of transplantation immunology has emerged with particular focus upon and investigation of the mechanisms of tolerance and whether tolerance can be induced in the transplanted host. Indeed, our understanding of tolerance has grown tremendously and has been the basis of clinical and preclinical studies developed in an attempt to induce true transplantation tolerance. True transplantation tolerance is measured by long-term graft acceptance due to a specific lack of immune response to the graft and without immunosuppression. While this Holy Grail of transplantation tolerance yet remains to be attained, many studies (some discussed later in this chapter) show promise that this goal is in the not too distant future and ultimately attainable.

The mechanisms operative in normal immune tolerance have direct relevance to the artificial acquisition of allogeneic graft tolerance. Essentially, for the latter to occur there has to be a variety of different interactions between introduced allogeneic cells and subpopulations of host immune cells. These interactions are not restricted to neonatal exposure and can be reproduced under the appropriate conditions in adult experimental animals. In order to understand these interactions it is important to get an overview of the means by which tolerance normally occurs in the host and to which cell populations.

II. Mechanisms of Central and Peripheral Immune Tolerance

A. The Central Compartment

The immune system is organized into two major subdivisions, the innate (nonspecific) immune system and the adaptive (specific) immune system [3, 4]. The innate immune system serves as a primary and major guard against invading organisms while the adaptive immune system affords specific secondary protection and can instill memory responses to the host that defend upon re-exposure to the offending pathogen or antigen. Cellular and humoral components are present in both of the arms of the immune system and there can be significant interaction between the two systems. Insofar as graft recognition and rejection, there is a role for the innate immune system in recognizing and promoting immunity to alloantigens [5], however, the principal system operative in the response to transplants is the adaptive immune system [6]. In contrast to the nonspecific, constitutive nature of the innate immune system, the adaptive component is antigen specific and exhibits immunological memory. These two latter features make the adaptive immune system a formidable hurdle that must be crossed in transplantation since allografts represent an introduction of foreign tissue. The adaptive system is exemplified by the actions of T cells and B cells in the immune response, essentially responsible for the specificity of cellular and humoral arms of the immune response, respectively. Antigen specificity by T cells and B cells is mediated through heterodimeric antigen receptors expressed on their surfaces. During the development of these cell lineages and the culmination of a series of molecular events, these receptors [T cell receptor (TCR) and B cell receptor (BCR)] [7, 8] are each instilled with a remarkable degree of intrinsic specificity for a particular ligand. The result is that there is a remarkable amount of diversity *between* these molecules and thus, the host upon encounter can identify a vast number of antigen epitopes.

The *generation* of T and B cells in the mammalian host results from central, regulated processes that provide the individual with latent immune cell populations that are capable of recognizing and responding to external antigens but that tend to ignore homologous or self molecules. Therefore, this *central* development of lymphoid cells is the period during which B and T cells are selected in a fashion that eliminates self-reacting cells but promotes those that recognize external antigens; a process characterized as *central tolerance*. T cells develop from hematopoietic stem cells that travel to the thymus. This development in the thymus requires interactions with stromal cells such as thymic epithelial cells (TECs), mesenchymal fibroblasts and bone marrow (BM)-derived dendritic cells (DCs). Signals are provided to these immature thymocytes (no expression of CD4 and CD8, i.e., double negative [DN] cells) to differentiate within distinct thymic anatomic sites [9]. As these cells move through the thymic cortex CD44 and subsequently CD25 are expressed. The two lineages of T cells—α/β and γ/δ separate at this stage, congruent with rearrangement of the T cell receptor (TCR). For α/β T cells there is the CD3, TCRβ, pre-TCRα chain (pTα) complex and for γ/δ T cells, there is the γ/δ/CD3 complex. CD4 and CD8 coreceptors are next expressed (double-positive [DP] thymocytes) and there is rearrangement of the TCR α locus. The specificity of the antigen receptor will then determine whether the cell survives through the process of positive and negative selection, the latter an important component of central tolerance. *Negative selection* is the mechanism by which T cells with unwanted reactivity to self-components are removed in the thymus. The DP thymocytes with high affinities or avidities to self-antigen result in the elimination of the cell (*clonal deletion*) [10]. Thymic *positive selection* of T cells is initiated by interaction of low affinity α/β TCR with self-MHC molecules, and involves rescue from programmed cell death (PCD), as well as induction of differentiation and maturation of certain precursors [11]. Thus, the process of whether a DP thymocyte is positively or negatively selected is determined by the overall avidity of the TCR with self-peptides presented by APC or epithelial cells in the thymus. There are many different molecules participating in these two processes and different pathways, however the ultimate result is that this provides a T-cell population that will respond to foreign antigenic peptides presented by self-major histocompatibility complex molecules. Ultimately, a small fraction of cells (less than 5%) will downregulate either CD4 or CD8, becoming either CD4 single positive (SP) or CD8 SP thereafter leaving the thymus as mature T cells.

Can *clonal deletion* of immune cells directed to given alloantigens be artificially accomplished in the host such that developing alloimmune T cells will no longer be in the repertoire and therefore no reaction to a transplant will take place? Essentially, the answer is yes with clonal deletion of allospecific T cells being one of several methods of achieving tolerance to donor alloantigens *in vivo*. The earliest observation that clonal deletion could be accomplished were the experiments performed in the 1950s by Billingham et al., [2] who first suggested that transplantation tolerance could be a result of neonatal exposure to donor cells. Indeed, there are other clinical examples where fetal and neonatal exposure to noninherited maternal HLA antigens may facilitate a level of lower reactivity in renal transplant recipients [12]. This phenomenon is now understood to be mediated by interactions between allogeneic antigen-presenting cells and responding T cells. These interactions are not limited to neonatal exposure and can be reproduced under the appropriate conditions in adult animals. The intrathymic presence of allogeneic cells or peptides under the appropriate conditions can result in a central deletion of these recipient alloreactive cells. In this regard, the induction of antigen-specific tolerance *within* the thymus has been accomplished but the techniques and results are complicated [13]. For some protein antigens, the use of a viral vector facilitates intrathymic injection and central tolerance induction with negative selection of effector T-cells and positive selection of regulatory T-cells [14]. In addition to the central compartment, chimeric donor strain cells can participate peripherally to clonally delete recipient effector cells [15]. Based on these observations, there have been many experimental systems [16-18] and clinical trials where there is an attempt to induce transplantation tolerance by infusing donor hematopoietic cells. Indeed, blood transfusions or donor bone marrow given before (or near) transplantation have sometimes resulted in enhanced graft survival and reduced responsiveness to donor-specific antigens [19]. Unfortunately, these results have been inconsistent [20] but they have laid foundation to the thought that central and peripheral clonal deletion of alloreactive clones is possible and represents one of the mechanisms by which the central T cell compartment can participate in transplantation tolerance acquisition.

The central compartment development of functional peripheral *B cells* is a regulated process that initiates with hematopoietic stem cells in the fetal liver before birth and afterward in the bone marrow. As with T cell development, there is a crucial role for TdT and recombinase (RAG-1 and RAG-2) synthesis in the maturation of B lymphoid progenitors [21]. Following D-J joining on the H chain chromosome is the development of early pro-B cells and after joining of a V segment to the D-J_H is accomplished is the late pro-B cell stage.

Subsequently, Pro-B cells become pre-B cells when they express membrane μ chains; another series of events develops surrogate light chains and the pre-B receptor [22]. There is a cytoplasmic signaling cascade (with μ chain expression) following antigen binding (the dividing large pre-B cell). Subsequently, non-dividing small pre-B cells productively synthesize light chain, which then (no longer dividing) undergo V-J joining on one L chain chromosome (immature B cell). If this latter cell type binds self-antigen in the bone marrow it will die. B cells not binding self antigen leave the marrow and become mature naive (resting) B cells with membrane IgD and IgM (mature naive B cells).

Concurrent with this process of B cell development is an appropriate regulation of self-reactive B cells. It is well known that as with T cells, there are notable proportions of antibodies (and the B cells that produce them) that bear reactivity to self amongst their vast repertoire of specificities. The levels of regulation of B cell differentiation from immature B cell to plasma cell in the central bone marrow compartment primarily involve an elimination of the immature autoreactive B cells that bear high avidity self reactive receptors following their interaction with self antigen. Following their encounter with antigen, these immature highly autoreactive B cells internalize the antigen and proceed to undergo antigen receptor light chain editing (i.e., BCR replacement) and developmental arrest that ultimately results in one of several fates [23]. The cell can now express a receptor that is no longer autoreactive whereupon the B cell undergoes apoptosis via alteration (essentially downregulation) of the Bcl-2 pathway and dies 1 or 2 days later. The other more frequently occurring alternative is that BCR editing results in a B cell with reduced or no autoreactivity; this cell now emigrates from the bone marrow and enters the secondary lymphoid circulation with the typical lifespan of a mature B cell [24].

B. The Peripheral Compartment

Mature T cells and B cells bearing their specific antigen receptors on their surface constitute an armada of cells that potentially can recognize and inactive a preponderance of the offending pathogens that a mammalian host potentially can face. The encounter and subsequent immune response to foreign antigen involves an intricate interplay of different cell populations, particularly antigen presenting cells (APCs) with the B and T cells. Possibly as the result of "danger" signals from tissue [25] containing pathogens, "professional", specialized APCs such as dendritic cells and different types of macrophages bind, process and present antigen via their major histocompatibility complex (MHC) molecules on their cell surface to T cells and B cells [26]. The T cells utilize their T cell receptor to recognize processed peptides of the foreign antigen; the latter presented by the APCs via their MHC molecules. Likewise, each B cell with its unique membrane-bound immunoglobulin B cell receptor protein can bind to one particular antigen. Once the T cell and B cell encounters and binds its cognate antigen by their antigen receptor, there are a multifarious series of biochemical events [27, 28] that ensue within these cells, and which are promoted and regulated by external cell populations (e.g., signals from helper T cells) and secreted cytokines. This activation process in T cells and B cells following antigen binding allows these cells to further differentiate into one of several potential cell types. In the case of the B cell it can become either a memory cell or plasma cell by hypermutation of the variable region of its immunoglobulin gene in an intermediate differentiation step (the germinal center reaction) or in direct fashion. In the case of the T cell, there are varying paths of activation depending on the cell subtype although the two-signal model is generally the best understood. There is an interaction between the TCR and specific MHC/antigen complexes on APCs and this represents signal 1 into the T cell. Signal 2 is a binding between costimulatory molecules such as CD28 on the T cell and B7 molecules on the APC [29]. In reality, there are various co-stimulatory and adhesive interactions between APCs and T cells that help to drive proliferative, proinflammatory cytokine and cytotoxic effector functions of T cells [30, 31]. Finally, there has been proposed a "signal 3", likely a soluble factor such as IL-12 [32] that is required for immune effector cell function. Importantly, without costimulation a T cell will become functionally inert or anergic.

Within the population of newly released mature single positive T cells from the thymus into the peripheral circulation are subpopulations of autoreactive cells that escaped central clonal deletion. An analogous deficiency in the selection of B cells leads to the presence of some cells in the periphery with autoreactive potential. The activity of these autoreactive T and B cell populations must be regulated to avoid autoimmune reactions and is the basis of *peripheral tolerance* mechanisms.

Self-reactive T cells that have escaped into the peripheral circulation can be further controlled by other tolerance mechanisms, some that have significant importance in transplantation tolerance. The first research suggesting that self-tolerance is established by way of T-cell mediated *control* of self-reactive T cells was conducted more than 30 years ago. In 1969, Nishizuka and Sakakura demonstrated that neonatal thymectomy of mice led to the destruction of the ovaries, which later was found to be caused by an autoimmune process [33]. Then, in 1973, Penhale et al. showed that thymectomy of adult rats followed by exposure to sublethal X-irradiation resulted in the development of autoimmune thyroiditis [34]. With inoculation of CD4+ T cells, disease was prevented. Thus, both groups thought that depletion of *suppressor T cells* may lead to autoimmune disorders. Additional studies have been performed suggesting that CD4+ T cells have autoimmune-inhibitory activity, including a study of rodents that developed type 1 diabetes mellitus. When inoculated with CD4+ T cells, diabetes was prevented. Likewise, Kilshaw, Brent and Pinto in 1975 recognized the role of suppressor cells in transplantation tolerance [35]. Suppressor T cells have since been renamed as *regulatory T cells* (Treg). Regulatory T cells (Treg) are critical players in the maintenance of peripheral tolerance and homeostasis of the immune system. Regulatory T cells are involved in the control of autoimmune diseases, transplantation tolerance, and anti-tumor immunity. Essentially, this diverse and pliable T-cell subpopulation serves to restrain T-cell activation and expansion.

Comparable to other T cells, regulatory T cells develop in the thymus. The large majority of Treg cells are (MHC) class II restricted CD4-expressing ($CD4^+$) cells (as are T helper cells) and express high levels of the interleukin-2 receptor alpha chain (CD25), similar to activated T cells. Unlike conventional CD4+ T cells, CD4+ regulatory T cells require high-affinity peptide-MHC class II interactions with agonist peptides that otherwise induce negative selection. However, Treg cells are further defined by expression of the forkhead family *transcription factor FOXP3* (forkhead box p3) (Foxp3 is not expressed on activated T cells). FOXP3 expression is required for regulatory T cell development and controls a genetic program specifying this cell fate [36]. In addition to the Foxp3-expressing $CD4^+CD25^+$ cells, there is also a minor population of MHC class I restricted $CD8^+$ Foxp3-expressing regulatory

T cells [37]. As defined by CD4 and CD25 expression, Treg cells comprise about 1-2% of $CD4^+$ helper T cells in humans.

$CD4^+CD25^+$ Foxp3+ regulatory T cells have also been referred to as "naturally-occurring" regulatory T cells to distinguish them from "suppressor" T cell populations that can be induced *in vitro* or *in vivo*. In fact, the "naturally-occurring" $CD4^+CD25^+$ regulatory T cell population is a subset of the total Foxp3-expressing regulatory T cell population. The regulatory T cell field is further complicated by reports of additional "suppressor" T cell populations, including Tr1, $CD8^+CD28^-$, NKT cells and Qa-1 restricted T cells [37, 38]. At this point, the contribution of these populations to self-tolerance and immune homeostasis is less well defined.

Currently, it appears that CD4+CD25+ regulatory T cells play a prominent role in transplantation tolerance [39]; in addition, CD8+, CD8+CD28-, T-cell receptor+CD4-CD8-, dendritic cells and natural killer T (NKT) cells have *also* been acknowledged to have the potential to downregulate immune responses [40, 41]. One of the issues with so many potential regulatory cell populations potentially operative during transplantation is our current inability to reliably identify these cells. Recently activated T cells, also known as effector T cells, express CD25 at lower levels and for a limited period of time, whereas CD4+ T cells with the greatest regulatory properties express CD25 at high levels continuously. A concern in using CD25 expression as a marker for regulatory T cells is that there have been several reports claiming regulatory activity in CD4+CD25- T cell populations following transplantation [37]. Therefore, other markers are necessary to further identify regulatory T cells after transplantation. This finding is particularly important for generating effective therapies targeted at achieving tolerance. Markers that are currently being investigated include CD45RB, cytotoxic T-lymphocyte antigen 4 (CTLA4; CD152), glucocorticoid-induced tumor necrosis factor receptor family-related gene (GITR; TNFRSF18), CD122, CD103, and FOXP3 [42, 43]. To date, no gene has fulfilled the criteria of exclusivity and stability.

It is has been known for several years that some T cells are incapable of becoming fully activated and moreover, they enter a state of hyporesponsiveness if rechallenged with the original antigen. This phenomenon known as *T cell anergy* [44] is a means of peripheral tolerance of autoreactive T cells and may also play a role in transplantation tolerance. There are several ways by which T cell anergy can be achieved [44]. The first manner is when there is *only* signal 1 (T cell receptor binds antigen and initiates intracellular biochemical cascade) in the *absence* of signal 2 (costimulation, e.g., the receptor CD28 on T cells binding to B7.1 [CD80] and B7.2 [CD86]). This scenario is present when resting APCs interact with T cells – deficient signal 2 results in T cell anergy [45]. This process requires induction of the transcription factor NF-AT [46] and protein synthesis [47]. Anergy may also result if altered peptide ligands are used to stimulate the T cells [48] even if there is sufficient signal 2 present. The exact mechanisms that place a T cell into the anergic state are unknown but one model proposes that in addition to T cell activation biochemical steps, there are also internal negative factors in the cells that shut down activation [44]. The role of anergic T cells is unclear but it may be a mechanism allowing T cells to respond to classical antigens preventing organ-specific responses that do not provide adequate signal 2. At this point, there are no anergy-promoting immunosuppressive agents – in fact, cyclosporine prevents T cell activation *and* the generation of anergy [47] since it binds to calcineurin and prevents NF-AT from working, the latter needed for the anergic state.

There have been other mechanisms of tolerance induction in T cells that have been described and that will be briefly mentioned here. *Clonal deletion* of T cells, as described above in the central compartment, can also occur in the peripheral circulation. Upon interaction with certain donor cell populations (e.g., certain dendritic cells) there can be an elimination of recipient alloreactive cells. This may be one of the mechanisms by which infused donor hematopoietic cells at the time of solid organ transplant promote the tolerance in experimental animal models. *Clonal ignorance* is felt to be a relatively rare mechanism of tolerance that involves the keeping the recipient's immune system "ignorant" of the presence of donor cells, and thus, an immune response is not mounted. For instance, encapsulating islet cells before being transplanted might allow the immune system to remain unresponsive [49, 50]. *Clonal exhaustion* can occur after episodes of repetitive stimulation of recipient T cells by alloantigen – this can lead to either deletion or inactivation of the immune effector T cells [15, 51]. This occurrence has been described following liver transplantation, where there are a significant number of donor antigen presenting cells that migrate from the liver to the surrounding lymphoid tissues [52]. Finally, many cytokines and other soluble factors are individually immunosuppressive to T cell function (e.g., IL-10) [53]. Any perturbation of their secretion and increase in their levels can markedly alter the surrounding milieu and dampen T cell function.

Some of the B cells that escape central bone marrow deletion and elimination do so because they possess low avidity autoreactive antigen receptors. These cells become *anergic*, a state similar to that with anergic T cells in which the cell undergoes innate biochemical alterations that prevents it from undergoing activation following antigen binding, thereby arresting further differentiation [54]. Alternatively, these anergic B cells in the peripheral circulation may require higher levels of the specific antigen in order to cross the threshold into the activated state [55]. At this point, the block in the activation pathway that occurs in B cell anergy is not well understood although it appears that NF-κB and toll-like receptor signaling via the BCR pathway are inhibited. Anergic B cells express reduced levels of B-cell activating factor (BAFF) receptor [56] ultimately making these cells less able to bind and utilize this crucial cytokine that is needed for B cell survival. Anergic B cells can potentially be reversed from this state of tolerance if the self antigen that induced anergy is no longer present (cessation of anergy signaling) or if the anergic B cell now encounters high avidity antigen in the presence of T cell help. Either of these latter situations may occur in graft transplantation. For example, a loss of donor chimeric cells may result in *reactivation* of anergic B cells since the tolerizing molecule is no longer sending the necessary signal to the B cell. In addition, exogenous antigens (e.g., infectious agents) may be encountered during graft rejection such that two immune responses are simultaneously occurring; in this way, the T cell involved in the response to the infection may provide the necessary help to break the anergic state of the B cell. This scenario could result in B cells that make anti-pathogen antibodies and recruitment of clones that now make anti-graft antibodies. Finally, during an active immune response in graft rejection, there may be a plethora of growth factors (e.g., BAFF) that can overcome the anergic B cell state.

Costimulation, as with T cells, is an important adjunct that can provide augmentation or inhibition of B cell activation following BCR signaling. There are several B cell molecules capable of behaving as inhibitory receptors [57] including CD22, CD23, and FcγRIIB1. The CD40:CD40 ligand (the latter on T cells) interaction is a potent stimulatory boost to B cell activation, followed by a release of cytokines that promote B cell activation and development.

One way in which B cells directed to alloantigens may be prevented from becoming activated is by a reduction or elimination of the T cell help (i.e., T cell tolerance to the same antigens). If CD4+ T cell tolerance to a particular alloantigen is overcome (by a variety of different means, including cross-reaction with other foreign peptides) then the alloreactive B cells against those same antigens can become activated.

Finally, if alloreactive B cells and alloantibodies (as seen with panel reactive antibodies [PRA]) are present in a transplanted patient this does not necessarily mean that injury will occur to the allograft. This phenomenon cannot be simply explained by the effects of immunosuppressive reagents and brings up the possibility that the *allograft itself* is capable of protecting itself to some degree from immune effector injury. For example, there could be concealing or downregulation of crucial alloantigen dominant epitopes seen by antibodies and effector T cells and inherent individual organ capacity to control inflammation. Future therapeutic agents may be able to promote these inherent immunosuppressive effects within the grafted organ. In this regard, *immune privilege* is a term used to describe specific organs that upon their transplantation into a host can *induce* tolerance or organs that upon receiving foreign tissue will *accept* the material due to the lack of an immune response to this antigenically disparate material [58]. The classical organ that can show both forms of immune privilege is the liver [59]. For example, livers that are orthotopically transplanted in several species are readily accepted in the absence of immunosuppression and despite MHC differences with the recipient [60]. In addition, livers can have foreign cells (e.g., pancreatic islets) injected under their capsule and there will not be any significant immune response; some infections in the liver are not exposed to any effective immune response. The anterior chamber of the eye is another example of a site where tissue is not recognized as foreign and has no effective immune response [61]; other sites with immune privilege include some areas of the central nervous system and the testis [62].

III. Tolerance in Human Solid Organ Transplantation

The modern day success story of clinical solid organ transplantation, now over 50 years old [63], is certainly one of the landmark achievements of medicine over the last century. The success of clinical transplantation has inexorably been allied with superior immunosuppression, improved surgical techniques and medical management, and a better understanding of donor and recipient characteristics that promote graft acceptance. In spite of an overall improvement in graft acceptance and patient survival in all forms of organ transplantation, there continue to be significant obstacles. Acute rejection and infections continue to beleaguer the post transplant course [64] of many patients and chronic rejection has been a consistent and unacceptably high hindrance to long term graft survival [65]. Moreover, the nonspecific nature of immunosuppression therapy induces a ubiquitous dampening of the immune response in the recipient that brings with it an array of potential side effects that can cause significant morbidity to the patient including, a higher risk of infections and malignancies [66, 67], increased risk of primary disease recurrence in the allograft, and direct toxic side effects of the immunosuppressive drugs [68]. Thus, there has been an increased focus in recent years from over- immunosuppression and towards achieving clinical immune tolerance. This would essentially allow the immune system to recognize the transplanted organ as if it were the native organ without the need for immunosuppressive agents. As compared to animal models however, achieving tolerance in humans has posed a greater challenge with only rare patients fitting the criteria for "true" immunological tolerance, the latter representing graft acceptance concomitant with a specific absence of immune reactivity to the transplant and therefore no immunosuppressive therapy. In spite of this, the use of new and different approaches and our recognition of underlying immune mechanisms have allowed us to consider that achieving tolerance in the transplant setting is a more realistic goal.

As opposed to "true" immunological tolerance, there have been multiple anecdotal cases of patients, particularly liver transplant recipients, who have been able to cease or be weaned of all immunosuppressive therapy with maintenance of long term graft function [69]. Episodes of acute rejection could still occur (implying an intact immune response to the allograft), but these episodes resolved spontaneously [70]. Patients who do well following cessation of immunosuppressive therapy typically have at least two years of post liver-transplantation follow-up, a low incidence of acute rejection prior to stopping therapy, and non-autoimmune primary liver disease [71]. These patients have been characterized as having *operational tolerance*, a clinical situation defined as stable graft function without clinical features of chronic rejection and in the absence of any immunosuppressive drugs, usually for more than one year [72]. In general it appears that well-selected patients who have been stable post-transplant make more suitable candidates for attempting to achieve operational tolerance. The limited clinical trials have involved a weaning from their immunosuppressive drug regimens with in some cases up to 20% of selected liver transplant recipients capable of full drug removal [73].

Another notion that been forwarded is that of partial or *prope tolerance* [74], a situation where patients sustain stable graft function with minimal immunosuppression. The approach for attaining prope tolerance is to have a powerful induction immunosuppressive regimen, followed by minimal immunosuppression. For example, transplantation can be performed soon after 1 to 2 doses of alemtuzumab (Campath 1H), a humanized anti-CD52 antibody and lytic agent for both T and B lymphocytes that produces a marked lymphopenia, are administered. The recipients are then treated with a low dose calcineurin inhibitor, without the need for additional immunosuppressive agents. This approach has had some success and provides an opportunity for the transplanted patient to receive lower drug doses; however, this is not true immunological tolerance. The underlying basis of prope tolerance is unknown but may be a selective expansion of T regulatory cells over T effector cells as lymphocyte populations are regenerated [75].

Although achieving operational tolerance or prope tolerance has met with some success in occasional liver transplant recipients, attaining tolerance in other solid organ transplant recipients has proven more difficult. In addition to weaning (operational) and induction/monotherapy (prope) approaches, there are other strategies that have been attempted to achieve tolerance in transplant patients. One approach of noteworthy interest is supplementation with infused donor cells to enhance donor hematopoietic chimerism. As described in the previous sections, this method has been very successful in inducing true immune tolerance in animal models for many years. In humans, creating hematopoietic chimerism has been attempted in multiple ways, including bone marrow ablative (eliminating the recipient's bone marrow) and nonablative techniques, as well donor blood transfusions

[76]. These cell infusions enhance the donor ("passenger") leucocytes that leave solid organs and populate the host [77]. These supplemental approaches to induce chimerism have met with mixed success and have not shown the striking results seen in animal models. Moreover, ablating and replacement with donor bone marrow is often not practical, frequently requiring powerful drugs and/or irradiation, both of which come with their own toxicities.

Clinical tolerance induction has also been attempted with strategies aimed to disrupt the normal *cooperation* of T cells in order to prevent rejection. Most of these techniques have utilized antibodies that either depletes host peripheral T cells or that temporarily block cell surface receptors. Rodent models have demonstrated that administering CD4 antibody combined with CD8 antibodies is quite successful at achieving a tolerant state [78]. Unfortunately, the high doses of antibodies required to achieve tolerance also have side-effects. CD40L antibodies, as well as antibodies against CD3 are currently being investigated and appear to have less severe side-effects [79]. With all of these approaches to tolerance induction, there is as of yet, no consistent set of reliable immunologic assays that can assess the likelihood of rejection or tolerance [80]. This latter issue is of paramount importance since the post transplant period needs to be carefully assessed with specific immunological assays rather than simple observation of long-term graft survival. These assays, yet to be determined, will hopefully be able to predict whether certain therapeutic regimens are leading to a successful attainment of tolerance, and the need for immunosuppressive therapy.

A. Kidney Transplantation

The overall progress in immunosuppressive therapy and optimizing recipient matching has improved short-term survival of renal allografts (as well as other allografts) by decreasing the frequency of acute rejections. Yet, the long-term survival of renal grafts has not notably improved with many transplanted kidneys having long-term failure as a result of chronic rejection [81]. Certainly, there have always been occasional patients that have had longstanding grafts with normal function and on minimal or no immunosuppression but this is a rare situation. The characteristics of these unusual patients who are seemingly tolerant (operational) of their kidney allografts are often not very different from other organ recipients. In 1992, Starzl et al, found that a group of long-term stable transplant patients (some 30 years post transplant) had multilineage chimeric cells of the donor in many lymphoid and non-lymphoid organs [82]. These and other studies implicated that the presence of donor chimeric cells was necessary for clinical tolerance to occur, although many since then have countered that acute rejection can occur in a host who has a high level of chimerism [83]. Nevertheless, many investigators maintain that the *presence* of chimeric cells is a prerequisite if some of the tolerance-inducing mechanisms (e.g., clonal deletion of immune effector cells) are to take place. A variety of tolerance-inducing strategies in renal transplant recipients have been attempted to enhance chimerism [84] and all have met with marginal or no consistent success [85]. There have been several trials that have been able to induce prope (or partial) tolerance in kidney transplant patients. For example, Cortesini, et al, showed that renal transplant patients could be maintained on minimal immunosuppression following irradiation and low doses of immunosuppression [86]. Roussey-Kesler, et al. [72] reported 10 cases of kidney transplant recipients who maintained operational tolerance for a period of 5 to 15 years. All but one recipient in the study received a kidney from a deceased mismatched donor, and most of the patients stopped taking immunosuppression over a long time period (typically non-compliance). Six patients out of eight transfused patients had low titers of anti-HLA antibodies (low PRA levels). Two of the patients' renal function declined after 9 to 13 years of stopping immunosuppressive agents and unfortunately five out of ten patients were clinically diagnosed with acute rejection during the follow-up. This latter point emphasizes that these patients *did* have a competent immune response to the donor and were therefore not truly tolerant. Some graft pathology of these patients included a moderate and focal infiltrate with an arteriolar intimal hyperplasia, suggestive of early chronic nephropathy, another with a focal interstitial infiltrate, and was described as normal. There have been other cases of operationally tolerant kidney transplants that have been described. Fudaba and colleagues [87] validated the use of nonmyeloablative bone marrow and kidney transplantation to treat patients with multiple myeloma and renal failure. HLA-Identical siblings were transplanted after undergoing nonmyeloablative conditioning, including cyclophosphamide (CP), peritransplant antithymocyte globulin and thymic irradiation. Cyclosporine (CyA) was given for approximately 2 months posttransplant, followed by donor leukocyte infusions. Interestingly, they concluded that long-term acceptance of renal allografts in this particular group of patients did not seem dependent on the persistence of hematopoietic chimerism.

The ability to have a simplified immunosuppressive regimen consisting of only one agent is highly advantageous to kidney transplant patients (Prope tolerance). Shapiro, et al, [88] described 150 renal transplant recipients who were pretreated with Thymoglobulin hours before transplantation, along with bolus doses of prednisone. Following transplantation, they were administered minimal immunosuppression consisting of tacrolimus monotherapy plus steroid pulses if rejection episodes occurred. Patients who had tolerated this treatment well were then weaned from their tacrolimus monotherapy at or after 4 months post-transplantation. Spaced weaning was initiated in 113 of 150 recipients. 23% of the weaned patients experienced acute rejection; however some of the patients were able to be weaned after the episodes of acute rejection subsided. One-year graft survival was 92% with 94 of the 150 patients subsequently taking tacrolimus in a spaced fashion. Only 7% needed long-term treatment with agents other than tacrolimus. Calne [89] studied thirty one patients with cadaveric renal transplants that were treated with Campath antibody on day 0 and 1 day post-transplantation. At 48 hours following transplantation, cyclosporine monotherapy was given with no additional immunosuppressants. The patients were then followed up for approximately 24 months. 30/31 patients were living, and 29 had functioning grafts and remained on low dose monotherapy with cyclosporine. Five patients developed rejection, which was treated with steroid pulses. One patient developed a recurrence of the original disease.

B. Liver Transplantation

As mentioned before, the liver is an immunoprivileged organ that has a lower susceptibility to rejection than other transplanted organs. Clinically, this is often reflected by successful transplants in the face of a positive cross-match, minimal importance of HLA matching, reduced incidence of hyperacute rejection, occasional spontaneous recovery following severe rejection, reduced incidence of chronic rejection, and the ability to sometimes reverse chronic rejection. Immunosuppression withdrawal or conversion to monotherapy is possible in certain liver transplant patients (see table 1). Often, these are patients who are non-compliant with their medications or ones with post transplant lymphoproliferative disorder (PTLD) that have had reduced levels of immunosuppressive drugs. There have been several experiences trying to induce tolerance in liver transplant patients. Some studies have attempted to induce tolerance shortly after transplantation, while in others a tolerance protocol is implemented many years following transplantation. This is a significant difference, considering that the longer an organ has been transplanted into a recipient, the more likely the organ will be tolerated. Mazariegos, et al at Pittsburgh [90] electively withheld immunosuppression in 95 recipients; of these 18 patients were able to be off all immunosuppressants and 37 patients were on spaced immunosuppression. Twenty eight patients experienced acute rejection and 12 were withdrawn from the protocol. The mean delay between the initiation of weaning and the biopsy-proven rejection was 13.2 months. All 18 patients off of immunosuppressive agents had a significantly improved health-related quality of life. Devlin, et al (King's College) discontinued immunosuppressive therapy in18 long-term, clinically stable liver transplant patients [91]. They found five (27%) of the patients who could stay off immunosuppressive therapy. The remaining 13 patients had elevated liver function tests and immunosuppression was started again. Four out of the 13 patients with elevated liver function tests had acute rejection on liver biopsy. The predictors of successful cessation of immunosuppression were lower incidence of early post liver transplantation rejection, good HLA matching, nonautoimmune and nonviral primary liver disease. The presence of donor microchimerism was not found to be a predictor of successful immunosuppressive cessation.

The Kyoto study [92] examined 26 pediatric living related liver transplant patients, having one HLA haplotype identity, in which immunosuppression was electively weaned. Six of the 26 patients (23%) were successfully weaned. 15.4% of the patients experienced an episode of acute rejection that resolved with either steroids or with Tacrolimus. In this study, neither the degree of HLA matching nor the early episodes of rejection were found to be indicative of success in weaning immunosuppressive therapy. They suggest that down regulation of intra-graft TH1 cytokines and increased numbers of peripheral blood regulatory CD4+CD25+ T cells are associated with an operationally tolerant state. As compared to long-term patients, Eason et al. [93] attempted to completely wean 18 patients (selected from a larger cohort of 280 patients) who were at least 6 months status-post liver transplantation and who had not experienced an episode of acute rejection. Only 1 patient (5.5%) was able to be completely weaned at one year. Tryphonopoulos, et al (Miami) had 20 out of 104 liver transplant patients who were able to be successfully weaned, regardless of whether or not they had received donor bone marrow infusions [94]. There were no significant differences in donor cell chimerism levels between those patients that were successfully weaned and those who developed graft rejection. The tolerant group had a lower incidence of renal dysfunction, malignancies and infections. Finally, Takatsuki et al. [95] studied 63 patients who were weaned from immunosuppressants. Twenty-four patients (38.1%) achieved a complete weaning with a median drug-free period of 23.5 months (range, 3-69 months).

Table 1. Clinical trials in organ transplantation attempting tolerance induction

Author	Patient no.	Type of Tolerance	Time between transplant and weaning (years)	Complete IS cessation	Acute/chronic rejection	Maintenance IS	Bone marrow	Follow-up time
Mazariegos(90)	95	Complete IS weaning	mean: 8.4	19%	26/0%	CsA, Aza, Tac	No	median:35.5 months, range: 10-58 months
Devlin (91)	18	Complete IS weaning	median: 7	16.70%	28/5.6%	CsA, Aza	No	>3 years
Takatsuki (92)	26	Complete IS weaning	>2	23.80%	12/0%	Tac	No	median: 21.9 months, range: 3-69 months
Pons (109)	9	Complete IS weaning	median: 5.2	23.80%	22/0%	CsA	No	range: 17-24 months
Eason (93)	18	Complete IS weaning	>0.5	5.60%	61/0%	Tac	No	1 year
Tryphonopoulos (94)	104	Complete IS weaning	mean: 4	19%	67/1.9%	Tac, CsA	45 patients received BM tspl.	median:25.9, range 11-36
Tisone (110)	34		mean: 5.25	23.40%	76.4/0%	CsA	No	mean: 45.5, range: 15-44
Takatsuki (95)	63	Complete IS weaning	>2	38.10%	25.50%	Tac	No	>69 months
De Ruvo (100)	22	Prope tolerance; Thymoglobulin, followed by low dose tacrolimus	4 months	N/A	37.00%	Tac	No	1 year

Table 1. (Continued).

Author	Patient no.	Type of Tolerance	Time between transplant and weaning (years)	Complete IS cessation	Acute/chronic rejection	Maintenance IS	Bone marrow	Follow-up time
Roussey-Kesler (72)	10	Complete IS weaning	7.8 +/- 4.3	80%	50% (acute)	Aza and CS, CsA	No	Median: 9.4 +/- 5.7 years
Shapiro (88)	150	Prope tolerance with Thymoglobulin, followed by Tac monotherapy	>4 months	0%/ 63% partially weaned	23% (acute)	Tac	No	6-21 months
Calne (89)	31	Prope tolerance; Campath 1H, followed by cyclosporine	Immediately following transplant	0%/94% remained on monotherapy	16%	Cya	No	2 years
Fudaba (87)	6	Complete IS weaning via nonmyeloablative conditioning, followed by Cyclosporine A and donor leukocyte infusions	Immediately following transplant	50%	17%	CyA	Nonmyeloablative BM transplant	1.3 to >7 years
Tzakis (104)	16	Prope tolerance: no steroids, tacrolimus at 1/2 normal dose	Immediately following transplant	N/A; 12/16 with functioning grafts	7 mild acute, 2 severe rejection, 3 moderate	Tac at approx. 1/2 dose normally given	No	Avg: 9 months

Abbreviations: CyA = Cyclosporine; Tac = tacrolimus; IS = immunosuppression; BM = bone marrow; Aza = Azathioprine.

A negative prognostic factor in the survival of transplant patients with Hepatitis C infection is an increased strength of immunosuppressants [96]. HCV RNA levels are related to the degree of immunosuppression, the higher the viral load, and the higher the degree of chronic hepatitis in the liver graft [97, 98]. Therefore, the level of induction of immunosuppression in an attempt to induce Prope tolerance (with monotherapy) has to be carefully considered. For example, a Pittsburgh study using Campath induction and tacrolimus monotherapy showed that liver transplant patients with hepatitis C had an increase in viral hepatitis in the Campath group (HCV) [99]. De Ruvo et al. [100] described a weaning protocol for HCV patients who received liver transplants due to HCV cirrhosis. Twenty-two patients received Thymoglobulin preoperatively and were given tacrolimus as maintenance therapy. Twelve of 22 patients treated with Thymoglobulin went through the planned weaning schedule; however, none of the patients were totally weaned off of immunosuppression. The recurrence rates of HCV infection in their study were not much different than those seen in patients treated with conventional therapy. There was a lower viral load in the patients in patients who were treated with tacrolimus and steroids. The authors ultimately concluded that although a longer follow up period is needed, Thymoglobulin given preoperatively in addition to tacrolimus monotherapy may be an effective therapy regimen in HCV-infected liver transplant recipients. These studies illustrate that tolerance induction in HCV liver transplant patients may be a difficult proposition at the current time.

C. Bowel Transplantation

Due to the large intrinsic lymphoid mass and immunogenic nature of the bowel, tolerance in intestinal transplantation has long been considered to be a difficult task to achieve. Bowel allografts are very susceptible to acute rejection, and these patients also experience a high risk of infection and PTLD [101]. An intertwining of sepsis, endotoxinemia, and rejection after intestinal transplantation is among reasons why the bowel is so highly immunogenic. Moreover, inflammation associated with intestinal transplantation may create a milieu that enables enterocytes to function as APCs. HLA mismatching is thought to play a role, based on studies in dogs that were less susceptible to rejection when MHC matching occurred [102], however, clinically this is not apparent.

Several clinical studies have been met with partial success in attempting to achieve tolerance in intestinal transplantation. In general, intestinal transplantation is now treated with smaller doses of immunosuppression than just several years ago and a goal of low dose monotherapy (i.e., Prope tolerance) is being actively pursued. A Pittsburgh study described progressively tapered tacrolimus monotherapy (following induction) with no observable compromise in graft function [103]. The University of Miami conducted a study of 21 adult patients receiving either intestinal or multivisceral transplants. They found that Campath induction therapy could be followed by Tacrolimus monotherapy, without the need for steroids and without causing frequent infections [104]. The liver is an immunoprivileged organ that may have a protective effect on other organs transplanted from the same donor as demonstrated in several experimental models [105, 106]. At this point, this has not translated into definitive success in humans. The mechanisms underlying this suppressive liver effect are likely multifactorial and may include soluble HLA molecule blocking factors, generation of Treg cells, induction of anergy and Th2 immune deviation. Multivisceral transplantation (with or without the liver) presents a massive donor antigenic challenge to the host with the potential to lead to exhaustion of the recipient's immune system [107]. This raises the possibility that transplant physicians may be able to take advantage and manipulate the large donor antigen challenge to decrease the anti-graft immune response. However, at this point, multivisceral transplantation still requires a vigorous regimen of immunosuppression to maintain graft function.

IV. Summary

There are many future challenges and budding opportunities in the field of clinical tolerance for autoimmunity, cancer and transplantation. In this regard, the National Institute on Allergy and Infectious Diseases (NIAID) convened an Expert Panel on Immune Tolerance that in 1997 ultimately established the Immune Tolerance Network (ITN) [108]. The goal of the ITN is to develop a collaborative approach to the clinical application of immune tolerance that encompasses a wide range of disease processes, including kidney and islet cell transplantation, autoimmune disease, and allergy and asthma. In addition, there are many other potential strategies for inducing immune tolerance that are at the experimental level and that may eventually be clinically applied in a safe and effective manner. The goal with tolerance in transplantation will be to achieve a specific lack of immune responsiveness to the graft, without immunosuppressive drugs and while maintaining other necessary immune functions. By combining our improved understanding of responses to the human allograft with the exciting possibility of new molecular targets and patient-tailored therapy we may finally be able to give credence to the notion that the upcoming years will let us attain the "Holy Grail" of transplantation tolerance.

References

[1] Owen RD. Immunogenic consequences of vascular anastomoses between bovine twins. *Science.* 102: 400-404, 1945.

[2] Billingham RE, Brent L, Medawar PB. Actively acquired tolerance of foreign cells. *Nature.* 172:603-606, 1953.

[3] Cohn M. The common sense of the self-nonself discrimination. *Springer Sem. Immunopath.* 27(1):3-17, 2005.

[4] Beutler B. Innate immunity: an overview. *Mol. Immunol.* 40(12):845-59, 2004.

[5] Andrade CF, Waddell TK, Keshavjee S, Liu M. Innate immunity and organ transplantation: the potential role of toll-like receptors. *Am. J. Transplant.* 5(5):969-975, 2005.

[6] Gould SJ, Hildreth JE, Booth AM. The evolution of alloimmunity and the genesis of adaptive immunity. *Quar. Rev. Biol.* 79(4):359-382, 2004.

[7] Garcia KC, Adams EJ. How the T cell receptor sees antigen--a structural view. *Cell.* 122(3):333-336, 2005.

[8] Pleiman CM, D'Ambrosio D, Cambier JC. The B-cell antigen receptor complex: structure and signal transduction. *Immunol. Today.* 15(9):393-399, 1994.

[9] He X, Kappes DJ. CD4/CD8 lineage commitment: light at the end of the tunnel? *Curr. Opin. Immunol.* 18(2):135-142, 2006.

[10] Siggs OM, Makaroff LE, Liston A. The why and how of thymocyte negative selection. *Curr. Opin. Immunol.* 18(2):175-183, 2006.

[11] Aliahmad P, Kaye J. Commitment issues: linking positive selection signals and lineage diversification in the thymus. *Immunol. Rev.* 209:253-273, 2006.

[12] Burlingham WJ, Grailer AP, Heisey DM, et al. Effect of tolerance to noninherited maternal HLA antigens on the survival of renal transplants from sibling donors. *N. Engl. J. Med.* 339:1657-1664, 1998.

[13] Attavar P, Budhai L, Kim BH, et al. Mechanisms of intrathymic tolerance induction to isolated rat hepatocyte allografts. *Hepatology.* 26(5):1287-1295, 1997.

[14] Marodon G, Fisson S, Levacher B, et al. Induction of antigen-specific tolerance by intrathymic injection of lentiviral vectors. *Blood.* 2006; 108: 2972 – 2978.

[15] Starzl TE. Chimerism and tolerance in transplantation. *PNAS* (USA) 101 Suppl. 2:14607-14614, 2004.

[16] Wekerle T, Sayegh MH, Chandraker A, et al. Role of peripheral clonal deletion in tolerance induction with bone marrow transplantation and costimulatory blockade. *Transplant. Proc.* 31(1-2):680, 1999.

[17] Ruiz P, Coffman TM, Howell DN, et al. Evidence that pretransplant donor blood transfusion prevents rat renal allograft dysfunction but not the in situ cellular alloimmune or morphologic manifestations of rejection. *Transplantation.* 45(1):1-7, 1988.

[18] Thomas JM, Neville DM, Contreras JL, et al. Preclinical studies of allograft tolerance in rhesus monkeys: a novel anti-CD3-immunotoxin given peritransplant with donor bone marrow induces operational tolerance to kidney allografts. *Transplantation.* 64(1):124-35, 1997.

[19] Marti HP, Henschkowski J, Laux G, et al. Effect of donor-specific transfusions on the outcome of renal allografts in the cyclosporine era. *Transplant. Internat.* 19(1):19-26, 2006.

[20] Hollander AA, de Waal LP, van Bockel HJ, et al. No tolerance induction with cryopreserved bone marrow cells after allogeneic kidney transplantation and antilymphocyte globulin in rhesus monkeys. *Transplant. Internat.* 10(3):249-50, 1997.

[21] Hagman J, Lukin K. Transcription factors drive B cell development. *Curr. Opin. Immunol.* 18(2):127-34, 2006.

[22] Louzoun Y, Fredman T, Luning Prak E, et al. Analysis of B cell receptor production and rearrangement. Part I. Light chain rearrangement. *Semin. Immunol.* 14:169-170, 2002.

[23] Nemazee D, Weigert M. Revising B cell receptors. *J. Exp. Med.* 191:1813-1817, 2000.

[24] Zhang M, Srivastava G, Lu L. The pre-B cell receptor and its function during B cell development. *Cell* Mol. Immunol. 1(2):89-94, 2004.

[25] Meylan E, Tschopp J, Karin M. Intracellular pattern recognition receptors in the host response. *Nature.* 442(7098):39-44, 2006.

[26] Hugues S, Boissonnas A, Amigorena S, Fetler L. The dynamics of dendritic cell-T cell interactions in priming and tolerance. *Curr. Opin. Immunol.* 18(4):491-495, 2006.

[27] Dorner T, Lipsky PE. Signalling pathways in B cells: implications for autoimmunity. *Curr. Top Microbiol. Immunol.* 305:213-240, 2006.

[28] Ashwell JD. The many paths to p38 mitogen-activated protein kinase activation in the immune system. *Nature Rev. Immunol.* 6(7):532-540, 2006.

[29] Greenwald RJ, et al. The B7 family revisited. *Annu. Rev. Immunol.* 23:515-548, 2005.

[30] Okazaki T, Iwai Y, Honjo T. New regulatory co-receptors: inducible co-stimulator and PD-1. *Curr. Opin. Immunol.* 14(6):779-782, 2002.

[31] Ortaldo JR, Young HA. IL-18 as critical co-stimulatory molecules in modulating the immune response of ITAM bearing lymphocytes. *Sem. Immunol.* 18(3):193-196, 2006.

[32] Brombacher F, Kastelein RA, Alber G. Novel IL-12 family members shed light on the orchestration of Th1 responses. *Trends Immunol.* 24(4):207-212, 2003.

[33] Nishizuka Y, Sakakura T. Thymus and reproduction: sex-linked dysgenesia of the gonad after neonatal thymectomy in mice. *Science.* 166(906):753-755, 1969.

[34] Penhale WJ, Farmer A, McKenna RP, Irvine WJ. Spontaneous thyroiditis in thymectomized and irradiated Wistar rats. *Clin. Exper. Immunol.* 15(2):225-236, 1973.

[35] Kilshaw PJ, Brent L, Pinto M. Suppressor T cells in mice made unresponsive to skin allografts. *Nature.* 255(5508):489-491, 1975.

[36] Sakaguchi, S: Naturally arising Foxp3-expressing CD25+CD4+ regulatory T cells in immunological tolerance to self and non-self. *Nat. Immunol.* 6:345-352, 2005.

[37] Jiang H, Chess L. Regulation of immune responses by T cells. *N. Engl. J. Med.* 354:1166-1176, 2006.

[38] Lohr J, Knoechel B, Abbas AK. Regulatory T cells in the periphery. *Immunol. Rev.* 212:149-162, 2006.

[39] Aluvihare VR, Betz AG. The role of regulatory T cells in alloantigen tolerance. *Immunol. Rev.* 212:330-43, 2006.

[40] McCurry KR, Colvin BL, Zahorchak AF, Thompson AW. Regulatory dendritic cell therapy in organ transplantation. *Transplant. Int.* 19:525-538, 2006.

[41] Kim HJ, Hwang SJ, Kim BK, et al. NKT cells play critical roles in the induction of oral tolerance by inducing regulatory T cells producing IL-10 and transforming growth factor beta, and by clonally deleting antigen-specific T cells. *Immunology.* 118(1):101-11, 2006.

[42] Marazuela M, Garcia-Lopez MA, Figueroa-Vega N, et al. Regulatory T cells in human autoimmune thyroid disease. *J. Clin. Endocrinol. Metab.* 91(9):3639-46, 2006.

[43] Uss E, Rowshani AT, Hooibrink B, et al. CD103 is a marker for alloantigen-induced regulatory CD8+ T cells. *J. Immunol.* 177(5):2775-83, 2006.

[44] Schwartz RH. Models of T cell anergy: is there a common molecular mechanism? *J. Exp. Med.* 184(1):1-8, 1996.

[45] Jenkins MK, Johnson JG. Molecules involved in T-cell costimulation. *Curr. Opin. Immunol.* 5:361-367, 2003.

[46] Macian F, Garcia-Cozar F, Im SH, Horton HR, et al. Transcriptional mechanisms underlying lymphocyte tolerance. *Cell.* 109:719-731, 2002.

[47] Jenkins MK, Chen CA, Jung G, Mueller DL, Schwartz RH. Inhibition of antigen-specific proliferation of type 1 murine T cell clones after stimulation with immobilized anti-CD3 monoclonal antibody. *J. Immunol.* 144(1):16-22, 1990.

[48] Sloan-Lancaster J, Evavold BD, Allen PM. Induction of T-cell anergy by altered T-cell receptor ligand on live antigen-presenting cells. *Nature.* 363:156-159, 1993.

[49] Wood K, Sakaguchi S. Regulatory T cells in transplantation tolerance. *Nature.* 3:199-209, 2003.

[50] Coulombe M. Gill RG. T lymphocyte indifference to extrathymic islet allografts. *J. Immunol.* 156(5):1998-2003, 1996.
[51] Welsh RM, McNally JM. Immune deficiency, immune silencing, and clonal exhaustion of T cell responses during viral infections. *Curr. Opin. Microbiol.* 2(4):382-387, 1999.
[52] Bishop G, Sun J, Sheil A, McCaughan G. High dose/activation-associated tolerance. *Transplantation.* 64: 1377-1382, 1997.
[53] Battaglia M, Gianfrani C, Gregori S, Roncarolo MG. IL-10-producing T regulatory type 1 cells and oral tolerance. *Ann. NY Acad. Sci.* 1029:142-153, 2004.
[54] Gauld SB, Merrell KT, Cambier JC. Silencing of autoreactive B cells by anergy: a fresh perspective. *Curr. Opin. Immunol.* 18(3):292-297, 2006.
[55] Melchers F, Rolink AR. B cell tolerance--how to make it and how to break it. *Curr. Top Microbiol. Immunol.* 305:1-23, 2006.
[56] Ait-Azzouzene D, Gavin AL, Skog P, Duong B. Nemazee D. Effect of cell:cell competition and BAFF expression on peripheral B cell tolerance and B-1 cell survival in transgenic mice expressing a low level of Ig kappa-reactive macroself antigen. *Eur. J. Immunol.* 36(4):985-996, 2006.
[57] Pritchard NR, Smith KG. B cell inhibitory receptors and autoimmunity. *Immunology.* 108(3):263-273, 2003.
[58] Streilein JW. Ocular immune privilege: therapeutic opportunities from an experiment of nature. *Nature Rev. Immunol.* 3(11):879-889, 2003.
[59] Crispe I, Giannandrea M, Klein I, et al. Cellular and molecular mechanisms of liver tolerance. *Immunol. Rev.* 213:101-118, 2006.
[60] Ruiz P, Harland R, Yamaguchi Y, Bollinger RR, Sanfilippo F. In situ and systemic cellular immunity associated with orthotopic rat liver allograft acceptance or rejection. *Transplant. Proc.* 21(1 Pt 1):416-420, 1989.
[61] Niederkorn JY. See no evil, hear no evil, do no evil: the lessons of immune privilege. *Nature Immunol.* 7(4):354-359, 2006.
[62] Schuppe HC, Meinhardt A. Immune privilege and inflammation of the testis. *Chem. Immunol. Allerg.* 88:1-14, 2005.
[63] Murray JE: The 50th anniversary of the first successful human organ transplant. *Rev. Invest. Clin.* 57(2): 118-119, 2005.
[64] Callaghan CJ. Bradley JA. Current status of renal transplantation. *Meth. Mol. Biol.* 333:1-28, 2006.
[65] Nankivell BJ, Chapman JR. Chronic allograft nephropathy: current concepts and future directions. *Transplantation.* 81(5):643-654, 2006.
[66] Hariharan S. BK virus nephritis after renal transplantation. *Kid. Int.* 69(4):655-662, 2006.
[67] Kauffman HM, Cherikh WS, McBride MA, Cheng Y, Hanto DW. Post-transplant de novo malignancies in renal transplant recipients: the past and present. *Transplant. Int.* 19(8):607-620, 2006.
[68] Wilkinson A, Pham PT. Kidney dysfunction in the recipients of liver transplants. *Liver Transplant.* 11(11 Suppl 2):S47-51, 2005.
[69] Calne R. Current status of clinical transplantation tolerance. *Curr. Opin. Org. Transplant.* 11:385-388, 2006.
[70] Calne R, Sells RA, Pena JR, Davis DR, Millard PR, Herbertson BM, *et al.*, Induction of immunological tolerance by porcine liver allografts. *Nature.* 223: 472–476, 1969.

[71] Sanchez-Fueyo A. Immunological tolerance and liver transplantation. *Gastroenterol. Hepatol.* 28(4):250-256, 2005.

[72] Roussey-Kesler G, Giral M, Moreau A, et al. Clinical operational tolerance after kidney transplantation. *Am. J. Transplant.* 6: 736-746, 2006.

[73] Lerut J, and Sanchez-Fueyo A. An appraisal of tolerance in liver transplantation. *Am. J. Transplant.* 6: 1774-1780, 2006.

[74] Calne R. "Prope" tolerance: induction, lymphocyte depletion with minimal maintenance.[comment]. *Transplantation.* 80(1):6-7, 2005.

[75] Suciu-Foca N, Manavalan JS, Cortesini R. Generation and function of antigen-specific suppressor and regulatory T cells. *Transplant. Immunol.* 11:235-244, 2003.

[76] Opelz G. The role of HLA matching and blood transfusions in the cyclosporine era. Collaborative Transplant Study. *Transplant. Proc.* 21(1 Pt 1):609-612, 1989.

[77] Morris PJ. Recognition of an allograft. *Nephrologie.* 7(3 Suppl):19-22, 1986.

[78] Wise M, Zelenika D, Bemelman F, Latinne D, Bazin H, Cobbold S, Waldmann H. CD4 T cells can reject major histocompatibility complex class I-incompatible skin grafts. *Eur. J. Immunol.* 29(1):156-167, 1999.

[79] Waldmann H. Transplantation tolerance—where do we stand? *Nature Med.* 5 (11): 1245-1248, 1999.

[80] Newell KA, Larsen CP. Toward transplantation tolerance: a large step on a long road. *Am. J. Transplant.* 6: 1989-1990, 2006.

[81] Nankivell BJ, Chapman JR. Chronic allograft nephropathy: current concepts and future directions. *Transplantation.* 81(5):643-654, 2006.

[82] Starzl TE, Demetris AJ, Murase N, Ildstad S, Ricordi C, Trucco M. Cell-migration, chimerism, and graft acceptance. *Lancet.* 339 (8809): 1579-1582, 1992.

[83] Lechler RI, Garden OA, Turka LA. The complementary roles of deletion and regulation in transplantation tolerance. *Nature Rev. Immunol.* 3(2):147-58, 2003.

[84] Guenther DA, Madsen JC. Advances in strategies for inducing central tolerance in organ allograft recipients. *Ped. Transplant.* 9(3):277-281, 2005.

[85] Garcia-Morales R, Esquenazi V, Zucker K, et al. An assessment of the effects of cadaver donor bone marrow on kidney allograft recipient blood cell chimerism by a novel technique combining PCR and flow cytometry. *Transplantation.* 62(8):1149-1160, 1996.

[86] Cortesini R, Renna-Molajoni E, Cinti P, Pretagostini R, Ho E, Rossi P, Suciu-Foca Cortesini N. Tailoring of immunosuppression in renal and liver allograft recipients displaying donor specific T-suppressor cells. *Hum. Immunol.* 63(11):1010-1018, 2002.

[87] Fudaba Y, Spitzer TR, Shaffer J, Kawai T, Fehr TI, Delmonico F, Preffer F, Tolkoff-Rubin N, Dey B, Saidman SL, Kraus A, Bonnefoix T, McAfee S, Kattleman K, Colvin RB, Sachs DH, Cosimi AB, Sykes M. Myeloma responses and tolerance following combined kidney and non-myeloablative marrow transplantation: in vivo and in vitro analyses. *Am. J. Transplant.* 6: 2121-2133, 2006.

[88] Shapiro R, Jordan M, Basu A, Scantlebury V, Potdar S, Tan H, Gray E, Randhawa P, Murase N, Zeevi A, Demetris A, Woodward J, Marcos A, Fung J, Starzl T. Kidney transplantation under a tolerogenic regimen of recipient pretreatment and low-dose postoperative immunosuppression with subsequent weaning. *Ann. Surg.* 238(4): 520–525, 2003.

[89] Calne R. Prope Tolerance: A step in the search for tolerance in the clinic. *World J. Surg.* 24(7): 793-796, 2000.

[90] Mazariegos GV, Reyes J, Marino IR et al. Weaning of immunosuppression in liver transplant recipients. *Transplantation.* 63:243-249. 1997.

[91] Devlin J, Doherty D, Thomson L, et al. Defining the outcome of immunosuppression withdrawal after liver transplantation. *Hepatology.* 27: 926-933, 1998.

[92] Takatsuki M, Uemoto S, Inomata Y et al. Analysis of alloreactivity and intragraft cytokine profiles in living donor transplant recipients with graft acceptance. *Transpl. Immunol.* 8: 279-286, 2001.

[93] Eason JD, Cohen AJ, Nair S, Alcantera T, Loss GE. Tolerance: is it worth the risk? *Transplantation.* 79(9):1157-1159, 2005.

[94] Tryphonopoulos P, Tzakis AG, Weppler D et al. The role of donor bone marrow infusions in withdrawal of immunosuppression in adult liver allotransplantation. *Am. J. Transplant.* 5: 608-613, 2005.

[95] Takatsuki M, Uemoto S, Inomata Y, Egawa H, Kiuchi T, Fujita S, Hayashi M, Kanematsu T, Tanaka K. Weaning of immunosuppression in living donor liver transplant recipients. *Transplantation.* 72(3):449-454, 2001.

[96] Berenguer M. Host and donor risk factor before and after liver transplantation that impact HCV recurrence. *Liver Transpl.* 9(11):S44-S47, 2003.

[97] Gane EJ, Naoumov NV, Qian KP, et al. A longitudinal analysis of hepatitis C virus replication following liver transplantation. *Gastroenterology.* 110: 167-177, 1996.

[98] Everson G. Impact of immunosuppressive therapy on recurrence of hepatitis C. *Liver Transpl.* 8(10): S19-S27, 2002.

[99] Marcos A, Eghtesad B, Fung JJ, et al. Use of alemtuzumab and tacrolimus monotherapy for cadaveric liver transplantation: with particular reference to hepatitis C virus. *Transplantation.* 78: 966-971, 2004.

[100] De Ruvo N, Cucchetti A, Lauro A, Masetti M, et al. Preliminary results of immunosuppression with thymoglobulin pretreatment and hepatitis C virus recurrence in liver transplantation. *Transplant. Proc.* 37: 2607-2608, 2005.

[101] Pirenne J, Kawai M. Tolerogenic protocols for intestinal transplantation. *Transplant. Immunology.* 13: 131-137, 2004.

[102] Meijssen MA, Heineman E, deBruin RW, Wolvekamp MC, Marquet RL, Molenaar JC. Long-term survival of DLA-matched segmental small-bowel allografts in dogs. *Transplantation.* 56(5):1062-1066, 1993.

[103] Starzl TE, Murase N, Abu-Elmagd K, et al. Tolerogenic immunosuppression for organ transplantation. *Lancet.* 361:1502-1510, 2003.

[104] Tzakis AG, Kato T, Nishida S, et al. Alemtuzumab (Campath 1H) combined with tacrolimus in intestinal and multivisceral transplantation. *Transplantation.* 75: 1512-1517, 2003.

[105] Calne RY, Sells RA, Pena JR, et al. Induction of immunological tolerance by porcine liver allografts. *Nature.* 223: 472-476, 1969.

[106] Kamada N, Wight DGD. Antigen-specific immunosuppression induced by liver transplantation in the rat. *Transplantation.* 38:217-221, 1984.

[107] Meyer D, Baumgardt S, Loeffeler S, et al. Apoptosis of T lymphocytes in liver and/or small bowel allografts during tolerance induction. *Transplantation.* 66(11)1530-1536, 1998.

[108] Bluestone J, Matthews J, Krensky A. The Immune Tolerance Network: The "Holy Grail" Comes to the Clinic. *J. Am. Soc. Nephrol.* 11: 2141-2146, 2000.

[109] Pons J, Yelamos J, Ramirez P et al. Endothelial cell chimerism does not influence allograft tolerance in liver transplantation patients after withdrawal of immunosuppression. *Transplantation.* 75:1045-1047, 2003.

[110] Tisone G, Orlando G, Palmieri G, et al. Complete weaning off immunosuppression in HCV liver transplant recipients is feasible and favourably impacts on the progression of disease recurrence. *J. Hepatol.* 44: 702-709, 2006.

In: Immune Tolerance Research Developments
Editor: Emile B. Pontell, pp. 117-150
ISBN: 978-1-60456-209-5

Chapter 6

Dendritic Cells and CD4$^+$CD25$^+$ T $_{Reg}$ Cells in Induction of Transplant Alloantigen-Specific Tolerance

Xunrong Luo[1,2], Joseph Leventhal[1] and Anat R. Tambur[1]
[1] Division of Organ Transplantation, Department of Surgery and
[2] Division of Nephrology and Hypertension, Department of Medicine
Northwestern University Feinberg School of Medicine, Chicago, IL

Abstract

The need for indefinite use of combinations of immunosuppressive drugs in organ transplantation may paradoxically impair long-term graft function. Tolerance induction may eliminate this need. One route for tolerance induction is to harness the power of dendritic cells (DCs) which are antigen presenting cells that have remarkable plasticity and the dichotomous function of directing immune responses toward either immunity or tolerance. It has also been recognized in recent years that a subtype regulatory T cells, the CD4$^+$CD25$^+$ T_{reg} cells, play a critical role in mediating allo-specific tolerance. More importantly, there appears to be bi-directional signaling between DCs and CD4$^+$CD25$^+$ T_{reg} cells. DCs mediate central as well as peripheral T_{reg} cell development and expansion. Conversely, T_{reg} cells may directly down-regulate the ability of DCs to stimulate effector T cells. Here we consider the specific characteristics of both DCs and CD4$^+$CD25$^+$ T_{reg} cells that are relevant to induction of transplant alloantigen-specific tolerance and discuss the therapeutic potential of DC or T_{reg} cell-based therapy in organ transplantation.

Introduction

The benefit of sustained and robust donor-specific tolerance would offer many benefits to transplant recipients. In the past half century, much effort has been devoted to understanding the cellular and molecular mechanisms of allograft rejection which has allowed the induction of tolerance possible in various animal models. The two cell types that have emerged to be critical players in tolerance induction are dendritic cells and regulatory T cells. Here, we will review recent advances in the understanding of the roles these two cell types play in transplant tolerance induction as well as their potentials as therapeutics in allogeneic transplant models.

Part I. Tolerogenic Dendritic Cells

Dendritic Cell Overview

Dendritic cells (DCs) were first discovered to derive from the bone marrow and share a common progenitor with macrophages and granulocytes[1]. They are uniquely equipped antigen presenting cells (APCs) whose primary function was originally thought to be initiation of innate and adaptive immunity in face of infectious organisms and other antigens such as allo-antigens from transplanted organs[2-5]. However, an expanding literature now suggests a critical role of DCs in induction of T cell tolerance[6, 7]. The dichotomy of DC functions is permitted possibly by the state of maturation DCs at which they are exposed to antigens, the type of DCs that encounter the antigen, and the context in which antigens are encountered.

State of Maturation

The conventional view states that DCs induce immunity or tolerance depending on their state of maturation, specifically, immature DCs induce T cell tolerance whereas mature DCs induce immunity. Many stimuli induce DC maturation. Ligands to Toll-like receptors (TLRs) are potent stimuli for DC maturation[8, 9]. These include microbial signals such as viral RNA and poly IC on TLR3, lipopolysaccharide (LPS) on TLR4, mycoplasma lipopeptide on TLR6, and CpG DNA (bacteria) on TLR9 among others. Several non-TLR pathway signals are also potent stimuli of DC maturation, such as TNF family members (TNF-α, FasL, CD40L) and type I interferons[10-12]. Upon maturation, DCs express higher levels of cell surface major histocompatibility complex (MHC) molecules as well as accessory molecules such as B7-family members (CD86, CD80, PD-L2/B7-DC, ICOS-L), TNF family members (CD137, CD124, CD70), and chemokine receptors (CCR5, CCR7)[13]. Matured DCs become potent stimulators of naïve $CD4^+$ and $CD8^+$ T cells. In contrast, immature DCs are poor stimulators of T cells at best. However, immature DCs are highly efficient in antigen uptake, processing, loading onto MHC class II molecules and transporting to cell surface, a feature that is to some degree dampened upon maturation[14]. The capacity for capturing and processing apoptotic cells by immature DCs is thought to be crucial in the maintenance of tolerance to self-antigens and non-inflammatory stimuli under steady-state conditions[6] It is therefore not surprising that experimental strategies for utilizing DCs to induce transplant tolerance center on blocking the DC maturation process. Approaches to "arrest" DC maturation can be broadly categorized into: 1) direct *in vivo* targeting of known cellular components of DC maturation pathway, and 2) *in vitro* generation of immature DCs under alternative culture conditions which result in alterations of accessory molecule expressions.

Targeting of Components of DC Maturation Pathway

Upregulation of costimulatory molecules upon DC maturation is in part dependent on NF-κB mediated gene transcription[15]. Strategies for blocking NF-κB signaling pathway have been studied to induce alloantigen specific tolerance. Lu *et al* described that bone marrow derived DCs treated with synthetic oligodexoynucleotides (ODN) containing consensus NF-κB binding sites showed decreased cell surface costimulatory molecules expression and induced allogeneic donor-specific hyporesponsiveness in mixed leukocyte reactions. When $2x10^6$ NF-κB ODN treated DCs were injected into full MHC mismatched recipients, they were able to prolong allogeneic heart graft survival from a mean survival time (MST) of 10 days to 27 days[16, 17]. Similarly, Benigni *et al* used an adenoviral vector encoding for a kinase-defective dominant negative form of IKK2 to block NF-κB activation and observed similar prolongation of allogeneic graft survival in a rat kidney transplantation model[18]. Blocking TNF-α signaling in DCs using a recombinant adenoviral vector expressing soluble TNF-α receptor type 1 (sTNFR1) has also been shown to result in resistance to LPS induced maturation and further impairment of DC chemotaxis[19]. Pre-treatment with donor DC-sTNFR1 led to marked prolongation of allogeneic heart transplantation (MST from 12 to 87 days).

A signaling pathway proximal to NF-κB that has recently gained significant attention in studies of transplant rejection is the Toll-like receptor (TLR) pathway. TLRs are pattern recognition receptors expressed on surface of APCs that are critical in the host detection and defense against microbial pathogens. Various TLRs, upon ligation, initiate a signaling pathway via their common signal adaptor protein MyD88 which eventually leads to the translocation of NF-κB and the DC maturation. Using an HY-incompatible skin transplant model, Lakkis *et al* has demonstrated that activation of TLR signal adaptor protein MyD88 is crucial for rejection of allogeneic transplants[20]. Engagement of a single TLR using CpG injections at the time of allogeneic transplant was sufficient to abolish tolerance mediated by co-stimulation blockade[21]. TLR activation in this model is associated with prevention of intragraft recruitment of $CD4^+Foxp3^+$ regulatory T cells. Clinical studies in renal transplant recipients are beginning to reveal an association between TLR polymorphisms and the development of acute rejection post-transplant[22]. These data not only underscored the importance of innate immunity in allograft rejection, but more importantly provided basis for future therapeutic strategies that target the TLR signal transduction pathway for transplant tolerance induction.

A downstream effect of DC maturation, namely enhanced cell surface expression of the B7 costimulatory molecules CD80 and CD86, and subsequent augmented CD28-B7 interaction, can be blocked by the fusion protein cytotoxic T lymphocyte Ag-immunoglobulin (CTLA4-Ig)[23]. This protein competes with CD28 for B7 ligation thereby blocking B7-CD28 mediated T cell activation. DCs retrovirally transduced with CTLA-Ig have been shown to induce alloantigen-specific T cell hyporesponsiveness *in vitro* and *in vivo*[24]. Pretreatment with CTLA4-Ig transduced DCs significantly prolonged allograft survival in a murine model of cardiac transplantation which could be further augmented by additional costimulation blockade using anti-CD40L mAb. Systemic treatment of recipients with CTLA4-Ig-coding adenoviral vector also led to long term allograft survival[25]. The protective effects appeared to be at least in part mediated by DC secreted soluble factor(s).

More recent data has shed light on a potential soluble factor, indoleamine 2,3-dioxygenase (IDO), a key enzyme in tryptophan catabolism[26]. It has been identified that CTLA4-Ig has a bidirectional signaling capacity: in addition to its negative effect on T cells (blocking CD28-mediated T cell activation), it also "reversely" signals the DCs through B7 molecules and promotes IDO production which in turn promotes T cell apoptosis[27]. This effect is paradoxically dependent on IFN-γ production[28]. This pathway provides an additional mechanism for DCs to maintain T cell homeostasis and self- tolerance by deletion.

In Vitro Generation of Immature DCs under Alternative Culture Conditions

Myeloid DCs can be derived from bone marrow progenitors in the presence of GM-CSF. Several natural cytokines have been exploited in altering DC differentiation and function. IL-10 is a multifunctional cytokine with diverse effects on many cell types. DCs that are exposed to IL-10 during differentiation or tranduced with viral vectors expressing IL-10 have been shown to display decreased levels of MHC II, CD80, and CD40, consistent with an immature state, and to induce antigen-specific T cell anergy *in vitro*[29]. *In vivo*, DCs engineered to express IL-10 alone did not significantly prolong allograft survival, but co-expression of another inhibitory cytokine TGF-β1[30] or the chemokine receptor CCR7[31] led to striking prolongation of allograft survival in heart transplant model.

Independent effects of TGF-β1 on DC differentiation and function have also been studied. DCs transduced to express TGF-β1 display a characteristic immature phenotype, exhibit poor allostimulaotry activity but enhance DC survival in allogeneic hosts[32]. Survival of allogeneic cardiac grafts could be prolonged in recipients injected with donor TGF-β1 transduced DCs prior to transplantation. TGF-β1 has also been shown to be crucial in $CD4^+CD25^+$ regulatory T cells induction and expansion[33], and a likely source of endogenous TGF-β1 is antigen presenting cells[34], the most efficient of which are the DCs. Most recently, it has been shown that DCs can be "licensed" by certain tumor cells to produce large quantities of TGF-β1 which then enable them to simulate $CD4^+CD25^+$ T_{reg} cell proliferation[35]. However, natural signals that stimulate DC TGF-β1 production remain to be determined.

DCs express high levels of vitamin D receptor (VDR)[36]. Results accumulated over the past two decades demonstrated that VDR ligands significantly modulate the phenotype and function of DCs (reviewed in[37]). Treatment of DCs with1,25-dihydroxyvitamin D_3, the active form of vitamin D, leads to downregulated expression of the costimulatory molecules and to decreased IL-12 and enhanced IL-10 production, resulting in decreased T cell activation[38, 39]. Interestingly, such VDR ligand treated DCs also seem to induce $CD4^+CD25^+$ T_{reg} cells, a mechanism that at least in part contribute to mediate transplant tolerance[40]. Direct *in vivo* tolerogenic effect of VDR ligand treated DCs has also been demonstrated by adoptive transfer of the treated DCs in allograft transplantation models[41]. Glucocorticoid is another agent that has been shown to arrest DC maturation with resulting down-regulation of costimulatory molecules and inflammatory cytokine secretions[42, 43]. Other pharmacological agents that have been studied in the process of DC maturation include LF15-0195[44, 45] and nacystelyn[46] which also target the NF-κB pathway as discussed above.

Though significant effort from the past has focused on immature DCs, it has been recently recognized that immature DCs generated *in vitro* as such may not be the ideal candidate for tolerance induction *in vivo*. They may have inefficient migratory capacity from lacking appropriate chemokine receptor[47] and they may also mature *in vivo* upon encountering proinflammatory stimuli in host microenvironment. Effort in recent years has been made to study partially activated types of DCs for transplant tolerance and the terms "alternatively activated" or "semi-mature" DCs have been coined to distinguish such DCs from immature DCs. Several alternative maturation protocols have been studied[19, 42, 48], which include TNF-α stimulation, LPS or CD40 ligation in combination with dexamethasone, among others. Such "semi-mature" DCs have unique profiles of costimulation molecule and chemokine receptor expressions as well as cytokine secretion (IL12/IL-10 ratio, TGF-β1), such that they may be more resistant to further maturation *in vivo* and are more efficient in induce long term allograft survival.

Role of DC Subsets in Transplant Tolerance

DC populations with distinct phenotype and function have been described both in humans and rodents. In mice, one subset of DCs is characterized by CD8α^+CD11b^{low} cell surface markers and is remarkably efficient in taking up apoptotic cells compared to CD8α^- DCs, the clearest differences in the functions of the CD8α^+ and CD8α^- subsets[49-51]. The CD8α^+ DCs have been called lymphoid DCs because they were initially thought to develop from lymphoid rather than myeloid progenitors. Subsequent adoptive transfer studies suggested that the CD8α^+ DCs may also develop from myeloid progenitors[52]. Evidence emerged to indicate that constitutive presentation of antigens acquired from dying cells by DCs in steady state led to deletion of naïve peripheral T cells and systemic antigen-specific tolerance[51]. The first report of the role of CD8α^+ DCs in allogeneic transplant tolerance studied both freshly isolated immature and over-night GM-CSF matured CD8α^+ DCs, and found that both immature as well as matured CD8α^+ DCs markedly prolong allogeneic heart graft survival[53]. This effect was associated with specific impairment of anti-donor T cell proliferative responses, which was not reversed by exogenous IL-2. This finding contrasts that seen with CD8α^- myeloid subset in that only the immature CD8α^- DCs were able to prolong transplant graft survival. A more recent study demonstrated that the CD8α^+ DCs may be highly efficient in expanding antigen-specific CD4$^+$CD25$^+$ Tregs from a polyclonal repertoire comparing to whole splenic DCs or bone marrow-derived DCs[54]. This unique capacity of the CD8α^+ DCs was attributed to a lower background stimulation originating from T cell autoreactivity, possibly related to the resemblance between the CD8α^+ DCs and thymic DCs which are involved in negative selection of highly atuoreactive T cells in the thymus.

Another subset of DCs that has been increasingly recognized to play an important role in immune tolerance is the plasmacytoid DCs (pDCs), a term that portrays their resemblance to plasma cells. Mouse pDCs characteristically express B220 and Ly6C on their cell surface, and are CD11c^{dim}, secrete large amounts of type I interferons upon exposure to viruses, and are thought to play an essential role in protecting the host against inflammatory responses in setting of harmless antigens[55]. Their development from hematopoietic stem cells in humans as well as in mice is uniquely promoted by fms-like tyrosine kinase 3 ligand (Flt-3L)[56, 57]. They express TLR9 and respond to stimulation with TLR9 ligand CpG-oligonucleotide with upregulation of B7 molecules[58]. Initial suggestion of the pDCs as "tolerogenic" DCs came from murine allogeneic BM transplant models where the presence of these cells correlated with stem cell engraftment and decreased occurrence of GVHD[59, 60]. The same authors have also shown that pDCs were able to induce durable tolerance to skin allografts. Examination of pDCs in vascularized organ allograft survival revealed that a single preoperative infusion of pDC of donor origin prolong heart graft survival significantly compared with untreated mice (MST 22 vs. 9 days, respectively)[61]. Corroborating with *in vitro* data suggesting that immature pDCs can induce T_{reg} cells, a recent study from Bromberg *et al* showed that alloantigen-presenting recipient pDCs home to local lymph nodes and induce generation of donor-specific $CD4^{+}CD25^{+}Foxp3^{+}$ regulatory T cells[62], a mechanism that at least in part contribute to tolerance induction by the well-characterized regimen using donor specific transfusion plus αCD40L. Depletion of pDCs in this model or prevention of pDC homing to LNs inhibit peripheral T_{reg} cell development and tolerance induction, whereas adoptive transfer of tolerized pDCs induce T_{reg} cell development and prolong cardiac graft survival. An alternative mechanism for pDC-induced tolerance has been proposed to be preferential induction of IDO expression upon ligation of a number of cell surface receptors[63]. As pointed out earlier, reverse signaling between CTLA4 and B7 upregulates IDO expression. This occurs with various degrees among different DC subsets, with the pDCs and the $CD8\alpha^{+}$ DCs being predominantly the subsets that express IDO upon CTLA4-Ig treatment. Classic myeloid DCs ($CD11c^{+}CD11b^{+}$) have much fewer IDO^{+} cells upon CTLA4-Ig treatment. More recently, another cell surface receptor, CD200R, which interacts with a broadly distributed cell surface glycoprotein CD200, has been identified to play an important role in the control of myeloid cellular activity and prevention of autoimmunity (reviewed in [64]). A fusion protein, CD200-Ig, has been shown to interact with CD200R expressed on murine pDCs. This can be further augmented by CpG oligodeoxynucleotide treatment. Ligation of CD200R on pDCs by CD200-Ig induces expression of IDO[65], which then initiates the tolerogenic pathway of tryptophan catabolism. As a result, pDCs are capable of suppressing antigen-specific responses *in vivo* when transferred into recipients after treatment with CD200-Ig. These studies underscore the novel functions and diverse mechanisms by which pDCs may be involved in host alloantigen-specific tolerance induction.

Indirect vs. Direct Pathway

In allogeneic transplantation, alloantigen directed immune responses are thought to be induced via two distinct pathways – the direct and the indirect pathways (reviewed in [66]). The direct pathway utilizes intact allogeneic MHC molecules on donor DCs to interact directly with recipient T cells, whereas the indirect pathway is driven by recipient DC-processed and self-MHC presented polymorphic sequences of allogeneic MHC molecules. This concept has two immediate implications: 1. As donor DCs are derived from the transplanted organ, they are limited in numbers as well as life span. Following their elimination over time, it is conceivable that the strength of direct anti-alloantigen specific response would diminish accordingly; and 2. Among the normal T cell repertoire, there is a higher frequency of T cells with direct allo-specificity compared to that of T cells with indirect allo-specificity implying that the direct allo-response dominates the early post-transplantation phase whereas the indirect pathway plays a more important role during later stages post-transplantation[67-69]. As a consequence, a paradigm has evolved whereby the direct allo-specific response is thought to mediate acute allograft rejection whereas the indirect allo-specific response is considered the major mediator of chronic allograft rejection. The relative contribution of either pathway to allograft rejection in vivo remains a subject of intense studies over the past two decades. Direct visualization of DC trafficking and interactions between recipient $CD4^+$ T cells with donor (direct) or recipient (indirect) DCs using immunofluorescent technique demonstrated differential kinetics of homing and lymphoid tissue localization of donor vs. recipient DCs during acute rejection or tolerance induction[70], further differentiating the importance of either pathways in allograft transplantation.

Targeting the Direct Pathway of Alloantigen Presentation

Depletion of donor leukocytes prior to allograft transplantation could prolong allograft survival in certain experimental conditions. Early studies showed that *in vitro* culture of allografts prior to allograft transplantation depletes donor bone marrow derived “passenger” leukocytes and prolongs graft survival[71, 72]. Later studies demonstrated that spontaneous acceptance of allografts could be achieved by “parking” the graft in an intermediate recipient before transplantation which again serves to deplete donor leukocytes. Reconstitution in such recipients with donor DCs, even in small numbers, precipitates rapid graft rejection[73]. These data demonstrated a key role of donor DCs during the initial phase of allo-responses and therefore a potential target for allo-specific tolerance induction. For instance, chemokine-dependent homing of donor dendritic cells to secondary lymphoid tissues is essential for host sensitization and acute allograft rejection. Allografts transplanted into the plt (*p*aucity of *l*ymph node *T* cell) recipients that are deficient in secondary lymphoid expression of the CCR7 ligands, CCL21 and CCL19, enjoy indefinite graft survival in a kidney capsule islet transplant model[74]. Likewise, donor DCs that lack the adhesion molecule ICAM-1 show substantially decreased level of T cell priming and at least in part contribute to prolonged $ICAM^{-/-}$ cardiac graft survival in allogeneic transplant model[75].

Targeting donor DCs using immunosuppressive cytokines or agents that block the NF-κB pathway with a consequence of diminishing alloantigen presentation have also been widely used to prolong allograft survival. For instance transducing IL-10 in donor derived dendritic cells and injecting the modified DCs 7 days prior to transplantation moderately prolonged allograft survival in a small intestine transplant model[76]. Donor DCs generated in the presence of TGF-β1 or engineered to express TGF-β1 retain immature phenotype and with further costimulation blockade by anti-CD40L mAb induce long-term allograft survival[77, 78]. Likewise, donor DCs treated with double-strand NF-κB decoy oligodeoxynucleotides prolonged liver allograft survival and regeneration[79]. Furthermore, donor DCs engineered to express FasL have been used to deliver apoptotic signals to Fas^+ T cells thereby downregulating donor-specific T cell responses[80]. In addition to donor-specific anergy and deletion, tolerogenic donor DCs have also been shown to induce and expand regulatory $CD4^+$ T cells in both the central and peripheral compartments.

Targeting the Indirect Pathway of Alloantigen Presentation

In contrast to the diminishing direct allo-specific response over time, a series of clinical studies have demonstrated that indirect allo-reponse increases over time, with increased frequencies of T cells bearing indirect allo-specificities[81]. As previously discussed, recipient DCs are well-equipped with the capacity to uptake, process, and present allogeneic MHC peptides in the context of recipient MHC molecules, therefore are central to indirect allospecific T cell activation. Conditions likely exist that allow recipient DCs to tolerize, rather than activate, indirect allospecific T cells. Indeed, in a model of heart transplantation, tolerance could not be achieved in recipients that were incapable of mounting indirect anti-donor responses[82], suggesting that indirect allorecognition is necessary to induce stable tolerance. As such, strategies for tolerance induction have placed significant emphasis on targeting the recipient DCs.

Initial observation that targeting the indirect pathway leads to spontaneous allograft acceptance came from early studies by Lechler *et al.* In a rat kidney semiallogeneic transplant model, the authors showed that when an F1 (AS x AUG) kidney was re-transplanted from an immunosuppressed parent recipient one month later to a second parent recipient of the same strain, the grafts were spontaneously accepted without the need for any immunosuppression therapy, whereas a fully allogneic kidney re-transplanted following the same protocol led to rejection[73]. The interpretation of the observation was that cells in the F1 graft co-expressing both AS and AUG MHC molecules developed the ability to silence AS T cells with indirect anti-AUG specificity. On the basis of these findings, the same authors tested the ability of F1 immature DCs to induce tolerance and regulation via the indirect pathway. Interestingly, injection of F1, but not donor, immature DCs was able to prolong allograft survival, confirming the privileged role of F1 DCs in the induction of indirect pathway regulation[83]. The protection was accompanied by donor-specific hyporesponsiveness by indirect presentation (tested with recipient DCs pulsed in vitro with allogeneic cell lysate). Furthermore, depletion of the $CD25^+$ T cell population unmasks a strong response to the donor antigen, suggesting the indirect regulation is in part mediated through development of regulatory T cells.

The above findings have obvious clinical relevance in tolerance induction in living related donor organ transplantations. However, other means for delivering donor antigens to recipient DCs are necessary to be investigated. Presentation of antigens from peripheral tissues by steady-state DCs in lymphoid organs has been shown to promote peripheral tolerance in mice. One strategy to deliver donor antigens to steady-state DCs with an inhibitory signal is by using donor cells undergoing apoptosis. Early studies using chemical cross-linking of soluble peptides to APCs by a chemical cross-linker 1-ethyl-3-(3'-dimethylaminopropyl)-carbodiimide (ECDI) have shown that such ECDI-coupled cells efficiently induce specific peptide tolerance and control autoimmunity[84]. Translating into alloantigen tolerance, subsequent studies using ECDI treated donor lymphocytes ("coupling" of cell surface MHC molecules to donor cells) have shown that i.v. injection of such cells prior to transplantation led to a transient but significant graft protection in full MHC-mismatched skin and heart transplant models[85, 86]. One possible mechanism underlying the protection of allografts may be induction of apoptosis by ECDI treatment and subsequent uptake of ECDI-fixed donor cells by host APCs[86]. *In vivo*, direct visualization by immunofluorescence revealed that recipient splenic $CD8\alpha^+$ DCs are most efficient in uptaking i.v. injected apoptotic donor cells, and that capturing apoptotic donor cells does not mature recipient DCs (which have similar levels of MHC-I/II, CD40, CD80 and CD86 compared to DCs that have not internalized apoptotic cells)[87]. Instead, it allows the recipient DCs to delete alloreactive cells. *In vitro*, recipient DCs loaded with donor-derived apoptotic cells are able to cross-tolerize recipient T cells, and direct infusion of such DCs prior to transplantation prolongs allograft survival[88]. Evidence also exists that recipient macrophages may play a role in apoptotic cell induced donor specific regulation and that TGF-β1-dependent regulatory T cell expansion may partially contribute to the regulation[89].

Semi-Direct Pathway of Alloantigen Presentation

More recently, a third pathway for allo-recognition has been proposed: the semi-direct pathway. This model proposes that intact donor MHC molecules can be transferred *in toto* from donor cells (for instance, donor endothelial cells or donor DCs) to recipient DCs which then prime recipient alloreactive T cells with donor MHCs[90]. One way of recipient DCs acquiring intact donor MHC (class I and class II) molecules is through exosomes secreted by other DCs[91]. This pathway was initially proposed to explain the observation of "unlinked help" in which $CD4^+$ T helper cells with indirect allospecificity appeared to be able to amplify an effector $CD8^+$ T cell response with direct allospecificity[92]. With the semi-direct pathway, recipient DCs acquire and present intact donor MHC class I molecule to direct allospecific $CD8^+$ T cells on the one hand and present processed donor MHC molecules as polymorphic peptides to indirect allospecific $CD4^+$ T cells on the other. Therefore it solves the conundrum of the "unlinked help" and provides a mechanism for "linked help". Likewise, "linked suppression" describes indirect allospecific $CD4^+$ regulatory T cells regulating effector $CD8^+$ T cells with direct allospecificity[93].

Part II. The Role of DCs in Expansion and Induction of $CD4^+CD25^+$ T_{reg} Cells

Regulatory T cells play a critical role in suppressing immune responses to a wide spectrum of antigens, therefore are emerging as key players in tolerance strategies in controlling autoimmune diseases and in allogeneic transplant rejections. Alloantigen-specific $CD4^+CD25^+$ cells are presumably generated in transplant recipients through multiple but not mutually exclusive pathways. There are several "types" of regulatory T cells. Tr1 and Th3 regulatory T cells depend on inhibitory cytokines IL-10 and TGF-β1 respectively for their function (reviewed in [94]). A different type referred to as the "natural" regulatory T cells (T_{reg}) develop in the thymus and are $CD4^+$ and $CD25^+$. They express the transcription factor Foxp3 which interacts with another calcium-regulated transcription factor NFAT to mediate their suppressive functions[95]. Recent data suggests a process of so-called "infectious tolerance", where CD4+CD25+ Treg in the periphery convert CD4+CD25- cells into T_{reg} cells [96] [97]. Foxp3 is upregulated in these "induced" T_{reg} cells. Whether these cells suppress in a cell-cell contact dependent or cytokine dependent manner remains to be determined. Both naturally and alloantigen-selected T_{reg} cells are expandable in the periphery by alloantigens and play important roles in controlling graft rejection and possibly lead to allograft tolerance. Numerous previously established tolerance protocols in rodents have focused upon generation and/or expansion of alloantigen-specific $CD4^{+}CD25^{+}$ cells using therapeutic manipulations in the transplant recipient. Examples of such tolerizing strategies include using monoclonal antibodies (mAb) specific for CD3, CD4 or CD154, a combination of 1,25-dihydroxyvitamin D3 with mycophenolate mofetil, pre-transplant donor blood transfusion, and administration of tolerogenic or regulatory dendritic cells [98-100]. Unfortunately, none of these approaches have been shown to expand $CD4^{+}CD25^{+}$ clones specifically and efficiently. Studies have shown that Treg can be effectively expanded *in vitro* (*ex vivo*) in the presence of immobilized anti-CD3 mAb plus IL-2 [101], or with antiCD3/CD28 coated microbeads and IL-2 [102]. This approach allows for expansion of the entire population of T_{reg} cells, while maintaining a diversified repertoire, so-called polyclonal regulatory cells. Infusion of *ex vivo* expanded polyclonal T_{reg} cells has been shown to delay or even prevent GVHD in mice [101, 103]. Alternatively, T_{reg} cells can be expanded and, at the same time, selected for their capacity to recognize allogeneic antigen, so that antigen specific T_{reg} cells can be obtained. Such antigen specific ex vivo expanded T_{reg} cells has also been shown to delay or prevent GVHD in mice [101, 104, 105]. In this section, we will focus on the role of DCs in peripheral expansion and generation of $CD4^{+}CD25^{+}$ $Foxp3^{+}$ T_{reg} cells.

The Role of DCs in In vitro Expansion of $CD4^{+}CD25^{+}$ T_{reg} Cells

Initial studies of the $CD4^{+}CD25^{+}$ $Foxp3^{+}$ T_{reg} cells revealed that they are "anergic" to TCR stimulation in culture[106]. Combined with the small percentages (5-10%) of such cells in the periphery, it makes their experimental studies and application in clinical conditions difficult. In a pioneer study by Yamazaki *et al*, it was demonstrated that the *in vitro* relative anergic state of the $CD4^{+}CD25^{+}$ $Foxp3^{+}$ T_{reg} cells was in part due to the suboptimal antigen presenting cells used in those studies that were largely in an immature functional state[107]. In contrast, when mature DCs were used to present antigens, the T_{reg} cells broke their apparent anergic state and underwent vigorous proliferation. This proliferation could be further augmented with exogenous IL-2. The DC-dependent T_{reg} cell expansion is contingent upon B7-CD28 costimulation. The expanded T_{reg} cells maintained high levels of CTLA-4 and GITR expression, and were functionally suppressive, suggesting that the proliferation did not come at the expense of regulatory function.

Subsequently, mature DC expanded antigen-specific T_{reg} cells have been studied both in autoimmune models as well as allogeneic transplant models[108]. In models of autoimmune diabetes, it was shown that mature DCs presenting a single β cell autoantigen peptide were able to expand islet antigen specific $CD4^{+}CD25^{+}$ T_{reg} cells *in vitro*, and that the expanded $CD4^{+}CD25^{+}$ T_{reg} cells showed enhanced suppressive function compared to freshly isolated T_{reg} cells and could effectively suppress diabetes in the NOD scid adoptive transfer model. Among the splenic $CD11c^{+}$ DCs, the $CD8\alpha^{+}$ subset induces the least degree of basal activation when co-cultured with a polyclonal pool of T cells[54]. Therefore, when pulsed with peptide or tissue antigens, the $CD11c^{+}$ $CD8\alpha^{+}$ DCs, among all DC subsets, allow the highest stimulation index of the co-cultured T cells compared to un-pulsed DCs. This feature makes the splenic $CD11c^{+}$ $CD8\alpha^{+}$ DCs an ideal DC population for selective expansion of T_{reg} cells of rare autoantigen specificities as only the T cells with engaged TCRs would be stimulated to proliferate. Indeed, when present at as low as 0.01% among wild-type polyclonal T cells, transgenic T cells expressing a TCR specific for an HA epitope could be selectively expanded over 500 fold by HA peptide pulsed CD8α$^+$ DCs. Furthermore, wild type T_{reg} cells with HA specificity could also be selectively expanded using CD11c$^+$ CD8α$^+$ DCs pulsed with either HA peptides or lysates of islet cells expressing HA as a neo-autoantigen. These selectively expanded HA-specific T_{reg} cells exert antigen-specific suppression *in vitro* after secondary stimulation, and more importantly suppress autoimmune diabetes in transgenic mice engineered to express HA in the pancreatic β cells.

With respect to alloantigen specific CD4$^+$CD25$^+$ T_{reg} cell expansion for transplant tolerance induction, allogeneic whole spleen APCs plus IL-2 was initially experimented by several groups, with the goal to increase the frequency of alloantigen-specific CD4$^+$CD25$^+$ T_{reg} cells from a polyclonal pool[104, 109-111]. Here, the initial frequency of alloreactive T cells is high in contrast to autoreactive T cells, presumably because of cross-reactivities between numerous allo-MHC peptide complexes and self-MHC molecules. These initial studies utilized skin graft transplantation or graft versus host disease (GVHD) models and demonstrate *in vivo* suppressive activity of the expanded T_{reg} cells. However, large numbers (10^6 to 10^7) of expanded T_{reg} cells were typically necessary to achieve alloantigen-specific suppression *in vivo*[104, 109, 110]. It was recently demonstrated that allogeneic mature DCs are much more efficient than whole splenic APCs at expanding alloantigen-specific CD4$^+$CD25$^+$ T_{reg} cells, with a three to five-fold expansion in cell numbers in 7-day mixed leukocyte reactions[112]. In addition, allogeneic DC expanded T_{reg} cells maintain higher levels of Foxp3 expression compared to whole spleen APCs, and can do so even in the absence of IL-2. The expanded T_{reg} cells show specific suppression of GVHD *in vivo*, whereas third party or syngeneic DC-expanded T_{reg} cells exhibit weaker suppression, indicating that an alloantigen-specific component of T_{reg} function has been induced following expansion with allogeneic DCs.

An alternative approach for expansion of the T_{reg} population is *de novo* induction CD4$^+$CD25$^+$Foxp3$^+$ T cells from the non-regulatory naïve CD4$^+$CD25$^-$Foxp3$^-$ T cells. This has been shown to be possible in the presence of nanomolar concentrations of TGF-β1[33]. Initial studies of *de novo* generation of CD4$^+$CD25$^+$Foxp3$^+$ T cells again utilized non-specific stimulation with mitogenic antibodies or bulk splenic APCs. We have recently shown that in contrast to expanding existing CD4$^+$CD25$^+$ T_{reg} cells, mature DCs are much less efficient in converting naïve CD4$^+$CD25$^-$Foxp3$^-$ T cells to CD4$^+$CD25$^+$Foxp3$^+$ T cells in the presence of TGF-β1 (X Luo and KV Tarbell, unpublished). Rather, freshly isolated splenic CD11c$^+$ DCs are able to induce Foxp3 expression in the presence of TGF-β1 in >90% of the resulting T cells that are initially Foxp3$^-$. Functionally, these *in vitro* DC-generated CD4$^+$CD25$^+$Foxp3$^+$ T cells show antigen-specific suppression *in vitro* and suppress autoimmune diabetes in NOD mice.

The Role of DCs in In Vivo Expansion of CD4$^+$CD25$^+$ T_{reg} Cells

In vivo, several transplant tolerance protocols have been shown to generate alloantigen-specific T_{reg} cells which might involve presentation of allogantigens by either donor or recipient DCs (reviewed in [96]). By using antigen conjugated to antibodies directed at the endocytic receptor DEC-205, which is expressed at high levels on DCs, Enk *et al* have shown that the targeted DCs were able to preferentially expand the number of CD4$^+$CD25$^+$ T_{reg} cells in intact lymphoid tissue[113]. Furthermore, von Boehmer *et al* showed that DCs delivered with low dose antigen by DEC-205 targeting were able to differentiate non-regulatory $CD4^-$ $CD25^+$ T cells into $CD4^+CD25^+$ $Foxp3^+$ T cells[114]. These observations suggest that *in vivo* renewal of $CD4^+CD25^+$ T_{reg} cells can occur in response to antigens presented by steady state DCs.

Part III. Transplant Tolerance: From Mouse to Human

Human DC Subsets

Human DCs are all bone marrow-derived leukocytes and are comprised of at least four different sub-types. Human peripheral blood displays two subsets of DC precursors: monocytes, which differentiate into immature myeloid DC (mDC) upon exposure to GM-CSF and to IL-4; and plasmacytoid cells (pDC), which display features of the lymphoid lineage and require IL-3 for their development into plasmacytoid DC (pDC)[115, 116]. These two cell types are present also in lymphoid and non-lymphoid tissues. In addition, there are the dermal/interstitial DCs (DDC-IDCs) and the Langerhans cells (LCs)[117], which will not be discussed in this current review.

The most accessible human DC precursor is the $CD14^+$ monocytes from peripheral blood. These cells can be differentiated into mDC that are $CD14^-$, $CD11c^+$, $CD83^{++}$, HLA-DR^{++} following incubation with GM-CSF and IL-4. mDC maturation can be achieved by the addition of a variety of stimuli to the culture (e.g., TNF-α, LPS) and is usually measured functionally by the production of IL-12[118].

Human pDC can also be generated from peripheral blood by exposing lineage negative, HLA-DR^{++}, BDCA-2^+, BDCA-4^+ and $CD123^{++}$ cells following FMS-like tyrosine kinase 3 ligand (Flt3-L) treatment[55, 119, 120]. Maturation of pDC is achieved by adding IL-3 in combination with CD154 (CD40L)[121]. Human pDC lack the mDC markers CD11c and CD33. For clinical vaccine trails the maturation cocktail usually contains a combination of IL-1, TNF-α, IL-6, and PGE_2[122]. pDC, upon exposure to viruses, produce very high levels of type I IFN, and are therefore considered the main link between the innate and adaptive immune systems[8]. Human mDC and pDC have been termed DC1 and DC2, respectively, due to their propensity to stimulate Th1 versus Th2 type responses. Current knowledge indicates that this is an oversimplification of the system, thus these terms will not be used in this review.

Effects of Pharmacological Agents on Human DCs

Many pharmacologic agents with known immunoregulatory effects, and specifically conventional immunosuppressant, have been investigated for their impact on human DC generation, maturation, and function. Immunosuppressive drugs can either indirectly target DC maturation and interfere with endocytosis developmentally or directly influence endocytosis irrespective of DC maturation.

Corticosteroids

Corticosteroids were shown to block *in vitro* differentiation of human monocytes into mDC[123]. *In vivo*, corticosteroids reduced the number and function of circulating human pDC as well as their numbers in tissues such as nasal and bronchial mucosae of atopic patients. Rozkova *et al.*[124] demonstrated that glucocorticoids dramatically impaired human monocyte differentiation, skewing the culture towards macrophage-like cells. The typical DC morphology was maintained, however, such that high levels of CD14 molecules were still present on the cell surface and costimulatory molecules were only mildly expressed. Glucocorticoid treated cells produced very low amounts of TNF and p70 IL-12 while producing higher amounts of IL-10 and retaining high endocytic activity. Interestingly, despite the fact that glucocorticoids increased the expression of Toll-like receptors TLR2, 3 and 4 on human DC, their stimulation with TLR-derived signals did not induce maturation[125, 126]. Hackstein *et al.*[127] studied the effect of immunosuppression, and in particular corticosteroid dosages, on DC precursor frequencies in peripheral blood of transplant recipients. Multivariate analysis revealed a significant negative impact that was dose dependent, mainly on the pDC sub-population. Functional studies performed by this group indicated a significant deficiency in IFN-α production after TLR7 and TLR9 stimulation, confirming the scarcity of pDCs in the circulation of these patients (Although TLR7 and TLR9 are expressed on cell types other than pDC, it is only the pDC that can secret IFN-α in response to their stimulation).

Calcineurin Inhibitors

FK506 (tacrolimus) inhibits the ability of human DC to allo-stimulate T-cells, but was reported to have heterogenous effects on DC maturation, depending on the stimuli used to trigger DC maturation[128]. The effects of Cyclosporine (CsA) however are rather controversial ranging from showing no effect on maturation or allostimulatory capacity of human mDC, to having a rather significant effect on DC maturation and function. Tajima *et al.*[129] presented data to support CsA inhibition on up-regulation of costimulatory molecules on both $CD11c^{+}$ mDC and $CD11c^{-}$ pDC subsets, with or without microbial stimuli and CD40L. They farther demonstrated that CsA negatively regulated the endocytic activity of mDCs during the immature state; and inhibited IL-12 production from mature mDC. CsA also reduced the IFN-α production from the pDCs. Schlichting *et al.*[130] investigated the impact of calcineurin inhibitors on DC binding and transmigration to allogeneic human microvascular endothelial cells (ECs) *in vitro*. Co-culture of DCs with ECs preincubated with CsA showed significant increased binding, whereas ECs preincubated with tacrolimus had minimal effect on DC binding. CsA effect was reversed using blocking antibodies to adhesion molecules such as VCAM-1. DC transmigration was also analyzed in this system demonstrating accelerated migration in the presence of CsA, as well as in the presence of high dose of tacrolimus. DC migration was significantly reduced in the tacrolimus treated group when PECAM-1 blocking antibodies were used. These data suggest different mechanisms associated with CsA and tacrolimus effects on DC binding and transmigration to allogeneic endothelial cells. This is in contrast to data from Szabo *et al.*[131] who showed that tacrolimus and CsA inhibit the allostimulatory capacity of *in vitro*-generated mDCs without significant effects on DC phenotypic maturation.

Sirolimus

Sirolimus (rapamycin; inhibits downstream signaling from the mammalian targets of rapamycin, mTOR) suppresses the generation of granulocyte–macrophage colony stimulating factor (GM-CSF) thus quantitatively reduces growth-factor-induced expansion of DC populations. Monti *et al.*[132] demonstrated that human DC in the presence of rapamycin express higher levels of CD1a, CD1b, and CD1c, and decreased levels of HLA class I, class II, CD40, CD80 and CD86. Consequently, CD40-ligand induced production of both IL-12 and IL-10 were reduced in rapamycin-treated DCs. Antigen uptake receptor expression (mannose receptor, CD32, CD46, CD91) was also reduced leading to impaired receptor-mediated and fluid phase endocytosis. Woltman *et al.*[133] have also shown that rapamycin induces apoptosis in monocyte-derived DCs while monocytes and macrophages are spared.

Aspirin

Hackstein *et al.*[134] reported that Aspirin, given in physiologic concentrations (1-3mM), was able to suppress the maturation and T cell-stimulatory function of human mDCs. It was speculated that the underlying molecular mechanism involves inhibitory effects on DCs maturation by inhibition of the p50 subunit of NF-κB. This pathway results in the inhibition of co-stimulatory molecules expression; e.g., CD40, CD80, CD83 and the MHC-II-complex [135]. Aspirin treated DCs retain their immature phenotype (round nucleus, prominent endocytic compartment compared) even if maturation is induced by lipopolysaccharide (LPS) stimulation; and exhibited decreased IL-12(p40) and IL10 secretion. In contrast TNF-α production was enhanced [136].

Vitamin D Receptor Analogues

DCs express the Vitamin D Receptor (VRD) on their cell surface, thereby becoming a key target to vitamin D and other VDR agonist [137]. The active metabolite of vitamin D, 1,25(OH)$_2$D3, and its analogs have been found to inhibit the differentiation of human CD1a+ monocyte-derived DCs, leading to reduced expression of costimulatory molecules and alloreactive capacity [138, 139]. Adorini, and colleagues [140] reported that incubation with 1,25(OH)$_2$D3 leads to a selective upregulation of ILT3 on immature as well as during maturation of DCs. pDCs, that express a priori high level of ILT3 obviously seems to be less affected than mDCs – which increase ILT3 expression considerably. Interestingly, ILT3 is selectively reduced by CD40 ligation on mDCs but not on pDCs. This selective responsiveness of ILT3 on the two DC cell populations suggests a novel mechanism for the immunomodulatory properties of this hormone that could play a role in the control of T-cell responses [141, 142].

Human Regulatory T Cells

During the last few years, researchers began to recognize the tolerizing function of the mDC and the pDC, as well as DCs in both immature and mature states. It has also become apparent that the tolerizing properties of DCs are likely linked to effects on regulatory T cells;

and that the unique ability of DCs to capture and cross-present antigens can be used to induce donor-specific tolerance under noninflammatory conditions. Importantly, a dialogue between regulatory T cells and tolerogenic DCs is crucial for the regulation of alloimmune responses. Several subsets of regulatory T cells have been described in human.

$CD4^+CD25^{bright}$ T_{reg} Cells

Center stage in immunological research of regulatory T cells is currently focused on $CD4^+CD25^{bright}$ T cells. Indeed, CD25 can be expressed also on recently activated non-regulatory T cells. Yet, such T cells usually express lower levels of CD25 on their cell surface compare with T_{reg} cells. The simultaneous presence of dim and bright CD25 molecules on the cell surface complicate the identification of truly regulatory T cells in human studies. Naturally occurring $CD4^+CD25^{bright}$ T_{reg} cells were first described as actively engaged in maintaining immunological self-tolerance. Deficiency in these cells in human leads to the X-linked immunodeficiency syndrome IPEX (immune dysregulation, polyendocrinopathy, enteropathy, X-linked syndrome) that is associated with an autoimmune disease syndrome that involves multiple endocrine organs, severe allergy, inflammatory bowel disease and fatal infection [143]. The natural occurring T_{reg} cells constitutively express GITR and CTLA-4 [144-147]. While they also express CD45RO, CD27, CD62L and CD122, these markers are also up-regulated upon T cell activation and therefore can not serve as specific markers to characterize T_{reg} cells. FOXP3, which is considered a more specific marker for T_{reg} cells in mouse, is also expressed by human T_{reg} cells, although it is not exclusive to this population as is reported for mice. It is accepted to refer to the human molecule in capital letters (FOXP3) to distinguish it from the rodent counterpart – Foxp3. Similar to mouse T_{reg} cells, human regulatory T cells do not proliferate when stimulated with anti-CD3 unless supplemented with high doses of IL-2 and are TLR ligation on DCs [148].

Costimulation of human naıve $CD4^+$ T cells with TGF-β induces the differentiation of $CD4^+CD25^+$ T_{reg} cells that exhibit contact-dependent and antigen-nonspecific suppressive activity [149]. Importantly, the suppressor function of human $CD4^+CD25^+$ T_{reg} cells is activation-dependent, requires protein synthesis; and can be inhibited by the presence of cycloheximide or monensin [150]. Furthermore, human $CD25^+$ T_{reg} cells down-regulate the proliferation of conventional $CD25^-$ T cells while inducing suppressive activity in tolerized $CD4^+$ T cells simultaneously - a phenomenon that has been termed infectious tolerance and is TGF-β dependent [150]. These studies have led to the speculation that the suppression of human $CD25^+$ T_{reg} cells is "spread" into conventional $CD4^+$ T cells and that this might be the mechanism by which induction and maintenance of peripheral tolerance is achieved.

In addition to targeting effector T cells directly; T_{reg} cells may also exert their suppressive activity by directly targeting DCs. For example, DCs may be rendered inefficient APCs following a cell-to-cell contact dependent interaction with $CD4^+CD25^+$ T_{reg} cells, despite pre-stimulation with CD40L[151, 152]. DCs co-cultured with $CD4^+CD25^+$ T_{reg} cells may also down-regulate the expression of costimulatory molecules, release high quantities of IL-10 and become unable to trigger T-cell activation properly [153, 154]. Houot and colleagues [155] studied the maturation of human mDC and pDC activated with TLR ligands in the presence of pre-activated T_{reg} cells *in vitro*. They showed that $CD4^+CD25^+$ T_{reg} cells modulate the expression of CCR7 and costimulatory molecules induced by TLR on mDC, but not on pDC.

It was also the TLR-activated mDC, but not the pDC, that were inhibited from secretion of proinflammatory cytokines following incubation with activated T_{reg} cells.

Another modulator of T_{reg} cells is IL-7. In a study reported by Rosenberg and colleagues [156], IL-7 was administrated to patients with lymphopenia due to HIV infection or cancer-related chemotherapy treatment. These patients showed selective increase in $CD4^+$ and $CD8^+$ non-regulatory T cells. Interestingly, using microarray analysis, Liu e*t al.* [157] demonstrated that the majority of T cells that down-regulated CD127 (IL-7 receptor) following activation - express FOXP3. FOXP3 expression, on the other hand, had no correlation to the level of CD25 expression on these cells membranes. More over, these $CD4^+CD127^{low/-}$ cells were anergic and were as suppressive as the "classical" $CD4^+CD25^{bright}$ cells. In fact, the authors proposed the use of CD127 as a biomarker to selectively enrich human T_{reg} cells. Seddiki and group [158] from Sydney, Australia corroborated this observation.

Human $CD4^+CD25^+$ T_{reg} cells display a polyclonal TCR-Vβ repertoire, suggesting potential recognition of a broad variety of antigens. However, while most $CD4^+CD25^+$ T_{reg} cells related publications discuss a suppressive effect of these cells in a non-antigen-specific manner, Levings and colleagues [159] showed that human non-proliferating $CD4^+CD25^+$ T_{reg} cells that up-regulate CLTA-4 expression and secrete IL-10 upon stimulation, decrease the proliferative responses of $CD4^+$ T cell to specific alloantigens *in vitro.* Jiang and coworkers were also able to identify allopeptide-specific human $CD4^+CD25^+$ T_{reg} cells [160, 161].

$CD8^+CD28^-$ Suppressor T Cells (Ts Cells)

A uniquely different family of human regulatory / suppressor T cells (Ts) was elegantly demonstrated by Suciu-Foca's group [162]. These cells express the $CD3^+CD8^+CD28^-FOXP3^+$ phenotype, both *in vitro* and *in vivo*. In culture, Ts cells can be generated by multiple priming of responding T cells with irradiated APCs from an allogeneic donor during a 2 week time period [163]. Once these cells are incubated with endothelial cells (sharing at least one HLA class I antigen with the priming APCs), they cause inhibition of co-stimulation by down regulating CD40 and CD58 and induce the up-regulation of the inhibitory receptors ILT3 and ILT4 [164]. More importantly, down regulation of activation markers (CD40, CD54, CD62L, CD83, CD106, HLA-DR) and up-regulation of the inhibitory markers were observed even if endothelial cells were previously treated with IFN-γ or TNF-α. The specificity of the suppressive reaction was demonstrated when responses were tested using endothelial cells that share no HLA antigens with the priming APCs [165]. Similar effects were demonstrated when Ts were incubated with DCs. Thus, the Ts effect is HLA class I allo-restricted. It was further shown that the suppressive effect requires a direct interaction between $CD8^+CD28^-$ Ts cells and the APCs for priming. This contact leads to inhibition of the CD40-mediated up-regulation of costimulatory molecules such as CD80 and CD86 on the APC; and eventually translates into inhibitory signals transmitted by means of the inhibitory immunoglobulin-like transcript ILT3 and ILT4 up-regulation to the $CD4^+$ Th cells that bind the same APC [166]. The unresponsiveness induced by $CD8^+CD28^-$ Ts cells treated APCs on the $CD4^+$ Th cells is characteristic of T cell anergy, since the lost of $CD4^+$ cell proliferation capacity is reversed by the addition of exogenous IL-2.

ILT3 and ILT4 are novel cell surface molecules of the immunoglobulin superfamily, which are selectively expressed by monocytes, macrophages, mDC and endothelial cells. ILT4 is expressed predominantly on mDC and binds HLA-A, HLA-B, HLA-C and HLA-G molecules. The ligand for ILT3 is still unknown, however, it is mainly expressed on pDCs. Functional studies showed that ILT3 is efficiently internalized upon cross-linking, and delivers its ligand to an intracellular compartment. The ligand is then processed and presented to specific T cells. Thus, ILT3 is involved in antigen capture and presentation. The expression of ILT on DCs is tightly controlled by inflammatory stimuli, cytokines, and growth factors, and is down-regulated following DC activation.

Up-regulation of ILT3 and ILT4 has also been shown to render monocytes and DCs tolerogenic in vivo. CD8+CD28- Ts cells obtained from stable heart transplant recipients were able to induce the up-regulation of ILT3 or ILT4 and inhibit CD40-signaling by donor APCs, thus suggesting the presence of allospecific Ts cells that may inhibit the direct recognition pathway involved in allograft rejection [167]. Up-regulation of ILT3 and ILT4 molecules on the surface of human mDC can also be induced by treatment of the cells with IL-10, as reported by Manavalan *et al.*[168]. Importantly, IL-10 treated DC induced T cell anergy is blocked by antibodies specific for ILT3 and ILT4. Interestingly, LPS stimulation of DCs can elicit the production of soluble, rather than membrane-bound, ILT4 molecules. Soluble ILT4 may competitively block T lymphocyte binding to the DC-membrane-bound ILT4, thereby favoring a stimulatory DC phenotype. If LPS stimulation is applied to IL-10 treated DCs, soluble ILT4 is not expressed and the tolerogenic capacity of the IL-10 treated DCs is thus promoted.

Other Types of Regulator T Cells

Apart from the naturally occurring T_{reg} cells and Ts cells, other distinct populations of regulatory T cells exist and are defined by their cytokine signature, such as secretion of high levels of IL-10 (Tr1) or TGF-β (Th3), depending on the route in which they encounter the antigen. For example, repeat stimulation of naïve T cells *in vitro* with immature DCs induced the generation of IL-10 producing Tr1 [169]. T-cell proliferation is not restored by the addition of IL-2. Tr1 cells inhibit the proliferation of Th_1 cells in a contact-dependent but antigen-nonspecific manner. *In vivo*, when human volunteers were immunized with a single subcutaneous injection of influenza peptide-pulsed immature DCs, as described by Dhodapkar *et al.*[170], a reduction of antigen-specific IFN-γ producing $CD8^+$ T cells was observed with a concomitant increase in IL-10 producing T cells. Th3 cells are inducible upon activation with an appropriate antigen or antibodies to CD3. These cells produce high levels of TGF-β and variable amounts of IL-4 and IL-10. Importantly, the loss of T-cell killing activity could not be attributed to deletion of effector cells but rather to modulation of the immune response.

A recent analysis revealed significant differences between the naturally occurring $CD4^+CD25^{bright}$ T_{reg} cells and IL-10-producing Tr1 cells. Specifically, suppressive $CD4^+CD25^{bright}$ T cell clones were shown to release TGF-β in the absence of IL-10 [171]. They inhibit the proliferation of bystander T cells irrespective of the presence of APCs, suggesting direct effects on effector T cells [172]. At variance with Tr1 cells, which expand in response to IL-2 and IL-15, $CD4^+CD25^{bright}$ T_{reg} cells failed to proliferate to these cytokines, either in combination or used alone. The observation that IL-15 can maintain Tr1 cell clones in culture for more than 30 days in the absence of TCR triggering suggests that IL-15, which is produced by several cell types during immune responses, might be involved in the long-term survival of Tr1 cells *in vivo* [173].

Effects of Pharmacological Agents on T_{reg} Cells

Valmori et al.[174] studied the effects of rapamycin in vitro on human circulating $CD4^+$ T cells, reporting that stimulation of these cells results in an increased suppressor activity in the cultures. Rapamycin delayed the differentiation of stimulated $CD4^+$ T cells, promoted an increase of $CD4^+CD25^{bright}$ T cells, and inhibited proliferation in cultures where suppressor cells were mixed with otherwise competent responder T cells. Interestingly, no increase in $FOXP3^+$ population correlated with rapamycin treatment in this study.

Over the last few years, the effect of immunosuppressive agents on the generation of Treg cells in vivo is extensively studied. San Segundo et al. [175] compared the effects of calcineurin inhibitors to those of rapamycin on T_{reg} cells in stable renal allograft recipients. T cells with the regulatory phenotype, $CD4^+CD25^{Bright}$, were decreased in stable renal transplant patients receiving calcineurin inhibitor immunosuppression compared with those receiving rapamycin therapy. Such differences were not observed with regard to $CD8^+CD28^-$ suppressor T cells. In this study only a modest association was observed between the presence of T_{reg} cells and renal function as measured by the delta serum creatinine.

A major concern was the potential effects of induction therapy with anti-CD25 (IL-2 receptor) monoclonal antibodies. Salama et al. [176] studied a cohort of 23 stable renal recipients and found a higher incidence of T_{reg} cells in patients with no history of acute rejection episodes compare to the group with history of rejection episodes. $CD4^+CD25^+$ regulatory cells were present in this study as early as 3 months post transplant, and the group concluded that induction treatment with anti-IL2R mAb did not prevent the development of T_{reg} cells. Game and colleagues [177] studied the effects of the rapamycin in combination with anti-CD25 monoclonal antibody basiliximab on the regulatory capacity of human $CD4^+CD25^+$ cells in vitro. They also concluded that $CD4^+CD25^+$ cells may still exert their effects in transplant recipients taking immunosuppression that interferes with IL-2 signaling.

Franske et al. [178], working with bone marrow transplant patients, have shown that G-CSF inhibit T-cell proliferative responses by eliciting the release of immunoregulatory soluble factors. Rutella and colleagues demonstrated that freshly isolated $CD4^+$ T cells, collected after clinical provision of G-CSF and challenged in vitro with alloantigens in the presence of autologous serum, were hyporesponsive in terms of proliferation and were polarized to a Tr1-like functional profile [179]. These cells acquired peculiar phenotypic features exhibiting reduced expression of CD62L and CD28, associated with high expression of the β chain (CD122) and γ chain (CD132) of the IL-2/IL-15 receptor complex, and were capable of suppressing bystander T cells through a mechanism that was largely cell contact-independent [179].

Ex-vivo Expansion of Human T_{reg} Cells

Naturally occurring $CD4^+CD25^+$ T_{reg} cells are instrumental for immunoregulation. Their roles in numerous fields including transplant rejection, cancer, vaccine, allergy, and autoimmune diseases, are well recognized. However, harnessing these cells for large cohort clinical applications in human have been hampered by the paucity of $CD4^+CD25^+$ T_{reg} cells in peripheral blood and the lack of appropriate ex-vivo expansion protocols. Only 1-2% or human peripheral blood lymphocytes are $CD4^+CD25^+$, translated to 3-5% of all $CD4^+$ T cells.

Additionally, human $CD25^+$ cells are composed of two overlapping populations of CD25, one dimmer than the other, but an exact distinction between the two populations is difficult to assign. It is only the brighter population that matches the characteristics of regulatory cells.

As previously discussed, regulatory T cells do not proliferate in response to any of the normal physiologic stimuli ex vivo. The cells show a G1/G0 cell cycle arrest and no production of IL-2, IL-4, or IFN-γ at either protein or mRNA levels. The anergic state of $CD4^+CD25^+$ T cells is not reversible by the addition of anti-CD3, anti-CD28, anti–CTLA-4, anti–transforming growth factor ß, or anti–IL-10 antibody. Jonuleit *et al.* [150]demonstrated that the refractory state of $CD4^+CD25^+$ freshly isolated human T cells was partially reversible by the addition of IL-2 or IL-4. However, it could not be reversed by the addition of anti-CD3 or anti-CD28. Dieckmann and colleagues [180], using $CD4^+CD25^+CD45RO^+$ cells from healthy adult volunteers, presented data to support a synergistic effect between IL-2 and IL-15 for reversing the anergic state of the T_{reg} cells, in the presence of an allogeneic stimulus, or a combination of immobilized anti-CD3 and anti-CD28. Following this protocol, Karakhanova and colleagues [181] used sorted CD4+CD25+ cells for further expansion. Activation was achieved by using paramagnetic beads coupled with anti-CD3 and anti-CD28. IL-2 and IL-15 were also added to the culture to farther augment the proliferation response to about 1000-fold after 2 cycles of re-stimulation.

Godfrey *et al.* [182] developed a method to propagate $CD4^+CD25^+$ T_{reg} cells in culture up to 100-fold expansion over the initial culture. To this aim they used cleavable microbeads coated with low levels of anti-CD25 – thus allowing for better purification of CD25+ cells. Ligation of CD3 and addition of IL-2 resulted in only 5-10 fold expansion, prompting the researchers to look for additional co-stimulation – provided by the use of cell-sized Dynabeads with anti-CD3 and anti-CD28 mAbs covalently attached. Lastly, to provide the proper cytokine milieu, irradiated $CD4^+CD25^-$ feeder cells were added at the initiation of T_{reg} cultures (1:1 ratio) culminating in a 100-fold ex-vivo expansion of the original culture. Importantly, the cultured T_{reg} cells were shown to maintain the suppressive capabilities when co-cultured with either activated or matured dendritic cell-driven.

While ex-vivo expansion of T_{reg} cells facilitates more in-depth studies of the intracellular signaling and mechanisms associated with their unique function, a much larger ex-vivo expansion is required to accelerate clinical applications. Hoffmann *et al.* [183] achieved a significant milestone shortly thereafter. As in the previous protocol, the anergic state of pure $CD4^+CD25^{high}$ T cells was abrogated after simultaneous stimulation via TCRs and CD28 in the presence of IL-2. Unique to the Hoffman's protocol is the addition of FcγRII (CD32)–bearing L cells in combination with stimulation via CD3 and CD28. Under these conditions T_{reg} cells expanded dramatically with an average 13 000-fold increase in cell numbers within 3 to 4 weeks. Using parallel cultures for several months, an ex-vivo expansion of up to 39,000 fold was established. Despite the long incubation, the expanded T_{reg} cells maintained high expression levels of both CD52L and CCR7, as well as their polyclonal repertoire of TCR Vβ.

The above-described methods for *in vitro* T_{reg} cell expansion have overcome the relative anergy of these cells. However, the expanded cells are polyclonal and antigen specificity has not been addressed. Evidence suggests that the *in vivo* efficacy of T_{reg}-based immuno-therapy is critically dependent on the specificity of the T_{reg} cells. Therefore the ability to expand T_{reg} cell populations with particular antigen specificities will allow using a lower number of cells to achieve the expected efficacy. By labeling freshly isolated $CD4^+CD25^+$ T_{reg} cells with

CFSE and stimulating them with HLA mismatched gamma-irradiated alloantigen along with IL-2 plus IL-15, Koenen and colleagues [184] were able to focus on the alloantigen-reactive dividing T_{reg} cells in a short term culture – choosing cells characterized by diluted CFSE. Cells were also selected based on their CD27 expression, indicating a memory T_{reg} cell population. This robust ex-vivo technique allowed purification of highly potent human monoclonal alloantigen-specific T_{reg} cells. The authors went on to demonstrate that these cells have a high-effector-suppressor potential – 500:1 for the $CD27^+$ T_{reg} cells. The use of Antigen-specific T_{reg} cells, as opposed to polyclonal expanded regulatory cells, has the potential of increased efficacy required of a T_{reg} cell-based immunotherapy. However, much has still to be learned about additional qualities of these $CD27^+$ T_{reg} cells, for example their *in vivo* trafficking patterns, their interactions with B cells, etc.

HLA-G as Natural Inducer of Immuno-Tolerance

HLA-G expression was demonstrated in vivo on epithelial cells of an "accepted" allograft tissue as well as on infiltrating mononuclear cells [185]. In fact, HLA-G expression was documented on tumor cells that escaped immune surveillance [186]. HLA-G is a non-classical HLA class I antigen that has restricted expression in extravillous cytotrohpoblasts, thymic epithelium and cornea under non-pathologic conditions. Its expression was reported to be crucial for protection of fetal cytotrophoblast from destruction by the maternal immune system, and is probably associated with the "privileged" status of the eye. During inflammation or other pathologic conditions, however, HLA-G can be expressed by infiltrating mononuclear cells and can inhibit NK cell and cytotoxic T cell function; as well as $CD4^+$ T cell allo-proliferation. HLA-G can be expressed as one of multiple isoforms generated by alternative splicing of a single message, and give rise to four membrane-bound isoforms (HLA-G1 through -4) and three soluble isoforms (HLA-G5, -G6, and -G7). HLA-G appears to be recognized mainly by immunoglobulin-like transcript (ILT) receptors, which are expressed by T and B lymphocytes, as well as by NK cells, macrophages and DCs [187]. Convincing evidence for an ability of HLA-G to influence T cells was first presented by Sanders et al. who showed that HLA-G-expressing cells bind to CD8α-expressing cells [188). HLA-G was also shown to modulate cytokine release from human allogeneic peripheral blood mononuclear cells in vitro [189] and to have a concentration-dependent effect on generation of an allogeneic CTL response [190]. As mentioned previously, an immune suppressive effect of HLA-G on APCs was documented by the finding that high levels of HLA-G proteins in the sera of heart transplant recipients with prolonged graft survival [191]. It has also been shown that HLA-G can be expressed by APCs themselves as a response inflammatory conditions during cytomegalovirus and other infections [192]. Since HLA-G exerts its effects via its interaction with the ILT-4 molecule on APCs [193, 194], it seems like HLA-G functions as a regulatory feed-back mechanism to control reactivity against noxious stimuli.

Concluding Remarks

A major goal in organ transplantation is to be able to harness tolerance processes so as to minimize the need for immunosuppressive drugs. Chronic immunosuppression is associated with increased risk of infection, malignancy, and aggregate impact of drug-specific toxicities. With respect to renal transplantation, the drugs cyclosporine and tacrolimus – current mainstays of most maintenance immunosuppressive protocols—are toxic to both native and transplanted kidneys. In addition, allografts are still at risk for development of chronic rejection, a process that currently limits the long-term survival of transplanted kidneys in many recipients. Transplantation tolerance is not only able to prevent acute or chronic rejection but also to avoid chronic immunosuppression and its associated complications. The clinical use of *ex vivo* expanded regulatory T cells to control GvHD and organ transplant rejection is a promising approach to modulate effector T cells, while preserving the beneficial effect mediated by other T cells. Results in preclinical models are promising, although efforts are required to optimize this procedure for clinical application regarding the number of T_{reg} cells to be used to obtain long-lasting beneficial effect. Moreover, the impact of T_{reg} cells on the reconstitution of the immune system still has to be completely unraveled. It still remains an open question, which is the most appropriate regulatory T-cell subset to be used. Although polyclonal $CD4^+CD25^+$ T_{reg} cells can be easily isolated and their *ex vivo* expansion is feasible, their undefined antigen specificity and the possible contamination with non-suppressor cells in the *ex vivo* expanded population might represent limiting factors to the use of these subset of regulatory T cells. Conversely, *ex vivo* induced antigen specific cells ensure the antigen specificity, but their low frequency obtained by short-term manipulation could limit their *in vivo* efficacy. Advances in understanding the molecular basis for the activation and expansion of T_{reg} cells together with the ongoing clinical trials will be crucial to dissect these issues and to unravel the therapeutic potential of regulatory T cells.

References

[1] Manz MG, Traver D, Miyamoto T, Weissman IL, Akashi K. 2001. Dendritic cell potentials of early lymphoid and myeloid progenitors. *Blood.* 97: 3333-41

[2] Guermonprez P, Valladeau J, Zitvogel L, Thery C, Amigorena S. 2002. Antigen presentation and T cell stimulation by dendritic cells. *Annu. Rev. Immunol.* 20: 621-67

[3] Pulendran B, Palucka K, Banchereau J. 2001. Sensing pathogens and tuning immune responses. *Science.* 293: 253-6

[4] Liu YJ. 2001. Dendritic cell subsets and lineages, and their functions in innate and adaptive immunity. *Cell.* 106: 259-62

[5] Rescigno M, Borrow P. 2001. The host-pathogen interaction: new themes from dendritic cell biology. *Cell.* 106: 267-70

[6] Steinman RM, Hawiger D, Nussenzweig MC. 2003. Tolerogenic dendritic cells. *Annu. Rev. Immunol.* 21: 685-711

[7] Barratt-Boyes B. 2003. The early history of cardiac surgery in New Zealand. *Heart Lung Circ.* 12 Suppl 1: S21-8

[8] Munz C, Steinman RM, Fujii S. 2005. Dendritic cell maturation by innate lymphocytes: coordinated stimulation of innate and adaptive immunity. *J. Exp. Med.* 202: 203-7

[9] Hemmi H, Akira S. 2005. TLR signalling and the function of dendritic cells. *Chem. Immunol. Allergy.* 86: 120-35

[10] Rescigno M, Piguet V, Valzasina B, Lens S, Zubler R, French L, Kindler V, Tschopp J, Ricciardi-Castagnoli P. 2000. Fas engagement induces the maturation of dendritic cells (DCs), the release of interleukin (IL)-1beta, and the production of interferon gamma in the absence of IL-12 during DC-T cell cognate interaction: a new role for Fas ligand in inflammatory responses. *J. Exp. Med.* 192: 1661-8

[11] Cella M, Scheidegger D, Palmer-Lehmann K, Lane P, Lanzavecchia A, Alber G. 1996. Ligation of CD40 on dendritic cells triggers production of high levels of interleukin-12 and enhances T cell stimulatory capacity: T-T help via APC activation. *J. Exp. Med.* 184: 747-52

[12] Luft T, Pang KC, Thomas E, Hertzog P, Hart DN, Trapani J, Cebon J. 1998. Type I IFNs enhance the terminal differentiation of dendritic cells. *J. Immunol.* 161: 1947-53

[13] Granucci F, Vizzardelli C, Virzi E, Rescigno M, Ricciardi-Castagnoli P. 2001. Transcriptional reprogramming of dendritic cells by differentiation stimuli. *Eur. J. Immunol.* 31: 2539-46

[14] Garrett WS, Chen LM, Kroschewski R, Ebersold M, Turley S, Trombetta S, Galan JE, Mellman I. 2000. Developmental control of endocytosis in dendritic cells by Cdc42. *Cell.* 102: 325-34

[15] Rescigno M, Martino M, Sutherland CL, Gold MR, Ricciardi-Castagnoli P. 1998. Dendritic cell survival and maturation are regulated by different signaling pathways. *J. Exp. Med.* 188: 2175-80

[16] Giannoukakis N, Bonham CA, Qian S, Chen Z, Peng L, Harnaha J, Li W, Thomson AW, Fung JJ, Robbins PD, Lu L. 2000. Prolongation of cardiac allograft survival using dendritic cells treated with NF-kB decoy oligodeoxyribonucleotides. *Mol. Ther.* 1: 430-7

[17] Chen Z, Lu L, Zhang H, Dean NM, Fung JJ, Qian S. 2003. Administration of antisense oligodeoxyribonucleotides targeting NF-kappaB prolongs allograft survival via suppression of cytotoxicity. *Microsurgery.* 23: 494-7

[18] Tomasoni S, Aiello S, Cassis L, Noris M, Longaretti L, Cavinato RA, Azzollini N, Pezzotta A, Remuzzi G, Benigni A. 2005. Dendritic cells genetically engineered with adenoviral vector encoding dnIKK2 induce the formation of potent CD4+ T-regulatory cells. *Transplantation.* 79: 1056-61

[19] Wang Q, Liu Y, Wang J, Ding G, Zhang W, Chen G, Zhang M, Zheng S, Cao X. 2006. Induction of allospecific tolerance by immature dendritic cells genetically modified to express soluble TNF receptor. *J. Immunol.* 177: 2175-85

[20] Goldstein DR, Tesar BM, Akira S, Lakkis FG. 2003. Critical role of the Toll-like receptor signal adaptor protein MyD88 in acute allograft rejection. *J. Clin. Invest.* 111: 1571-8

[21] Thornley TB, Brehm MA, Markees TG, Shultz LD, Mordes JP, Welsh RM, Rossini AA, Greiner DL. 2006. TLR agonists abrogate costimulation blockade-induced prolongation of skin allografts. *J. Immunol.* 176: 1561-70

[22] Ducloux D, Deschamps M, Yannaraki M, Ferrand C, Bamoulid J, Saas P, Kazory A, Chalopin JM, Tiberghien P. 2005. Relevance of Toll-like receptor-4 polymorphisms in renal transplantation. *Kidney Int.* 67: 2454-61

[23] Larsen CP, Ritchie SC, Hendrix R, Linsley PS, Hathcock KS, Hodes RJ, Lowry RP, Pearson TC. 1994. Regulation of immunostimulatory function and costimulatory

molecule (B7-1 and B7-2) expression on murine dendritic cells. *J. Immunol.* 152: 5208-19

[24] Takayama T, Morelli AE, Robbins PD, Tahara H, Thomson AW. 2000. Feasibility of CTLA4Ig gene delivery and expression in vivo using retrovirally transduced myeloid dendritic cells that induce alloantigen-specific T cell anergy in vitro. *Gene Ther.* 7: 1265-73

[25] Laumonier T, Potiron N, Boeffard F, Chagneau C, Brouard S, Guillot C, Soulillou JP, Anegon I, Le Mauff B. 2003. CTLA4Ig adenoviral gene transfer induces long-term islet rat allograft survival, without tolerance, after systemic but not local intragraft expression. *Hum. Gene Ther.* 14: 561-75

[26] Fallarino F, Grohmann U, Vacca C, Bianchi R, Orabona C, Spreca A, Fioretti MC, Puccetti P. 2002. T cell apoptosis by tryptophan catabolism. *Cell Death Differ.* 9: 1069-77

[27] Munn DH, Sharma MD, Mellor AL. 2004. Ligation of B7-1/B7-2 by human CD4+ T cells triggers indoleamine 2,3-dioxygenase activity in dendritic cells. *J. Immunol.* 172: 4100-10

[28] Grohmann U, Orabona C, Fallarino F, Vacca C, Calcinaro F, Falorni A, Candeloro P, Belladonna ML, Bianchi R, Fioretti MC, Puccetti P. 2002. CTLA-4-Ig regulates tryptophan catabolism in vivo. *Nat. Immunol.* 3: 1097-101

[29] Zhang M, Wang Q, Liu Y, Sun Y, Ding G, Fu Z, Min Z, Zhu Y, Cao X. 2004. Effective induction of immune tolerance by portal venous infusion with IL-10 gene-modified immature dendritic cells leading to prolongation of allograft survival. *J. Mol. Med.* 82: 240-9

[30] Gorczynski RM, Bransom J, Cattral M, Huang X, Lei J, Xiaorong L, Min WP, Wan Y, Gauldie J. 2000. Synergy in induction of increased renal allograft survival after portal vein infusion of dendritic cells transduced to express TGFbeta and IL-10, along with administration of CHO cells expressing the regulatory molecule OX-2. *Clin. Immunol.* 95: 182-9

[31] Takayama T, Morelli AE, Onai N, Hirao M, Matsushima K, Tahara H, Thomson AW. 2001. Mammalian and viral IL-10 enhance C-C chemokine receptor 5 but down-regulate C-C chemokine receptor 7 expression by myeloid dendritic cells: impact on chemotactic responses and in vivo homing ability. *J. Immunol.* 166: 7136-43

[32] Lee WC, Zhong C, Qian S, Wan Y, Gauldie J, Mi Z, Robbins PD, Thomson AW, Lu L. 1998. Phenotype, function, and in vivo migration and survival of allogeneic dendritic cell progenitors genetically engineered to express TGF-beta. *Transplantation.* 66: 1810-7

[33] Chen W, Jin W, Hardegen N, Lei KJ, Li L, Marinos N, McGrady G, Wahl SM. 2003. Conversion of peripheral CD4+CD25- naive T cells to CD4+CD25+ regulatory T cells by TGF-beta induction of transcription factor Foxp3. *J. Exp. Med.* 198: 1875-86

[34] Marie JC, Letterio JJ, Gavin M, Rudensky AY. 2005. TGF-beta1 maintains suppressor function and Foxp3 expression in CD4+CD25+ regulatory T cells. *J. Exp. Med.* 201: 1061-7

[35] Ghiringhelli F, Puig PE, Roux S, Parcellier A, Schmitt E, Solary E, Kroemer G, Martin F, Chauffert B, Zitvogel L. 2005. Tumor cells convert immature myeloid dendritic cells into TGF-{beta}-secreting cells inducing CD4+CD25+ regulatory T cell proliferation. *J. Exp. Med.* 202: 919-29

[36] Griffin MD, Lutz W, Phan VA, Bachman LA, McKean DJ, Kumar R. 2001. Dendritic cell modulation by 1alpha,25 dihydroxyvitamin D3 and its analogs: a vitamin D receptor-dependent pathway that promotes a persistent state of immaturity in vitro and in vivo. *Proc. Natl. Acad. Sci. U S A.* 98: 6800-5

[37] Griffin MD, Kumar R. 2003. Effects of 1alpha,25(OH)2D3 and its analogs on dendritic cell function. *J. Cell Biochem.* 88: 323-6

[38] Penna G, Adorini L. 2000. 1 Alpha,25-dihydroxyvitamin D3 inhibits differentiation, maturation, activation, and survival of dendritic cells leading to impaired alloreactive T cell activation. *J. Immunol.* 164: 2405-11

[39] Adorini L, Penna G, Giarratana N, Roncari A, Amuchastegui S, Daniel KC, Uskokovic M. 2004. Dendritic cells as key targets for immunomodulation by Vitamin D receptor ligands. *J. Steroid Biochem. Mol. Biol.* 89-90: 437-41

[40] Adorini L, Penna G, Giarratana N, Uskokovic M. 2003. Tolerogenic dendritic cells induced by vitamin D receptor ligands enhance regulatory T cells inhibiting allograft rejection and autoimmune diseases. *J. Cell Biochem.* 88: 227-33

[41] Gregori S, Casorati M, Amuchastegui S, Smiroldo S, Davalli AM, Adorini L. 2001. Regulatory T cells induced by 1 alpha,25-dihydroxyvitamin D3 and mycophenolate mofetil treatment mediate transplantation tolerance. *J. Immunol.* 167: 1945-53

[42] Emmer PM, van der Vlag J, Adema GJ, Hilbrands LB. 2006. Dendritic cells activated by lipopolysaccharide after dexamethasone treatment induce donor-specific allograft hyporesponsiveness. *Transplantation.* 81: 1451-9

[43] Roelen DL, Schuurhuis DH, van den Boogaardt DE, Koekkoek K, van Miert PP, van Schip JJ, Laban S, Rea D, Melief CJ, Offringa R, Ossendorp F, Claas FH. 2003. Prolongation of skin graft survival by modulation of the alloimmune response with alternatively activated dendritic cells. *Transplantation.* 76: 1608-15

[44] Beriou G, Peche H, Guillonneau C, Merieau E, Cuturi MC. 2005. Donor-specific allograft tolerance by administration of recipient-derived immature dendritic cells and suboptimal immunosuppression. *Transplantation.* 79: 969-72

[45] Min WP, Zhou D, Ichim TE, Xia X, Zhang X, Yang J, Huang X, Garcia B, Dutartre P, Jevnikar AM, Strejan GH, Zhong R. 2003. Synergistic tolerance induced by LF15-0195 and anti-CD45RB monoclonal antibody through suppressive dendritic cells. *Transplantation.* 75: 1160-5

[46] Vosters O, Neve J, De Wit D, Willems F, Goldman M, Verhasselt V. 2003. Dendritic cells exposed to nacystelyn are refractory to maturation and promote the emergence of alloreactive regulatory t cells. *Transplantation.* 75: 383-9

[47] Emmanouilidis N, Guo Z, Dong Y, Newton-West M, Adams AB, Lee ED, Wang J, Pearson TC, Larsen CP, Newell KA. 2006. Immunosuppressive and trafficking properties of donor splenic and bone marrow dendritic cells. *Transplantation.* 81: 455-62

[48] Lan YY, Wang Z, Raimondi G, Wu W, Colvin BL, de Creus A, Thomson AW. 2006. "Alternatively activated" dendritic cells preferentially secrete IL-10, expand Foxp3+CD4+ T cells, and induce long-term organ allograft survival in combination with CTLA4-Ig. *J. Immunol.* 177: 5868-77

[49] Huang FP, Platt N, Wykes M, Major JR, Powell TJ, Jenkins CD, MacPherson GG. 2000. A discrete subpopulation of dendritic cells transports apoptotic intestinal epithelial cells to T cell areas of mesenteric lymph nodes. *J. Exp. Med.* 191: 435-44

[50] Iyoda T, Shimoyama S, Liu K, Omatsu Y, Akiyama Y, Maeda Y, Takahara K, Steinman RM, Inaba K. 2002. The CD8+ dendritic cell subset selectively endocytoses dying cells in culture and in vivo. *J. Exp. Med.* 195: 1289-302

[51] Liu K, Iyoda T, Saternus M, Kimura Y, Inaba K, Steinman RM. 2002. Immune tolerance after delivery of dying cells to dendritic cells in situ. *J. Exp. Med.* 196: 1091-7

[52] Traver D, Akashi K, Manz M, Merad M, Miyamoto T, Engleman EG, Weissman IL. 2000. Development of CD8alpha-positive dendritic cells from a common myeloid progenitor. *Science.* 290: 2152-4

[53] O'Connell PJ, Li W, Wang Z, Specht SM, Logar AJ, Thomson AW. 2002. Immature and mature CD8alpha+ dendritic cells prolong the survival of vascularized heart allografts. *J. Immunol.* 168: 143-54

[54] Fisson S, Djelti F, Trenado A, Billiard F, Liblau R, Klatzmann D, Cohen JL, Salomon BL. 2006. Therapeutic potential of self-antigen-specific CD4+ CD25+ regulatory T cells selected in vitro from a polyclonal repertoire. *Eur. J. Immunol.* 36: 817-27

[55] Liu YJ. 2005. IPC: professional type 1 interferon-producing cells and plasmacytoid dendritic cell precursors. *Annu. Rev. Immunol.* 23: 275-306

[56] Brawand P, Fitzpatrick DR, Greenfield BW, Brasel K, Maliszewski CR, De Smedt T. 2002. Murine plasmacytoid pre-dendritic cells generated from Flt3 ligand-supplemented bone marrow cultures are immature APCs. *J. Immunol.* 169: 6711-9

[57] Gilliet M, Boonstra A, Paturel C, Antonenko S, Xu XL, Trinchieri G, O'Garra A, Liu YJ. 2002. The development of murine plasmacytoid dendritic cell precursors is differentially regulated by FLT3-ligand and granulocyte/macrophage colony-stimulating factor. *J. Exp. Med.* 195: 953-8

[58] Boonstra A, Asselin-Paturel C, Gilliet M, Crain C, Trinchieri G, Liu YJ, O'Garra A. 2003. Flexibility of mouse classical and plasmacytoid-derived dendritic cells in directing T helper type 1 and 2 cell development: dependency on antigen dose and differential toll-like receptor ligation. *J. Exp. Med.* 197: 101-9

[59] Fugier-Vivier IJ, Rezzoug F, Huang Y, Graul-Layman AJ, Schanie CL, Xu H, Chilton PM, Ildstad ST. 2005. Plasmacytoid precursor dendritic cells facilitate allogeneic hematopoietic stem cell engraftment. *J. Exp. Med.* 201: 373-83

[60] Huang Y, Kucia M, Rezzoug F, Ratajczak J, Tanner MK, Ratajczak MZ, Schanie CL, Xu H, Fugier-Vivier I, Ildstad ST. 2006. Flt3-ligand-mobilized peripheral blood, but not Flt3-ligand-expanded bone marrow, facilitating cells promote establishment of chimerism and tolerance. *Stem Cells.* 24: 936-48

[61] Abe M, Wang Z, de Creus A, Thomson AW. 2005. Plasmacytoid dendritic cell precursors induce allogeneic T-cell hyporesponsiveness and prolong heart graft survival. *Am. J. Transplant.* 5: 1808-19

[62] Ochando JC, Homma C, Yang Y, Hidalgo A, Garin A, Tacke F, Angeli V, Li Y, Boros P, Ding Y, Jessberger R, Trinchieri G, Lira SA, Randolph GJ, Bromberg JS. 2006. Alloantigen-presenting plasmacytoid dendritic cells mediate tolerance to vascularized grafts. *Nat. Immunol.* 7: 652-62

[63] Munn DH, Sharma MD, Baban B, Harding HP, Zhang Y, Ron D, Mellor AL. 2005. GCN2 kinase in T cells mediates proliferative arrest and anergy induction in response to indoleamine 2,3-dioxygenase. *Immunity.* 22: 633-42

[64] Gorczynski RM. 2005. CD200 and its receptors as targets for immunoregulation. *Curr. Opin. Investig. Drugs.* 6: 483-8

[65] Fallarino F, Asselin-Paturel C, Vacca C, Bianchi R, Gizzi S, Fioretti MC, Trinchieri G, Grohmann U, Puccetti P. 2004. Murine plasmacytoid dendritic cells initiate the immunosuppressive pathway of tryptophan catabolism in response to CD200 receptor engagement. *J. Immunol.* 173: 3748-54

[66] Jiang S, Herrera O, Lechler RI. 2004. New spectrum of allorecognition pathways: implications for graft rejection and transplantation tolerance. *Curr. Opin. Immunol.* 16: 550-7

[67] Lindahl KF, Wilson DB. 1977. Histocompatibility antigen-activated cytotoxic T lymphocytes. I. Estimates of the absolute frequency of killer cells generated in vitro. *J. Exp. Med.* 145: 500-7

[68] Lindahl KF, Wilson DB. 1977. Histocompatibility antigen-activated cytotoxic T lymphocytes. II. Estimates of the frequency and specificity of precursors. *J. Exp. Med.* 145: 508-22

[69] Suchin EJ, Langmuir PB, Palmer E, Sayegh MH, Wells AD, Turka LA. 2001. Quantifying the frequency of alloreactive T cells in vivo: new answers to an old question. *J. Immunol.* 166: 973-81

[70] Ochando JC, Krieger NR, Bromberg JS. 2006. Direct versus indirect allorecognition: Visualization of dendritic cell distribution and interactions during rejection and tolerization. *Am. J. Transplant.* 6: 2488-96

[71] Talmage DW, Dart G, Radovich J, Lafferty KJ. 1976. Activation of transplant immunity: effect of donor leukocytes on thyroid allograft rejection. *Science.* 191: 385-8

[72] Bowen KM, Andrus L, Lafferty KJ. 1980. Successful allotransplantation of mouse pancreatic islets to nonimmunosuppressed recipients. *Diabetes.* 29 Suppl 1: 98-104

[73] Lechler RI, Batchelor JR. 1982. Restoration of immunogenicity to passenger cell-depleted kidney allografts by the addition of donor strain dendritic cells. *J. Exp. Med.* 155: 31-41

[74] Wang L, Han R, Lee I, Hancock AS, Xiong G, Gunn MD, Hancock WW. 2005. Permanent survival of fully MHC-mismatched islet allografts by targeting a single chemokine receptor pathway. *J. Immunol.* 175: 6311-8

[75] Zhang QW, Kish DD, Fairchild RL. 2003. Absence of allograft ICAM-1 attenuates alloantigen-specific T cell priming, but not primed T cell trafficking into the graft, to mediate acute rejection. *J. Immunol.* 170: 5530-7

[76] Zhu M, Wei MF, Liu F, Shi HF, Wang G. 2003. Interleukin-10 modified dendritic cells induce allo-hyporesponsiveness and prolong small intestine allograft survival. *World J. Gastroenterol.* 9: 2509-12

[77] Takayama T, Kaneko K, Morelli AE, Li W, Tahara H, Thomson AW. 2002. Retroviral delivery of transforming growth factor-beta1 to myeloid dendritic cells: inhibition of T-cell priming ability and influence on allograft survival. *Transplantation.* 74: 112-9

[78] Lu L, Li W, Fu F, Chambers FG, Qian S, Fung JJ, Thomson AW. 1997. Blockade of the CD40-CD40 ligand pathway potentiates the capacity of donor-derived dendritic cell progenitors to induce long-term cardiac allograft survival. *Transplantation.* 64: 1808-15

[79] Xu MQ, Suo YP, Gong JP, Zhang MM, Yan LN. 2004. Augmented regeneration of partial liver allograft induced by nuclear factor-kappaB decoy oligodeoxynucleotides-modified dendritic cells. *World J. Gastroenterol.* 10: 573-8

[80] Min WP, Gorczynski R, Huang XY, Kushida M, Kim P, Obataki M, Lei J, Suri RM, Cattral MS. 2000. Dendritic cells genetically engineered to express Fas ligand induce

donor-specific hyporesponsiveness and prolong allograft survival. *J. Immunol.* 164: 161-7

[81] Hornick PI, Mason PD, Baker RJ, Hernandez-Fuentes M, Frasca L, Lombardi G, Taylor K, Weng L, Rose ML, Yacoub MH, Batchelor R, Lechler RI. 2000. Significant frequencies of T cells with indirect anti-donor specificity in heart graft recipients with chronic rejection. *Circulation.* 101: 2405-10

[82] Yamada A, Chandraker A, Laufer TM, Gerth AJ, Sayegh MH, Auchincloss H, Jr. 2001. Recipient MHC class II expression is required to achieve long-term survival of murine cardiac allografts after costimulatory blockade. *J. Immunol.* 167: 5522-6

[83] Mirenda V, Berton I, Read J, Cook T, Smith J, Dorling A, Lechler RI. 2004. Modified dendritic cells coexpressing self and allogeneic major histocompatability complex molecules: an efficient way to induce indirect pathway regulation. *J. Am. Soc. Nephrol.* 15: 987-97

[84] Miller SD, Wetzig RP, Claman HN. 1979. The induction of cell-mediated immunity and tolerance with protein antigens coupled to syngeneic lymphoid cells. *J. Exp. Med.* 149: 758-73

[85] Elliott C, Wang K, Miller S, Melvold R. 1994. Ethylcarbodiimide as an agent for induction of specific transplant tolerance. *Transplantation.* 58: 966-8

[86] Kaneko K, Morelli AE, Wang Z, Thomson AW. 2003. Alloantigen presentation by ethylcarbodiimide-treated dendritic cells induces T cell hyporesponsiveness, and prolongs organ graft survival. *Clin. Immunol.* 108: 190-8

[87] Wang Z, Larregina AT, Shufesky WJ, Perone MJ, Montecalvo A, Zahorchak AF, Thomson AW, Morelli AE. 2006. Use of the inhibitory effect of apoptotic cells on dendritic cells for graft survival via T-cell deletion and regulatory T cells. *Am. J. Transplant.* 6: 1297-311

[88] Xu DL, Liu Y, Tan JM, Li B, Zhong CP, Zhang XH, Wu CQ, Tang XD. 2004. Marked prolongation of murine cardiac allograft survival using recipient immature dendritic cells loaded with donor-derived apoptotic cells. *Scand. J. Immunol.* 59: 536-44

[89] Kleinclauss F, Perruche S, Masson E, de Carvalho Bittencourt M, Biichle S, Remy-Martin JP, Ferrand C, Martin M, Bittard H, Chalopin JM, Seilles E, Tiberghien P, Saas P. 2006. Intravenous apoptotic spleen cell infusion induces a TGF-beta-dependent regulatory T-cell expansion. *Cell Death Differ.* 13: 41-52

[90] Huang JF, Yang Y, Sepulveda H, Shi W, Hwang I, Peterson PA, Jackson MR, Sprent J, Cai Z. 1999. TCR-Mediated internalization of peptide-MHC complexes acquired by T cells. *Science.* 286: 952-4

[91] Andre F, Chaput N, Schartz NE, Flament C, Aubert N, Bernard J, Lemonnier F, Raposo G, Escudier B, Hsu DH, Tursz T, Amigorena S, Angevin E, Zitvogel L. 2004. Exosomes as potent cell-free peptide-based vaccine. I. Dendritic cell-derived exosomes transfer functional MHC class I/peptide complexes to dendritic cells. *J. Immunol.* 172: 2126-36

[92] Lee RS, Grusby MJ, Glimcher LH, Winn HJ, Auchincloss H, Jr. 1994. Indirect recognition by helper cells can induce donor-specific cytotoxic T lymphocytes in vivo. *J. Exp. Med.* 179: 865-72

[93] Wise MP, Bemelman F, Cobbold SP, Waldmann H. 1998. Linked suppression of skin graft rejection can operate through indirect recognition. *J. Immunol.* 161: 5813-6

[94] Lan RY, Ansari AA, Lian ZX, Gershwin ME. 2005. Regulatory T cells: development, function and role in autoimmunity. *Autoimmun. Rev.* 4: 351-63

[95] Wu Y, Borde M, Heissmeyer V, Feuerer M, Lapan AD, Stroud JC, Bates DL, Guo L, Han A, Ziegler SF, Mathis D, Benoist C, Chen L, Rao A. 2006. FOXP3 controls regulatory T cell function through cooperation with NFAT. *Cell.* 126: 375-87

[96] Wood KJ, Sakaguchi S. 2003. Regulatory T cells in transplantation tolerance. *Nat. Rev. Immunol.* 3: 199-210

[97] Tarbell KV, Yamazaki S, Steinman RM. 2006. The interactions of dendritic cells with antigen-specific, regulatory T cells that suppress autoimmunity. *Semin. Immunol.* 18: 93-102

[98] van Maurik A, Herber M, Wood KJ, Jones ND. 2002. Cutting edge: CD4+CD25+ alloantigen-specific immunoregulatory cells that can prevent CD8+ T cell-mediated graft rejection: implications for anti-CD154 immunotherapy. *J. Immunol.* 169: 5401-4

[99] Sanchez-Fueyo A, Weber M, Domenig C, Strom TB, Zheng XX. 2002. Tracking the immunoregulatory mechanisms active during allograft tolerance. *J. Immunol.* 168: 2274-81

[100] Graca L, Thompson S, Lin CY, Adams E, Cobbold SP, Waldmann H. 2002. Both CD4(+)CD25(+) and CD4(+)CD25(-) regulatory cells mediate dominant transplantation tolerance. *J. Immunol.* 168: 5558-65

[101] Taylor PA, Lees CJ, Blazar BR. 2002. The infusion of ex vivo activated and expanded CD4(+)CD25(+) immune regulatory cells inhibits graft-versus-host disease lethality. *Blood.* 99: 3493-9

[102] Tang Q, Henriksen KJ, Bi M, Finger EB, Szot G, Ye J, Masteller EL, McDevitt H, Bonyhadi M, Bluestone JA. 2004. In vitro-expanded antigen-specific regulatory T cells suppress autoimmune diabetes. *J. Exp. Med.* 199: 1455-65

[103] Taylor PA, Panoskaltsis-Mortari A, Swedin JM, Lucas PJ, Gress RE, Levine BL, June CH, Serody JS, Blazar BR. 2004. L-Selectin(hi) but not the L-selectin(lo) CD4+25+ T-regulatory cells are potent inhibitors of GVHD and BM graft rejection. *Blood.* 104: 3804-12

[104] Cohen JL, Trenado A, Vasey D, Klatzmann D, Salomon BL. 2002. CD4(+)CD25(+) immunoregulatory T Cells: new therapeutics for graft-versus-host disease. *J. Exp. Med.* 196: 401-6

[105] Jones SC, Murphy GF, Korngold R. 2003. Post-hematopoietic cell transplantation control of graft-versus-host disease by donor CD425 T cells to allow an effective graft-versus-leukemia response. *Biol. Blood Marrow Transplant.* 9: 243-56

[106] Takahashi T, Kuniyasu Y, Toda M, Sakaguchi N, Itoh M, Iwata M, Shimizu J, Sakaguchi S. 1998. Immunologic self-tolerance maintained by CD25+CD4+ naturally anergic and suppressive T cells: induction of autoimmune disease by breaking their anergic/suppressive state. *Int. Immunol.* 10: 1969-80

[107] Yamazaki S, Iyoda T, Tarbell K, Olson K, Velinzon K, Inaba K, Steinman RM. 2003. Direct expansion of functional CD25+ CD4+ regulatory T cells by antigen-processing dendritic cells. *J. Exp. Med.* 198: 235-47

[108] Tarbell KV, Yamazaki S, Olson K, Toy P, Steinman RM. 2004. CD25+ CD4+ T cells, expanded with dendritic cells presenting a single autoantigenic peptide, suppress autoimmune diabetes. *J. Exp. Med.* 199: 1467-77

[109] Trenado A, Charlotte F, Fisson S, Yagello M, Klatzmann D, Salomon BL, Cohen JL. 2003. Recipient-type specific CD4+CD25+ regulatory T cells favor immune reconstitution and control graft-versus-host disease while maintaining graft-versus-leukemia. *J. Clin. Invest.* 112: 1688-96

[110] Nishimura E, Sakihama T, Setoguchi R, Tanaka K, Sakaguchi S. 2004. Induction of antigen-specific immunologic tolerance by in vivo and in vitro antigen-specific expansion of naturally arising Foxp3+CD25+CD4+ regulatory T cells. *Int. Immunol.* 16: 1189-201

[111] Joffre O, Gorsse N, Romagnoli P, Hudrisier D, van Meerwijk JP. 2004. Induction of antigen-specific tolerance to bone marrow allografts with CD4+CD25+ T lymphocytes. *Blood.* 103: 4216-21

[112] Yamazaki S, Patel M, Harper A, Bonito A, Fukuyama H, Pack M, Tarbell KV, Talmor M, Ravetch JV, Inaba K, Steinman RM. 2006. Effective expansion of alloantigen-specific Foxp3+ CD25+ CD4+ regulatory T cells by dendritic cells during the mixed leukocyte reaction. *Proc. Natl. Acad. Sci. U S A.* 103: 2758-63

[113] Mahnke K, Qian Y, Knop J, Enk AH. 2003. Induction of CD4+/CD25+ regulatory T cells by targeting of antigens to immature dendritic cells. *Blood.* 101: 4862-9

[114] Kretschmer K, Apostolou I, Hawiger D, Khazaie K, Nussenzweig MC, von Boehmer H. 2005. Inducing and expanding regulatory T cell populations by foreign antigen. *Nat. Immunol.* 6: 1219-27

[115] Robinson SP, Patterson S, English N, Davies D, Knight SC, Reid CD. 1999. Human peripheral blood contains two distinct lineages of dendritic cells. *Eur. J. Immunol.* 29: 2769-78

[116] MacDonald KP, Munster DJ, Clark GJ, Dzionek A, Schmitz J, Hart DN. 2002. Characterization of human blood dendritic cell subsets. *Blood.* 100: 4512-20

[117] Caux C, Massacrier C, Vanbervliet B, Dubois B, Durand I, Cella M, Lanzavecchia A, Banchereau J. 1997. CD34+ hematopoietic progenitors from human cord blood differentiate along two independent dendritic cell pathways in response to granulocyte-macrophage colony-stimulating factor plus tumor necrosis factor alpha: II. Functional analysis. *Blood.* 90: 1458-70

[118] Romani N, Reider D, Heuer M, Ebner S, Kampgen E, Eibl B, Niederwieser D, Schuler G. 1996. Generation of mature dendritic cells from human blood. An improved method with special regard to clinical applicability. *J. Immunol. Methods.* 196: 137-51

[119] Curti A, Fogli M, Ratta M, Biasco G, Tura S, Lemoli RM. 2001. Dendritic cell differentiation from hematopoietic CD34+ progenitor cells. *J. Biol. Regul. Homeost. Agents.* 15: 49-52

[120] McKenna HJ. 2001. Role of hematopoietic growth factors/flt3 ligand in expansion and regulation of dendritic cells. *Curr. Opin. Hematol.* 8: 149-54

[121] Dauer M, Obermaier B, Herten J, Haerle C, Pohl K, Rothenfusser S, Schnurr M, Endres S, Eigler A. 2003. Mature dendritic cells derived from human monocytes within 48 hours: a novel strategy for dendritic cell differentiation from blood precursors. *J. Immunol.* 170: 4069-76

[122] Lee AW, Truong T, Bickham K, Fonteneau JF, Larsson M, Da Silva I, Somersan S, Thomas EK, Bhardwaj N. 2002. A clinical grade cocktail of cytokines and PGE2 results in uniform maturation of human monocyte-derived dendritic cells: implications for immunotherapy. *Vaccine.* 20 Suppl 4: A8-A22

[123] Matyszak MK, Citterio S, Rescigno M, Ricciardi-Castagnoli P. 2000. Differential effects of corticosteroids during different stages of dendritic cell maturation. *Eur. J. mmunol.* 30: 1233-42

[124] Rozkova D, Horvath R, Bartunkova J, Spisek R. 2006. Glucocorticoids severely impair differentiation and antigen presenting function of dendritic cells despite upregulation of Toll-like receptors. *Clin. Immunol.* 120: 260-71

[125] Mazzoni A, Segal DM. 2004. Controlling the Toll road to dendritic cell polarization. *J. Leukoc. Biol.* 75: 721-30

[126] Reis e Sousa C. 2006. Dendritic cells in a mature age. *Nat. Rev. Immunol.* 6: 476-83

[127] Hackstein H, Renner FC, Bohnert A, Nockher A, Frommer T, Bein G, Weimer R. 2005. Dendritic cell deficiency in the blood of kidney transplant patients on long-term immunosuppression: results of a prospective matched-cohort study. *Am. J. Transplant.* 5: 2945-53

[128] Schlichting CL, Schareck WD, Nickel T, Weis M. 2005. Dendritic cells as pharmacological targets for the generation of regulatory immunosuppressive effectors. New implications for allo-transplantation. *Curr. Med. Chem.* 12: 1921-30

[129] Tajima K, Amakawa R, Ito T, Miyaji M, Takebayashi M, Fukuhara S. 2003. Immunomodulatory effects of cyclosporin A on human peripheral blood dendritic cell subsets. *Immunology.* 108: 321-8

[130] Schlichting CL, Schareck WD, Weis M. 2005. Dendritic cell adhesion is enhanced on endothelial cells preexposed to calcineurin inhibitors. *J. Cardiovasc. Pharmacol.* 46: 250-4

[131] Szabo G, Gavala C, Mandrekar P. 2001. Tacrolimus and cyclosporine A inhibit allostimulatory capacity and cytokine production of human myeloid dendritic cells. *J. Investig. Med.* 49: 442-9

[132] Monti P, Mercalli A, Leone BE, Valerio DC, Allavena P, Piemonti L. 2003. Rapamycin impairs antigen uptake of human dendritic cells. *Transplantation.* 75: 137-45

[133] Woltman AM, van der Kooij SW, Coffer PJ, Offringa R, Daha MR, van Kooten C. 2003. Rapamycin specifically interferes with GM-CSF signaling in human dendritic cells, leading to apoptosis via increased p27KIP1 expression. *Blood.* 101: 1439-45

[134] Hackstein H, Morelli AE, Larregina AT, Ganster RW, Papworth GD, Logar AJ, Watkins SC, Falo LD, Thomson AW. 2001. Aspirin inhibits in vitro maturation and in vivo immunostimulatory function of murine myeloid dendritic cells. *J. Immunol.* 166: 7053-62

[135] Matasic R, Dietz AB, Vuk-Pavlovic S. 2001. Maturation of human dendritic cells as sulfasalazine target. *Croat. Med. J.* 42: 440-5

[136] Ho LJ, Chang DM, Shiau HY, Chen CH, Hsieh TY, Hsu YL, Wong CS, Lai JH. 2001. Aspirin differentially regulates endotoxin-induced IL-12 and TNF-alpha production in human dendritic cells. *Scand. J. Rheumatol.* 30: 346-52

[137] Piemonti L, Monti P, Sironi M, Fraticelli P, Leone BE, Dal Cin E, Allavena P, Di Carlo V. 2000. Vitamin D3 affects differentiation, maturation, and function of human monocyte-derived dendritic cells. *J. Immunol.* 164: 4443-51

[138] Adorini L. 2002. 1,25-Dihydroxyvitamin D3 analogs as potential therapies in transplantation. *Curr. Opin. Investig. Drugs.* 3: 1458-63

[139] Griffin MD, Xing N, Kumar R. 2003. Vitamin D and its analogs as regulators of immune activation and antigen presentation. *Annu. Rev. Nutr.* 23: 117-45

[140] Adorini L, Giarratana N, Penna G. 2004. Pharmacological induction of tolerogenic dendritic cells and regulatory T cells. *Semin. Immunol.* 16: 127-34

[141] Penna G, Vulcano M, Roncari A, Facchetti F, Sozzani S, Adorini L. 2002. Cutting edge: differential chemokine production by myeloid and plasmacytoid dendritic cells. *J. Immunol.* 169: 6673-6

[142] Penna G, Roncari A, Amuchastegui S, Daniel KC, Berti E, Colonna M, Adorini L. 2005. Expression of the inhibitory receptor ILT3 on dendritic cells is dispensable for induction of CD4+Foxp3+ regulatory T cells by 1,25-dihydroxyvitamin D3. *Blood.* 106: 3490-7

[143] Bennett CL, Ochs HD. 2001. IPEX is a unique X-linked syndrome characterized by immune dysfunction, polyendocrinopathy, enteropathy, and a variety of autoimmune phenomena. *Curr. Opin. Pediatr.* 13: 533-8

[144] Shevach EM, DiPaolo RA, Andersson J, Zhao DM, Stephens GL, Thornton AM. 2006. The lifestyle of naturally occurring CD4+ CD25+ Foxp3+ regulatory T cells. *Immunol. Rev.* 212: 60-73

[145] Lehmann J, Huehn J, de la Rosa M, Maszyna F, Kretschmer U, Krenn V, Brunner M, Scheffold A, Hamann A. 2002. Expression of the integrin alpha Ebeta 7 identifies unique subsets of CD25+ as well as CD25- regulatory T cells. *Proc. Natl. Acad. Sci. U S A.* 99: 13031-6

[146] Takahashi T, Tagami T, Yamazaki S, Uede T, Shimizu J, Sakaguchi N, Mak TW, Sakaguchi S. 2000. Immunologic self-tolerance maintained by CD25(+)CD4(+) regulatory T cells constitutively expressing cytotoxic T lymphocyte-associated antigen 4. *J. Exp. Med.* 192: 303-10

[147] Shimizu J, Yamazaki S, Takahashi T, Ishida Y, Sakaguchi S. 2002. Stimulation of CD25(+)CD4(+) regulatory T cells through GITR breaks immunological self-tolerance. *Nat. Immunol.* 3: 135-42

[148] Xu D, Liu H, Komai-Koma M. 2004. Direct and indirect role of Toll-like receptors in T cell mediated immunity. *Cell. Mol. Immunol.* 1: 239-46

[149] Yamagiwa S, Gray JD, Hashimoto S, Horwitz DA. 2001. A role for TGF-beta in the generation and expansion of CD4+CD25+ regulatory T cells from human peripheral blood. *J. Immunol.* 166: 7282-9

[150] Jonuleit H, Schmitt E, Stassen M, Tuettenberg A, Knop J, Enk AH. 2001. Identification and functional characterization of human CD4(+)CD25(+) T cells with regulatory properties isolated from peripheral blood. *J. Exp. Med.* 193: 1285-94

[151] Cobbold SP, Adams E, Graca L, Waldmann H. 2003. Serial analysis of gene expression provides new insights into regulatory T cells. *Semin. Immunol.* 15: 209-14

[152] Cobbold SP, Nolan KF, Graca L, Castejon R, Le Moine A, Frewin M, Humm S, Adams E, Thompson S, Zelenika D, Paterson A, Yates S, Fairchild PJ, Waldmann H. 2003. Regulatory T cells and dendritic cells in transplantation tolerance: molecular markers and mechanisms. *Immunol. Rev.* 196: 109-24

[153] Misra N, Bayry J, Lacroix-Desmazes S, Kazatchkine MD, Kaveri SV. 2004. Cutting edge: human CD4+CD25+ T cells restrain the maturation and antigen-presenting function of dendritic cells. *J. Immunol.*172: 4676-80

[154] Cederbom L, Hall H, Ivars F. 2000. CD4+CD25+ regulatory T cells down-regulate co-stimulatory molecules on antigen-presenting cells. *Eur. J. Immunol.* 30: 1538-43

[155] Houot R, Perrot I, Garcia E, Durand I, Lebecque S. 2006. Human CD4+CD25high regulatory T cells modulate myeloid but not plasmacytoid dendritic cells activation. *J. Immunol.* 176: 5293-8

[156] Rosenberg SA, Sportes C, Ahmadzadeh M, Fry TJ, Ngo LT, Schwarz SL, Stetler-Stevenson M, Morton KE, Mavroukakis SA, Morre M, Buffet R, Mackall CL, Gress RE. 2006. IL-7 administration to humans leads to expansion of CD8+ and CD4+ cells but a relative decrease of CD4+ T-regulatory cells. *J. Immunother.* 29: 313-9

[157] Liu W, Putnam AL, Xu-Yu Z, Szot GL, Lee MR, Zhu S, Gottlieb PA, Kapranov P, Gingeras TR, Fazekas de St Groth B, Clayberger C, Soper DM, Ziegler SF, Bluestone JA. 2006. CD127 expression inversely correlates with FoxP3 and suppressive function of human CD4+ T reg cells. *J. Exp. Med.* 203: 1701-11

[158] Seddiki N, Santner-Nanan B, Martinson J, Zaunders J, Sasson S, Landay A, Solomon M, Selby W, Alexander SI, Nanan R, Kelleher A, Fazekas de St Groth B. 2006. Expression of interleukin (IL)-2 and IL-7 receptors discriminates between human regulatory and activated T cells. *J. Exp. Med.* 203: 1693-700

[159] Levings MK, Sangregorio R, Roncarolo MG. 2001. Human cd25(+)cd4(+) t regulatory cells suppress naive and memory T cell proliferation and can be expanded in vitro without loss of function. *J. Exp. Med.* 193: 1295-302

[160] Jiang S, Camara N, Lombardi G, Lechler RI. 2003. Induction of allopeptide-specific human CD4+CD25+ regulatory T cells ex vivo. *Blood.* 102: 2180-6

[161] Jiang S, Lechler RI. 2003. Regulatory T cells in the control of transplantation tolerance and autoimmunity. *Am. J. Transplant.* 3: 516-24

[162] Vlad G, Cortesini R, Suciu-Foca N. 2005. License to heal: bidirectional interaction of antigen-specific regulatory T cells and tolerogenic APC. *J. Immunol.* 174: 5907-14

[163] Suciu-Foca N, Manavalan JS, Cortesini R. 2003. Generation and function of antigen-specific suppressor and regulatory T cells. *Transpl. Immunol.* 11: 235-44

[164] Chang CC, Ciubotariu R, Manavalan JS, Yuan J, Colovai AI, Piazza F, Lederman S, Colonna M, Cortesini R, Dalla-Favera R, Suciu-Foca N. 2002. Tolerization of dendritic cells by T(S) cells: the crucial role of inhibitory receptors ILT3 and ILT4. *Nat. Immunol.* 3: 237-43

[165] Manavalan JS, Kim-Schulze S, Scotto L, Naiyer AJ, Vlad G, Colombo PC, Marboe C, Mancini D, Cortesini R, Suciu-Foca N. 2004. Alloantigen specific CD8+CD28- FOXP3+ T suppressor cells induce ILT3+ ILT4+ tolerogenic endothelial cells, inhibiting alloreactivity. *Int. Immunol.* 16: 1055-68

[166] Suciu-Foca N, Manavalan JS, Scotto L, Kim-Schulze S, Galluzzo S, Naiyer AJ, Fan J, Vlad G, Cortesini R. 2005. Molecular characterization of allospecific T suppressor and tolerogenic dendritic cells: review. *Int. Immunopharmacol.* 5: 7-11

[167] Colovai AI, Mirza M, Vlad G, Wang S, Ho E, Cortesini R, Suciu-Foca N. 2003. Regulatory CD8+CD28- T cells in heart transplant recipients. *Hum. Immunol.* 64: 31-7

[168] Manavalan JS, Rossi PC, Vlad G, Piazza F, Yarilina A, Cortesini R, Mancini D, Suciu-Foca N. 2003. High expression of ILT3 and ILT4 is a general feature of tolerogenic dendritic cells. *Transpl. Immunol.* 11: 245-58

[169] Jonuleit H, Schmitt E, Schuler G, Knop J, Enk AH. 2000. Induction of interleukin 10-producing, nonproliferating CD4(+) T cells with regulatory properties by repetitive stimulation with allogeneic immature human dendritic cells. *J. Exp. Med.* 192: 1213-22

[170] Dhodapkar MV, Steinman RM, Krasovsky J, Munz C, Bhardwaj N. 2001. Antigen-specific inhibition of effector T cell function in humans after injection of immature dendritic cells. *J. Exp. Med.* 193: 233-8

[171] Levings MK, Bacchetta R, Schulz U, Roncarolo MG. 2002. The role of IL-10 and TGF-beta in the differentiation and effector function of T regulatory cells. *Int. Arch. Allergy Immunol.* 129: 263-76

[172] Levings MK, Sangregorio R, Sartirana C, Moschin AL, Battaglia M, Orban PC, Roncarolo MG. 2002. Human CD25+CD4+ T suppressor cell clones produce transforming growth factor beta, but not interleukin 10, and are distinct from type 1 T regulatory cells. *J. Exp. Med.* 196: 1335-46

[173] Bacchetta R, Sartirana C, Levings MK, Bordignon C, Narula S, Roncarolo MG. 2002. Growth and expansion of human T regulatory type 1 cells are independent from TCR activation but require exogenous cytokines. *Eur. J. Immunol.* 32: 2237-45

[174] Valmori D, Tosello V, Souleimanian NE, Godefroy E, Scotto L, Wang Y, Ayyoub M. 2006. Rapamycin-mediated enrichment of T cells with regulatory activity in stimulated CD4+ T cell cultures is not due to the selective expansion of naturally occurring regulatory T cells but to the induction of regulatory functions in conventional CD4+ T cells. *J. Immunol.* 177: 944-9

[175] Segundo DS, Ruiz JC, Fernandez-Fresnedo G, Izquierdo M, Gomez-Alamillo C, Cacho E, Benito MJ, Rodrigo E, Palomar R, Lopez-Hoyos M, Arias M. 2006. Calcineurin Inhibitors Affect Circulating Regulatory T Cells in Stable Renal Transplant Recipients. *Transplant. Proc.* 38: 2391-3

[176] Salama AD, Najafian N, Clarkson MR, Harmon WE, Sayegh MH. 2003. Regulatory CD25+ T cells in human kidney transplant recipients. *J. Am. Soc. Nephrol.* 14: 1643-51

[177] Game DS, Hernandez-Fuentes MP, Lechler RI. 2005. Everolimus and basiliximab permit suppression by human CD4+CD25+ cells in vitro. *Am. J. Transplant.* 5: 454-64

[178] Franzke A, Piao W, Lauber J, Gatzlaff P, Konecke C, Hansen W, Schmitt-Thomsen A, Hertenstein B, Buer J, Ganser A. 2003. G-CSF as immune regulator in T cells expressing the G-CSF receptor: implications for transplantation and autoimmune diseases. *Blood.* 102: 734-9

[179] Rutella S, Pierelli L, Bonanno G, Sica S, Ameglio F, Capoluongo E, Mariotti A, Scambia G, d'Onofrio G, Leone G. 2002. Role for granulocyte colony-stimulating factor in the generation of human T regulatory type 1 cells. *Blood.* 100: 2562-71

[180] Dieckmann D, Plottner H, Berchtold S, Berger T, Schuler G. 2001. Ex vivo isolation and characterization of CD4(+)CD25(+) T cells with regulatory properties from human blood. *J. Exp. Med.* 193: 1303-10

[181] Karakhanova S, Munder M, Schneider M, Bonyhadi M, Ho AD, Goerner M. 2006. Highly efficient expansion of human CD4+CD25+ regulatory T cells for cellular immunotherapy in patients with graft-versus-host disease. *J. Immunother.* 29: 336-49

[182] Godfrey WR, Ge YG, Spoden DJ, Levine BL, June CH, Blazar BR, Porter SB. 2004. In vitro-expanded human CD4(+)CD25(+) T-regulatory cells can markedly inhibit allogeneic dendritic cell-stimulated MLR cultures. *Blood.* 104: 453-61

[183] Hoffmann P, Eder R, Kunz-Schughart LA, Andreesen R, Edinger M. 2004. Large-scale in vitro expansion of polyclonal human CD4(+)CD25high regulatory T cells. *Blood.* 104: 895-903

[184] Koenen HJ, Fasse E, Joosten I. 2005. CD27/CFSE-based ex vivo selection of highly suppressive alloantigen-specific human regulatory T cells. *J. Immunol.* 174: 7573-83

[185] Creput C, Durrbach A, Menier C, Guettier C, Samuel D, Dausset J, Charpentier B, Carosella ED, Rouas-Freiss N. 2003. Human leukocyte antigen-G (HLA-G) expression in biliary epithelial cells is associated with allograft acceptance in liver-kidney transplantation. *J. Hepatol.* 39: 587-94

[186] Lefebvre S, Antoine M, Uzan S, McMaster M, Dausset J, Carosella ED, Paul P. 2002. Specific activation of the non-classical class I histocompatibility HLA-G antigen and expression of the ILT2 inhibitory receptor in human breast cancer. *J. Pathol.* 196: 266-74

[187] Allan DS, McMichael AJ, Braud VM. 2000. The ILT family of leukocyte receptors. *Immunobiology.* 202: 34-41

[188] Sanders SK, Giblin PA, Kavathas P. 1991. Cell-cell adhesion mediated by CD8 and human histocompatibility leukocyte antigen G, a nonclassical major histocompatibility complex class 1 molecule on cytotrophoblasts. *J. Exp. Med.* 174: 737-40

[189] Kanai T, Fujii T, Kozuma S, Yamashita T, Miki A, Kikuchi A, Taketani Y. 2001. Soluble HLA-G influences the release of cytokines from allogeneic peripheral blood mononuclear cells in culture. *Mol. Hum. Reprod.* 7: 195-200

[190] Kapasi K, Albert SE, Yie S, Zavazava N, Librach CL. 2000. HLA-G has a concentration-dependent effect on the generation of an allo-CTL response. *Immunology.* 101: 191-200

[191] Lila N, Amrein C, Guillemain R, Chevalier P, Latremouille C, Fabiani JN, Dausset J, Carosella ED, Carpentier A. 2002. Human leukocyte antigen-G expression after heart transplantation is associated with a reduced incidence of rejection. *Circulation.* 105: 1949-54

[192] Onno M, Pangault C, Le Friec G, Guilloux V, Andre P, Fauchet R. 2000. Modulation of HLA-G antigens expression by human cytomegalovirus: specific induction in activated macrophages harboring human cytomegalovirus infection. *J. Immunol.* 164: 6426-34

[193] Colonna M, Navarro F, Bellon T, Llano M, Garcia P, Samaridis J, Angman L, Cella M, Lopez-Botet M. 1997. A common inhibitory receptor for major histocompatibility complex class I molecules on human lymphoid and myelomonocytic cells. *J. Exp. Med.* 186: 1809-18

[194] LeMaoult J, Rouas-Freiss N, Carosella ED. 2005. Immuno-tolerogenic functions of HLA-G: relevance in transplantation and oncology. *Autoimmun. Rev.* 4: 503-9

In: Immune Tolerance Research Developments
Editor: Emile B. Pontell, pp. 151-166
ISBN: 978-1-60456-209-5

Chapter 7

Recent Advances in Immune Tolerance in Stem Cells

B. Linju Yen[1], Men-Luh Yen[2], Ko-Jiunn Liu[3] and Ray Chu-Jeng Chiu[4,*]

[1]Stem Cell Research Center, National Health Research Institute, Zhunan, Taiwan
[2]Departments of Primary Care Medicine and Obstetrics/Gynecology, College of Medicine, National Taiwan University, Taipei, Taiwan
[3]Institute of Cancer Research, National Health Research Institute, Zhunan, Taiwan
[4]McGill University Health Center, Montreal, Canada

Introduction

The burst of interest and activity in stem cell research in recent years, which foretells the dawn of regenerative therapy for many diseases, has been accompanied by a number of moral and ethical controversies. One of such issues is the strategy to use cloned human embryonic stem cells in order to avoid immune rejection by the recipient of the stem cell therapy. It had been taken for granted that the stem cells will be subjected to immune surveillance like any other cells, such that only autologous cells will be immunologically tolerated and accepted.

As it turned out, it is now known that stem cells derived from a number of sources exhibit unique immune tolerance, both in the *in vitro* and *in vivo* studies. Their ability to circumvent immune surveillance allows them to be chosen as "universal donor cells" for therapeutic use, with vast clinical and logistic advantages. Such development should be able to circumvent these ethical/moral controversies, thus accelerate the advance and realization of regenerative therapies.

* E-mail address: ray.chiu@mcgill.ca; Room C9-169, 1650 Cedar Avenue, Montreal, PQ, Canada (Corresponding author)

The Proliferating Sources of Stem Cells

Stem cells are specialized cells capable of self-renewal and multilineage differentiation. Advances in stem cell biology within the past few years have fueled the hope of using these versatile cells as curative therapy for degenerative diseases. Based on their origin, stem cells are often categorized into embryonic (ESC) or adult stem cells (ASCs). ESCs are derived from the inner cell mass of pre-implantation embryos, and are able to differentiate into all tissue types including germ cells. The derivation of mouse ESCs over 20 years ago was a landmark achievement [1],[2], and is the foundation on which mammalian transgenic animal research is based on. The isolation of the human counterpart has lagged behind and was not successfully achieved until 1998 by Thomson [3], mostly due to technical difficulties but also ethical concerns of embryo destruction. These pluripotent—if not totipotent—stem cells can be propagated indefinitely and are capable of differentiating into tissues from all three germ layers [3], [4]. Although tests of totipotency in terms of chimera formation and germline transmission are ethically not possible for human ESCs, it is inferred from ESCs of other species that human ESCs represent the widest proliferative and differentiation capacity of any human stem cells. Therefore, although known to generate teratomas—a benign germ cell tumor—when injected into SCID mice, human ESCs are considered a possible source for cell therapy, and active research is on-going in this area with clinical trials planned for the future [5], [6].

The other category of stem cells is ASCs, long thought to have only limited differentiation potential. Also known as somatic stem cells, the first ASCs to be identified were hematopoeitic stem cells (HSCs) from the bone marrow (BM), and most of our knowledge regarding ASCs has been derived from studies of this population of post-natal stem cells [7]. First discovered over 40 years ago, HSCs give rise to all cells of the hematopoeitic system and are able to reconstitute an organism's entire hemtaopoeitic system. Since then, ASCs have increasingly been isolated from many organs—i.e. skin, gut—as well as sites previously not thought to have regenerative capacity, including the pancreas and the brain [8]. Moreover, in recent years, many reports have shown that some ASCs, in addition to being able to repopulate its organ of origin, also possess unexpected plasticity, differentiating into other tissue types [9-12], . Because ASCs do not have the ethical or tumorgenicity problems of ESCs, the findings of plasticity have generated much excitement, giving hope to the therapeutic use of ASCs in a wide range of diseases. A number of these transdifferentiation findings were reported for bone marrow mesenchymal stem cells (MSCs) [13-18]. First identified over 20 years ago, BMMSCs were previously known as stromal cells and thought only to provide support for HSC growth and development [19], [20]. It has now been shown that BMMSCs are the precursor cells for components of the skeleton, including bone, cartilage, muscle, and adipose tissue [21], [22], and may additionally be able to differentiate into extra-mesodermal lineages including neural and endodermal cell types [16], [17], [23].

Increasingly, MSCs have been found in adult tissues other than the bone marrow, including fat and bone [24-26]. Although without many of the problems of ESCs, BMMSC numbers decrease significantly with the age of the individual [27], and cells obtained from any adult sources still require invasive procedures. Thus, the search for easily accessible and abundant sources of multipotent stem cells have led many groups to look into fetal-source tissue, and MSCs have been successfully isolated from various mid-gestational fetal tissue, including amniotic fluid [28-30], first-trimester fetal tissues [31], and second-trimester fetal tissues [32-34]. Multipotent cells have also been isolated from the placenta and associated tissues, including umbilical cord blood (UCB) [35-38], umbilical cord mesenchyme [39],[40], and the placenta itself [41-44]. The human placenta is a fetomaternal organ, formed by both fetal and maternal tissue. Its successful formation is a critical process in embryogenesis, and the normal development and function of the placenta is crucial to the well-being of the fetus [45]. This remarkable organ is discarded postpartum, after having performed its necessary function of supporting the embryo/fetus. Except for the decidua, the other layers and components of the placenta are derived from the embryo/fetus. The advantages of stem cells isolated from fetal-source tissues are multiple. Although unlikely to have the differentiation and proliferative potential of ESCs, fetal-source stem cells (FSCs) are more immature than ASCs and may be superior to ASCs in many aspects. Indeed, in addition to demonstrating multilineage differentiation capacity, various laboratories have reported finding ESC markers in a number of FSCs [29], [30], [38], [44], [46]. Moreover, the use of term fetal tissues—i.e. placenta, UCB—would not require invasive procedures nor generate ethical conflicts, since these components would have otherwise been discarded. In terms of tumorigenicity of FSCs, there have been no reports in the literature so far. Thus, FSCs, along with BMMSCs and other adult somatic stem cells, appear to be possible sources of stem cells for future clinical use.

Graft-Versus-Host Disease (Gvhd) in HSC Transplantation

The therapeutic use of stem cells is not a new concept. The use of HSCs from the BM for treatment of hematopoietic malignancies has been established for several decades. As with any transplantation paradigm, donor and recipient must be matched as to histocompatilibity. Patients are matched for histocompatibility for a BM donor from which HSCs are harvested. The patient, or recipient, undergo BM ablation and subsequently are infused with the matched donor's BM HSCs. These donor-derived HSCs are able to reconsistitute the recipient's entire hematopoietic system. Overall, HSC therapy has saved numerous lives. However, the appearance of graft-versus-host disease (GVHD) continues to be a major barrier to successful allogeneic HSC transplantation [47]. GVHD is an immunologically mediated disease that is induced primarily by cytotoxic effector cells from the transplanted graft population. Despite much progress in the understanding of the mechanism behind GVHD, successful treatment has remained elusive, with most patients who develop the severe manifestations of GVHD succumbing to it or to complications of therapy [48].

In the last decade or so, UCB has emerged as a source of HSCs for clinical use [49], [50]. Previously discarded, UCB is now known to contain HSCs and other immature hematopoeitic precursors [51]. Easy to obtain and store, UCBHSC transplantation is increasingly viewed as an alternative to BMHSC transplantation in many situations. Data from the United States show that only about 30% of eligible patients with leukemia have a related histocompatible donor, and of the remainder patients, only 20% receive a transplant from an unrelated donor or an HLA-mismatched related donor [52]. Patients who undergo transplantation of grafts from unrelated donors or related donors with partially matched HLA antigens are at increased risk of chronic GVHD [53-55]. UCBHSC transplantation from unrelated donors have been successful, primarily in children but also increasingly for adults as well [49], [50], [56], [57]. While stem cell numbers are more limited with UCB and engraftment is slower, the incidence of GVHD and other immune-related complications appears to be decreased [56], [58-60]. The exact reasons remain unclear but it may be that UCB cells are immunologically more naive than their adult counterpart, and functional differences in UCB lymphoid cells compared to adult cells can be seen (for review, see [61]). The overall favorable clinical outcome for both pediatric and adult patients who have received mismatched UCB HSC transplantation has prompted continued research into increasing the indications for this easily accessible source of HSCs [62].

Table 1. Comparison of immunosuppressive mechanisms for various types of stem cells.

Mechanisms	BMMSCs	ESCs	FSCs
Increase surface HLA-DR expression to IFN-γ	Strongly, in 2 days	Not seen *stimulated for 2 days	In 7 days
Inhibit T cell proliferation	√	√	√
Soluble cytokines: TGF-β	√		√
IDO and tryptophan metabolism	√		√
Increase Tregs	√		√
Resistant to unactivated NK	√	√	√
Decrease NK production of IFN-γ	√	√	√
In vivo immune modulation	√	√	

Immunosuppressive Properties of MSCs

It is the hope that, as with HSCs, other newly isolated types of stem cells can also have therapeutic applications. Indeed, clinical studies using autologous MSCs or same-donor MSCs from previously HLA-matched HSC transplantation have proven successful, although patient numbers remain small [63-67]. While such results are promising, autologous and same-donor use limits prevalent application of such versatile cells. Allogeneic use of non-HSC populations would strongly increase the range of use of such cells, but immunological rejection is a major concern. Even with HSC transplantation, an established clinical treatment, immune complications still occur, resulting in such lethal complications as GVHD. In solid organ transplantation, besides the lack of donor organs, the other major problem for patients is the survival of the transplanted organ in the recipient. Post-transplantation, recipients depend on immunosuppressive therapy to suppress host immune responses toward the foreign tissue. Although immunosuppression is necessary to avoid rejection, these drugs also increase susceptibility to infection and malignancy, two of the leading causes of mortality in transplant patients [68].

Recent research is revealing that one population of ASCs, the MSCs, not only do not elicit host immune responses, but in fact suppress immune reactivity of allogeneic lymphocytes, both *in vitro* and *in vivo*. Just as with the findings of transdifferentiation, the immunosuppression data challenge current scientific dogma, but evidence continues to accumulate. Allogeneic BMMSCs from humans, baboons, and mice have been shown to decrease the immune response of lymphocytes *in vitro* [69-73]. The inhibitory effects of BMMSCs appear to work via a number of mechanisms, some of which have been elucidated. Most reports find that the immunosuppressive properties are broad, effective whether the stimulation is specific or non-specific [69], [70], [72], [73], across species [69], [71], [74], and across different populations of lymphocytes [74-76]. The majority of studies to date show that cell-cell contact is not necessary for the inhibitory effects of human BMMSCs, implicating a role for secreted soluble factors at work with the most likely candidates being transforming growth factor (TGF-) β, hepatocyte growth factor, and interleukin (IL-) 10 (reviewed in [77]). In addition to *in vitro* data, *in vivo* data show that skin engraftment in mice is improved with concurrent transplantation of MSCs [69], and histocompatibility mismatched MSCs can be tolerated without immunosuppression in fully immunocompetent adult rodents [78-81]. The immunosuppressive effects of BMMSCs have resulted in the therapeutic application of these stem cells for GVHD. In 2005, a pediatric patient with severe, acute GVHD refractory to standard drug regimen was treated with haploidentical BMMSCs from his mother with subsequent recovery [82]. Currently, a multi-center, prospective clinical trial investigating the use of ex vivo expanded mesenchymal stem cells for GVHD has been started in Europe [83].

Immunosuppressive Properties of FSCs and ESCs

The decreased incidence of immune-related complications seen in UCBHSC transplantation has led us to hypothesize that ESCs and FSCs may show less immune reaction than ASCs. Moreover, the paradoxical survival of the fetal allograft during pregnancy is living proof of the "immune-privileged" status of embryonic and fetal cells. A multitude of theories have been put forth to explain this phenomenon, which has long fascinated immunologists. More recently, research has begun to shed light on some of these mechanisms. These include the expression of nonclassical MHC molecules by trophoblast cells [84], tryptophan catabolism by the enzyme indoleamine 2, 3-dioxygenase (IDO) [85], and alterations to the complement system [86], a part of the innate immune system. Studies have also documented a role for regulatory T cells (Tregs) [87], a sub-population of T cells which are CD4+CD25bright and have immune-tolerant properties Sakaguchi S, Sakaguchi N Shimizu. More recent data also show that the T lymphocyte inhibitory costimulatory molecule, programmed death ligand 1 (PD-L1), also play a role in maintenance of fetomaternal tolerance [88]. Interestingly, a few of these fetomaternal tolerance mechanisms actually have been implicated in the immunosuppressive effects of BMMSCs, including the expression of IDO [89] and the generation of Tregs [90], [91].

While the immune characteristics of BMMSCs are increasingly being studied, there are only a few reports regarding the immune properties of the more developmentally primitive stem cells, ESCs and FSCs. The few studies using ESCs—both human and mouse—have documented that these stem cells are also immunosuppressive towards T lymphocytes *in vitro*, and may be tolerated *in vivo* after transplantation in immunocompetent mice [92-94]. There is, however, one report that shows human ESCs being rejected after transplantation in wild type mice [95]. One explanation for these divergent results is the difference in the experimental models used. Such discrepancies highlight the need for further research using a variety of systems and experimental models to clarify results and mechanisms. Nevertheless, the consistent finding across all these studies show that once ESCs are differentiated into teratomas, rejection occurs [92-95]. Regardless of the source of stem cells—whether adult, fetal or embryonic—the immunosuppressive results using *in vitro* mixed lymphocyte cultures and against T cells have been qualitatively similar. ESCs and FSCs also prominently suppress allogeneic peripheral blood mononuclear cell (PBMC) and T lymphocyte proliferation [92-94], [96], with immunosuppressive effects involving the generation of Tregs and soluble factors such as TGF-β [97]. However, there are some important differences in the immunobiology of ESCs and FSCs versus BMMSCs. In our comparative study using placenta-derived multipotent cells (PDMCs) and BMMSCs, we found that PDMCs suppress both mitogen- and alloantigen-stimulated PBMC proliferation to a greater extent than BMMSCs [97]. Human ESCs and most FSCs are positive for MHC I molecules but express little or no MHC II or costimulatory molecules, similar to BMMSCs [98], [99]. However, BMMSCs upregulate HLA-DR expression strongly after 48 hours of stimulation with interferon-γ (IFN-γ) but hESCs do not [92], [98], even after up to 7 days of stimulation [95]. A similar trend is seen with FSCs; we found that PDMCs do not express HLA-DR even after 2 days of IFN-γ stimulation [97], while others have found that fetal liver MSCs require 7 days of stimulation before expression of surface HLA-DR [100]. FSCs derived from the placenta also show some placenta-specific tolerance mechanisms not found in BMMSCs. We saw the expression of HLA-G, a placenta-specific MHC-I antigen critical to the immune tolerant state of pregnancy in PDMCs but not BMMSCs. Moreover, after IFN-γ stimulation, PDMCs but not BMMSCs show increased expression of the inhibitory molecule PD-L1 [97].

The Role of Natural Killer Lymphocytes (NKs)

The focus in stem cell immunobiology has so far been mainly centered on interactions with T cells, since with regards to transplantation immunology, these lymphocytes are arguably the most important subpopulation. More recently, the innate arm of the immune system—very critical in mediating maternal-fetal tolerance—has been found to be important in transplantation immunology as well, and natural killer lymphocytes (NKs) play a particularly prominent role in these interactions [101]. While derived from the same lymphoid precursor, NKs, unlike B and T cells, are not activated by specific antigen on target cells, but rather mount effector cytolytic responses to the "missing self," or absence of self-MHC molecules [102]. In transplantation immunology, the role of NKs has been believed to be limited to BM transplantation. However, recent data show that these lymphocytes participate in crosstalk with the adaptive arm of the immune response and in rejection of solid organs [103]. Research on the immune interactions of this important population of lymphocytes with MSCs is still scarce. Although it does appear that MSCs also suppress some effector responses of NKs, the immunosuppressive effects are not as profound nor as clearly defined as for T cells. BMMSCs are resistant to cytolysis of freshly isolated NK but not cytokine-stimulated NKs [104-106]. The production of IFN-γ by NKs is reduced in the presence of BMMSCs [99], [104-107]. However, reports on the ability of BMMSCs to inhibit NK cytolysis towards its target cells are contradictory [104], [107].

Due to their earlier developmental origin, ESCs and FSCs may have different interactions with NKs than BMMSCs. Indeed, although undifferentiated human ESCs express rather low levels of MHC I, they are not effectively recognized or lysed by NKs, as expected [98]. In the placenta, the expression of non-classical MHC I molecules including HLA-G on trophoblasts is thought to confer a protective effect against maternal NK cells by taking the place of classical MHC I antigens [101]. It also appears that, under the influence of locally produced hormones and factors, maternal NK cells of the uterus are inherently altered. During pregnancy, decidualization of the uterus occurs under the influence of progesterone and is associated with leukocyte infiltration; 70% of the infiltrating CD45+ cells are NK cells, with some macrophages and very few T cells [108]. Uterine NK cells have phenotypic and functional properties which are different than peripheral populations of NK cells. The role of uterine NKs in pregnancy is still being debated, but they appear functionally to be less cytotoxic than peripheral NKs. The preponderance of NK cells in the uterus and decidua during pregnancy along with a number of other mechanisms points to the importance of the innate immune system in modulating feto-maternal tolerance. This makes sense teleologically; a successful pregnancy is key to the survival of the species and a top priority evolutionarily, so should not be delegated to the adaptive immune system, which was evolved much later than the innate immune system and found only in jawed vertebrates. It will be interesting to see if stem cells from embryonic and fetal sources have distinctive interactions with the innate immune system that are different than adult BMMSCs.

Mechanisms of Stem Cell Immune Tolerance

BMMSCs, ESCs, and FSCs all have prominent immunosuppressive effects, but detailed mechanisms and effects towards specific subpopulations of lymphocytes may differ. It is yet unclear why these stem cell populations would have such effects, and the reasons may be quite divergent. FSCs and ESCs may harbor such effects because of the legacy of maternal-fetal tolerance, but this argument does not apply to BMMSCs. It may be that the "HSC-feeder" function of BMMSCs requires the maintenance of a locally immuno-privileged niche for HSCs to mature in, avoiding premature exposure to antigenic "noise" before functional competency of differentiated cells are acquired. This establishment of a locally immuno-privileged environment actually shares some analogy to the current working hypothesis for the maternal-fetal model of tolerance; that a local alteration in the uterus is generally enough, which allows systemic immune functions of the pregnant woman to remain intact. This may also explain why some of the mechanisms at work in the immunosuppressive effects of BMMSCs and maternal-fetal tolerance are so similar. It does appear that the local immunosuppressive environment is established to a great extent by the embryonic/fetal cells or BMMSCs, in other words, that the immunosuppressive properties of these stem cells are intrinsic. This would explain why extra-uterine pregnancies ouside of the reproductive tract are tolerated. Furthermore, recent experimental studies indicate that BMMSCs transplanted out of their usual bone marrow "niche", into various organs of allo-109, 110 or even xeno-geneic111 recipients can survive without being rejected.

One speculates perhaps the immune tolerance of BMMSCs represents the manifestation of what we may call "immunological homeostasis". The major signalling molecules for BMMSC tolerance are various anti-inflammatory cytokines such as IL-10. When there is a tissue injury, such as in acute myocardial infarction, inflammatory immune cells are mobilized to the injury site and pro-inflammatory cytokines (such as IL-1b, TNF-a, INF-r etc) expressed, preventing infection and removing necrotic debries. However, it has been shown that excessive inflammatory response can be detrimental to heart, aggravating the ventricular remodelling process causing cardiac dilatation and dysfunction112. Mobilization of the anti-inflammatory cells such as BMMSCs activates T-reg cells and secrete anti-inflammatory cytokines (such as IL-10, bFGF, TGF-a etc)113, thus restore a measure of "immunological homeostasis", avoiding excessive inflammatory damage. Since such BMMSCs are multi-potent stem cells, they may differentiate into various cardiac cells *in situ* to provide a measure of repair by cellular regeneration114. These may be the evolutionary roles of such immune tolerant adult stem cells, namely to contain excessive inflammatory response to acute injury, and to participate in the repair process. Of course this hypothesis is highly speculative at present. However, the recent clinical reports indicating patients who suffered from coronary artery disease would have better prognosis if their anti-inflammatory/pro-inflammatory cytokine ratio is higher in their blood115, appear to be consistent with such a hypothesis. Clearly the immunobiology of various sources of stem cells merits further investigation.

Differentiation of the Stem Cells and Immune Tolerance

One issue which had not been addressed in the discussions above is the question why these stem cells, even after they underwent subsequent differentiation and fully expressed their HLA-mismatch in allo- or xeno-geneic evironment, could continue to show immune tolerance and avoid rejection. By applying Paula Matzinger's "Danger Model" theory116, one of us (RCJC) proposed a "Stealth Immune Tolerance" hypothesis to explain this phenomenon117. In essence, this is based on the understanding that the T cell activation rquires two signals from the APCs, namely a recognition signal (HLA) and an activation signal. The latter is provided by evidence that the host tissue has been damaged or stressed. The proteins signaling presence of such "danger" are processed through TLR rceptors of the innate immune system118. In an organ transplant, the surgical damage incurred during the transplant procedure will provide such danger signal. In contrast, by the time an immune tolerant stem cell has differentiated in vivo which may take many days and weeks, the danger signal generated by the surgical trauma of cell implant procedure have subsided, thus avoiding rejection. Although this hypothesis requires further confirmation, it may explain phenomena such as the maternal microchimera119, in which mis-matched cells of fetal origin can be found to survive for decades in the maternal blood and tissue, and even undergo differentiation *in situ*.

Preliminary Translational and Clinical Studies to Exploit Stem Cell Immune Tolerance for Regenerative Therapy

One of the fantastic therapeutic potential of immune tolerant stem cells is their use as universal donor cells for regenerative therapy of damaged tissues and organs. Autologous cells are immune tolerant, but in senile and/or debilitated patients, their autologous stem cells such as BMMSCs could be few and dysfunctional120. The autologous cells need to be isolated and processed patient by patient, which is both time consuming and expensive. Availability of universal donor cells obtained from young healthy donors will be therapeutically more effective and logistically superior, as they will be obtainable "off the shelf"! In view of such obvious advantages, translational animal studies and early clinical trials are being undertaken. For example, using allogeneic BMMSCs for the therapy of myocardial infarction had been undertaken in porcine and in rodent models109, 110, demonstrating survival and differentiation of implanted cells without any immunosuppression. Most importantly, improvement in cardiac functions were observed. Xenotransplantation of mouse BMMSCs into infarcted rat myocardium had been reported to show similar results111. Recently Multicenter Phase I clinical trial (Osiris) approved by the FDA of the United States had been carried out, in which un-matched human BMMSCs were given intravenously, without immunosuppression, to patients with acute myocardial infaction. Further trials for other organ diseases can also be expected.

Conclusion

Further understanding of the mechanisms of stem cell immune tolerance may yield insights into the enduring immunological mystery of the fetal allograft, as well as help us to find a way to achieve transplant tolerance, which remains the holy grail of the emerging regenerative therapy for wide range of diseases.

References

[1] Evans MJ, Kaufman MH. Establishment in culture of pluripotential cells from mouse embryos. *Nature.* Jul 9 1981;292(5819):154-156.

[2] Martin GR. Isolation of a pluripotent cell line from early mouse embryos cultured in medium conditioned by teratocarcinoma stem cells. *Proc Natl Acad Sci* U S A. Dec 1981;78(12):7634-7638.

[3] Thomson JA, Itskovitz-Eldor J, Shapiro SS, et al. Embryonic stem cell lines derived from human blastocysts. *Science.* Nov 6 1998;282(5391):1145-1147.

[4] Reubinoff BE, Pera MF, Fong CY, Trounson A, Bongso A. Embryonic stem cell lines from human blastocysts: somatic differentiation in vitro. *Nat Biotechnol.* Apr 2000;18(4):399-404.

[5] Cloutier F, Siegenthaler MM, Nistor G, Keirstead HS. Transplantation of human embryonic stem cell-derived oligodendrocyte progenitors into rat spinal cord injuries does not cause harm. *Regen Med.* Jul 2006;1(4):469-479.

[6] Faulkner J, Keirstead HS. Human embryonic stem cell-derived oligodendrocyte progenitors for the treatment of spinal cord injury. *Transpl Immunol.* Dec 2005;15(2):131-142.

[7] Orkin SH. Diversification of haematopoietic stem cells to specific lineages. *Nat Rev Genet.* Oct 2000;1(1):57-64.

[8] Korbling M, Estrov Z. Adult stem cells for tissue repair - a new therapeutic concept? *N Engl J Med.* Aug 7 2003;349(6):570-582.

[9] Petersen BE, Bowen WC, Patrene KD, et al. Bone marrow as a potential source of hepatic oval cells. *Science.* May 14 1999;284(5417):1168-1170.

[10] Eglitis MA, Mezey E. Hematopoietic cells differentiate into both microglia and macroglia in the brains of adult mice. *Proc Natl Acad Sci* U S A. Apr 15 1997;94(8):4080-4085.

[11] Brazelton TR, Rossi FM, Keshet GI, Blau HM. From marrow to brain: expression of neuronal phenotypes in adult mice. *Science.* Dec 1 2000;290(5497):1775-1779.

[12] Theise ND, Badve S, Saxena R, et al. Derivation of hepatocytes from bone marrow cells in mice after radiation-induced myeloablation. *Hepatology.* Jan 2000;31(1):235-240.

[13] Kopen GC, Prockop DJ, Phinney DG. Marrow stromal cells migrate throughout forebrain and cerebellum, and they differentiate into astrocytes after injection into neonatal mouse brains. *Proc Natl Acad Sci* U S A. Sep 14 1999;96(19):10711-10716.

[14] Liechty KW, MacKenzie TC, Shaaban AF, et al. Human mesenchymal stem cells engraft and demonstrate site-specific differentiation after in utero transplantation in sheep. *Nat Med.* Nov 2000;6(11):1282-1286.

[15] Dezawa M, Ishikawa H, Itokazu Y, et al. Bone marrow stromal cells generate muscle cells and repair muscle degeneration. *Science.* Jul 8 2005;309(5732):314-317.

[16] Sanchez-Ramos J, Song S, Cardozo-Pelaez F, et al. Adult bone marrow stromal cells differentiate into neural cells in vitro. *Exp Neurol.* Aug 2000;164(2):247-256.

[17] Woodbury D, Schwarz EJ, Prockop DJ, Black IB. Adult rat and human bone marrow stromal cells differentiate into neurons. *J Neurosci Res.* Aug 15 2000;61(4):364-370.

[18] Oswald J, Boxberger S, Jorgensen B, et al. Mesenchymal stem cells can be differentiated into endothelial cells in vitro. *Stem Cells.* 2004;22(3):377-384.

[19] Friedenstein AJ, Ivanov-Smolenski AA, Chajlakjan RK, et al. Origin of bone marrow stromal mechanocytes in radiochimeras and heterotopic transplants. *Exp Hematol.* May 1978;6(5):440-444.

[20] Friedenstein A. Stromal mechanisms of bone marrow: cloning in vitro and retransplantation in vivo. *Berlin: Springer-Verlag*; 1980.

[21] Prockop DJ. Marrow stromal cells as stem cells for nonhematopoietic tissues. *Science.* Apr 4 1997;276(5309):71-74.

[22] Pittenger MF, Mackay AM, Beck SC, et al. Multilineage potential of adult human mesenchymal stem cells. *Science.* Apr 2 1999;284(5411):143-147.

[23] Moriscot C, de Fraipont F, Richard MJ, et al. Human bone marrow mesenchymal stem cells can express insulin and key transcription factors of the endocrine pancreas developmental pathway upon genetic and/or microenvironmental manipulation in vitro. *Stem Cells.* Apr 2005;23(4):594-603.

[24] Sakaguchi Y, Sekiya I, Yagishita K, Ichinose S, Shinomiya K, Muneta T. Suspended cells from trabecular bone by collagenase digestion become virtually identical to mesenchymal stem cells obtained from marrow aspirates. *Blood.* Nov 1 2004;104(9):2728-2735.

[25] Noth U, Osyczka AM, Tuli R, Hickok NJ, Danielson KG, Tuan RS. Multilineage mesenchymal differentiation potential of human trabecular bone-derived cells. *J Orthop Res.* Sep 2002;20(5):1060-1069.

[26] Zuk PA, Zhu M, Mizuno H, et al. Multilineage cells from human adipose tissue: implications for cell-based therapies. *Tissue Eng.* Apr 2001;7(2):211-228.

[27] Rao MS, Mattson MP. Stem cells and aging: expanding the possibilities. *Mech Ageing Dev.* May 31 2001;122(7):713-734.

[28] De Coppi P, Bartsch G, Jr., Siddiqui MM, et al. Isolation of amniotic stem cell lines with potential for therapy. *Nat Biotechnol.* Jan 2007;25(1):100-106.

[29] Miki T, Lehmann T, Cai H, Stolz DB, Strom SC. Stem cell characteristics of amniotic epithelial cells. *Stem Cells.* Nov-Dec 2005;23(10):1549-1559.

[30] Tsai MS, Lee JL, Chang YJ, Hwang SM. Isolation of human multipotent mesenchymal stem cells from second-trimester amniotic fluid using a novel two-stage culture protocol. *Hum Reprod.* Jun 2004;19(6):1450-1456.

[31] Campagnoli C, Roberts IA, Kumar S, Bennett PR, Bellantuono I, Fisk NM. Identification of mesenchymal stem/progenitor cells in human first-trimester fetal blood, liver, and bone marrow. *Blood.* Oct 15 2001;98(8):2396-2402.

[32] Almeida-Porada G, El Shabrawy D, Porada C, Zanjani ED. Differentiative potential of human metanephric mesenchymal cells. *Exp Hematol.* Dec 2002;30(12):1454-1462.

[33] Hu Y, Liao L, Wang Q, et al. Isolation and identification of mesenchymal stem cells from human fetal pancreas. *J Lab Clin Med.* May 2003;141(5):342-349.

[34] in 't Anker PS, Noort WA, Scherjon SA, et al. Mesenchymal stem cells in human second-trimester bone marrow, liver, lung, and spleen exhibit a similar immunophenotype but a heterogeneous multilineage differentiation potential. *Haematologica.* Aug 2003;88(8):845-852.

[35] Goodwin HS, Bicknese AR, Chien SN, Bogucki BD, Quinn CO, Wall DA. Multilineage differentiation activity by cells isolated from umbilical cord blood: expression of bone, fat, and neural markers. *Biol Blood Marrow Transplant.* 2001;7(11):581-588.

[36] Kogler G, Sensken S, Airey JA, et al. A new human somatic stem cell from placental cord blood with intrinsic pluripotent differentiation potential. *J Exp Med.* Jul 19 2004;200(2):123-135.

[37] Lee OK, Kuo TK, Chen WM, Lee KD, Hsieh SL, Chen TH. Isolation of multipotent mesenchymal stem cells from umbilical cord blood. *Blood.* Mar 1 2004;103(5):1669-1675.

[38] McGuckin CP, Forraz N, Baradez MO, et al. Production of stem cells with embryonic characteristics from human umbilical cord blood. *Cell Prolif.* Aug 2005;38(4):245-255.

[39] Romanov YA, Svintsitskaya VA, Smirnov VN. Searching for alternative sources of postnatal human mesenchymal stem cells: candidate MSC-like cells from umbilical cord. *Stem Cells.* 2003;21(1):105-110.

[40] Wang HS, Hung SC, Peng ST, et al. Mesenchymal stem cells in the Wharton's jelly of the human umbilical cord. *Stem Cells.* 2004;22(7):1330-1337.

[41] Fukuchi Y, Nakajima H, Sugiyama D, Hirose I, Kitamura T, Tsuji K. Human placenta-derived cells have mesenchymal stem/progenitor cell potential. *Stem Cells.* 2004;22(5):649-658.

[42] In 't Anker PS, Scherjon SA, Kleijburg-van der Keur C, et al. Isolation of mesenchymal stem cells of fetal or maternal origin from human placenta. *Stem Cells.* 2004;22(7):1338-1345.

[43] Wulf GG, Viereck V, Hemmerlein B, et al. Mesengenic progenitor cells derived from human placenta. *Tissue Eng.* Jul-Aug 2004;10(7-8):1136-1147.

[44] Yen BL, Huang HI, Chien CC, et al. Isolation of multipotent cells from human term placenta. *Stem Cells.* 2005;23(1):3-9.

[45] Georgiades P, Ferguson-Smith AC, Burton GJ. Comparative developmental anatomy of the murine and human definitive placentae. *Placenta.* Jan 2002;23(1):3-19.

[46] Zhao Y, Wang H, Mazzone T. Identification of stem cells from human umbilical cord blood with embryonic and hematopoietic characteristics. *Exp Cell Res.* Aug 1 2006;312(13):2454-2464.

[47] Vogelsang GB, Lee L, Bensen-Kennedy DM. Pathogenesis and treatment of graft-versus-host disease after bone marrow transplant. *Annu Rev Med.* 2003;54:29-52.

[48] Lee SJ. New approaches for preventing and treating chronic graft-versus-host disease. *Blood.* Jun 1 2005;105(11):4200-4206.

[49] Kurtzberg J, Laughlin M, Graham ML, et al. Placental blood as a source of hematopoietic stem cells for transplantation into unrelated recipients. *N Engl J Med.* Jul 18 1996;335(3):157-166.

[50] Wagner JE, Rosenthal J, Sweetman R, et al. Successful transplantation of HLA-matched and HLA-mismatched umbilical cord blood from unrelated donors: analysis of engraftment and acute graft-versus-host disease. *Blood.* Aug 1 1996;88(3):795-802.

[51] Mayani H, Lansdorp PM. Biology of human umbilical cord blood-derived hematopoietic stem/progenitor cells. *Stem Cells.* 1998;16(3):153-165.

[52] Bone marrow transplants: despite recruitment successes national programs may be underutilized. In: Office GA, ed; 2002.

[53] McGlave P, Bartsch G, Anasetti C, et al. Unrelated donor marrow transplantation therapy for chronic myelogenous leukemia: initial experience of the National Marrow Donor Program. *Blood.* Jan 15 1993;81(2):543-550.

[54] Hansen JA, Gooley TA, Martin PJ, et al. Bone marrow transplants from unrelated donors for patients with chronic myeloid leukemia. *N Engl J Med.* Apr 2 1998;338(14):962-968.

[55] Szydlo R, Goldman JM, Klein JP, et al. Results of allogeneic bone marrow transplants for leukemia using donors other than HLA-identical siblings. *J Clin Oncol.* May 1997;15(5):1767-1777.

[56] Rocha V, Cornish J, Sievers EL, et al. Comparison of outcomes of unrelated bone marrow and umbilical cord blood transplants in children with acute leukemia. *Blood.* May 15 2001;97(10):2962-2971.

[57] Laughlin MJ, Eapen M, Rubinstein P, et al. Outcomes after transplantation of cord blood or bone marrow from unrelated donors in adults with leukemia. *N Engl J Med.* Nov 25 2004;351(22):2265-2275.

[58] Barker JN, Davies SM, DeFor T, Ramsay NK, Weisdorf DJ, Wagner JE. Survival after transplantation of unrelated donor umbilical cord blood is comparable to that of human leukocyte antigen-matched unrelated donor bone marrow: results of a matched-pair analysis. *Blood.* May 15 2001;97(10):2957-2961.

[59] Rocha V, Labopin M, Sanz G, et al. Transplants of umbilical-cord blood or bone marrow from unrelated donors in adults with acute leukemia. *N Engl J Med.* Nov 25 2004;351(22):2276-2285.

[60] Takahashi S, Ooi J, Tomonari A, et al. Comparative single-institute analysis of cord blood transplantation from unrelated donors with bone marrow or peripheral blood stem-cell transplants from related donors in adult patients with hematologic

malignancies after myeloablative conditioning regimen. *Blood.* Feb 1 2007;109(3):1322-1330.

[61] Barker JN, Wagner JE. Umbilical cord blood transplantation: current practice and future innovations. *Crit Rev Oncol Hematol.* Oct 2003;48(1):35-43.

[62] Sanz MA. Cord-blood transplantation in patients with leukemia--a real alternative for adults. *N Engl J Med.* Nov 25 2004;351(22):2328-2330.

[63] Bang OY, Lee JS, Lee PH, Lee G. Autologous mesenchymal stem cell transplantation in stroke patients. *Ann Neurol.* Jun 2005;57(6):874-882.

[64] Chen SL, Fang WW, Qian J, et al. Improvement of cardiac function after transplantation of autologous bone marrow mesenchymal stem cells in patients with acute myocardial infarction. *Chin Med J (Engl).* Oct 2004;117(10):1443-1448.

[65] Koc ON, Day J, Nieder M, Gerson SL, Lazarus HM, Krivit W. Allogeneic mesenchymal stem cell infusion for treatment of metachromatic leukodystrophy (MLD) and Hurler syndrome (MPS-IH). *Bone Marrow Transplant.* Aug 2002;30(4):215-222.

[66] Koc ON, Gerson SL, Cooper BW, et al. Rapid hematopoietic recovery after coinfusion of autologous-blood stem cells and culture-expanded marrow mesenchymal stem cells in advanced breast cancer patients receiving high-dose chemotherapy. *J Clin Oncol.* Jan 2000;18(2):307-316.

[67] Mazzini L, Fagioli F, Boccaletti R, et al. Stem cell therapy in amyotrophic lateral sclerosis: a methodological approach in humans. *Amyotroph Lateral Scler Other Motor Neuron Disord.* Sep 2003;4(3):158-161.

[68] Merion RM. Preface: 2003 SRTR Report on the State of Transplantation. *Am J Transplant.* Nov 2004;4(Suppl 9):5-6.

[69] Bartholomew A, Sturgeon C, Siatskas M, et al. Mesenchymal stem cells suppress lymphocyte proliferation in vitro and prolong skin graft survival in vivo. *Exp Hematol.* Jan 2002;30(1):42-48.

[70] Di Nicola M, Carlo-Stella C, Magni M, et al. Human bone marrow stromal cells suppress T-lymphocyte proliferation induced by cellular or nonspecific mitogenic stimuli. *Blood.* May 15 2002;99(10):3838-3843.

[71] Djouad F, Plence P, Bony C, et al. Immunosuppressive effect of mesenchymal stem cells favors tumor growth in allogeneic animals. *Blood.* Nov 15 2003;102(10):3837-3844.

[72] Krampera M, Glennie S, Dyson J, et al. Bone marrow mesenchymal stem cells inhibit the response of naive and memory antigen-specific T cells to their cognate peptide. *Blood.* May 1 2003;101(9):3722-3729.

[73] Tse WT, Pendleton JD, Beyer WM, Egalka MC, Guinan EC. Suppression of allogeneic T-cell proliferation by human marrow stromal cells: implications in transplantation. *Transplantation.* Feb 15 2003;75(3):389-397.

[74] Glennie S, Soeiro I, Dyson PJ, Lam EW, Dazzi F. Bone marrow mesenchymal stem cells induce division arrest anergy of activated T cells. *Blood.* Apr 1 2005;105(7):2821-2827.

[75] Beyth S, Borovsky Z, Mevorach D, et al. Human mesenchymal stem cells alter antigen-presenting cell maturation and induce T-cell unresponsiveness. *Blood.* Mar 1 2005;105(5):2214-2219.

[76] Le Blanc K, Rasmusson I, Gotherstrom C, et al. Mesenchymal stem cells inhibit the expression of CD25 (interleukin-2 receptor) and CD38 on phytohaemagglutinin-activated lymphocytes. *Scand J Immunol.* Sep 2004;60(3):307-315.

[77] Rasmusson I. Immune modulation by mesenchymal stem cells. *Exp Cell Res.* Jul 15 2006;312(12):2169-2179.

[78] Amado LC, Saliaris AP, Schuleri KH, et al. Cardiac repair with intramyocardial injection of allogeneic mesenchymal stem cells after myocardial infarction. *Proc Natl Acad Sci* U S A. Aug 9 2005;102(32):11474-11479.

[79] Dai W, Hale SL, Martin BJ, et al. Allogeneic mesenchymal stem cell transplantation in postinfarcted rat myocardium: short- and long-term effects. *Circulation.* Jul 12 2005;112(2):214-223.

[80] MacDonald DJ, Luo J, Saito T, et al. Persistence of marrow stromal cells implanted into acutely infarcted myocardium: observations in a xenotransplant model. *J Thorac Cardiovasc Surg.* Oct 2005;130(4):1114-1121.

[81] Saito T, Kuang JQ, Bittira B, Al-Khaldi A, Chiu RC. Xenotransplant cardiac chimera: immune tolerance of adult stem cells. *Ann Thorac Surg.* Jul 2002;74(1):19-24; discussion 24.

[82] Le Blanc K, Rasmusson I, Sundberg B, et al. Treatment of severe acute graft-versus-host disease with third party haploidentical mesenchymal stem cells. *Lancet.* May 1 2004;363(9419):1439-1441.

[83] Ringden O, Uzunel M, Rasmusson I, et al. Mesenchymal stem cells for treatment of therapy-resistant graft-versus-host disease. *Transplantation.* May 27 2006;81(10):1390-1397.

[84] Ishitani A, Sageshima N, Lee N, et al. Protein expression and peptide binding suggest unique and interacting functional roles for HLA-E, F, and G in maternal-placental immune recognition. *J Immunol.* Aug 1 2003;171(3):1376-1384.

[85] Munn DH, Zhou M, Attwood JT, et al. Prevention of allogeneic fetal rejection by tryptophan catabolism. *Science.* Aug 21 1998;281(5380):1191-1193.

[86] Hsi BL, Hunt JS, Atkinson JP. Differential expression of complement regulatory proteins on subpopulations of human trophoblast cells. *J Reprod Immunol.* Apr 1991;19(3):209-223.

[87] Aluvihare VR, Kallikourdis M, Betz AG. Regulatory T cells mediate maternal tolerance to the fetus. *Nat Immunol.* Mar 2004;5(3):266-271.

[88] Guleria I, Khosroshahi A, Ansari MJ, et al. A critical role for the programmed death ligand 1 in fetomaternal tolerance. *J Exp Med.* Jul 18 2005;202(2):231-237.

[89] Meisel R, Zibert A, Laryea M, Gobel U, Daubener W, Dilloo D. Human bone marrow stromal cells inhibit allogeneic T-cell responses by indoleamine 2,3-dioxygenase-mediated tryptophan degradation. *Blood.* Jun 15 2004;103(12):4619-4621.

[90] Maccario R, Podesta M, Moretta A, et al. Interaction of human mesenchymal stem cells with cells involved in alloantigen-specific immune response favors the differentiation of CD4+ T-cell subsets expressing a regulatory/suppressive phenotype. *Haematologica.* Apr 2005;90(4):516-525.

[91] Prevosto C, Zancolli M, Canevali P, Zocchi MR, Poggi A. Generation of CD4+ or CD8+ regulatory T cells upon mesenchymal stem cell-lymphocyte interaction. *Haematologica.* Jul 2007;92(7):881-888.

[92] Drukker M, Katchman H, Katz G, et al. Human embryonic stem cells and their differentiated derivatives are less susceptible to immune rejection than adult cells. *Stem Cells.* Feb 2006;24(2):221-229.

[93] Bonde S, Zavazava N. Immunogenicity and engraftment of mouse embryonic stem cells in allogeneic recipients. *Stem Cells.* Oct 2006;24(10):2192-2201.

[94] Li L, Baroja ML, Majumdar A, et al. Human embryonic stem cells possess immune-privileged properties. *Stem Cells.* 2004;22(4):448-456.

[95] Grinnemo KH, Kumagai-Braesch M, Mansson-Broberg A, et al. Human embryonic stem cells are immunogenic in allogeneic and xenogeneic settings. *Reprod Biomed Online.* Nov 2006;13(5):712-724.

[96] Li CD, Zhang WY, Li HL, et al. Mesenchymal stem cells derived from human placenta suppress allogeneic umbilical cord blood lymphocyte proliferation. *Cell Res.* Jul 2005;15(7):539-547.

[97] Chang CJ, Yen ML, Chen YC, et al. Placenta-derived multipotent cells exhibit immunosuppressive properties that are enhanced in the presence of interferon-gamma. *Stem Cells.* Nov 2006;24(11):2466-2477.

[98] Drukker M, Katz G, Urbach A, et al. Characterization of the expression of MHC proteins in human embryonic stem cells. *Proc Natl Acad Sci* U S A. Jul 23 2002;99(15):9864-9869.

[99] Aggarwal S, Pittenger MF. Human mesenchymal stem cells modulate allogeneic immune cell responses. *Blood.* Feb 15 2005;105(4):1815-1822.

[100] Gotherstrom C, Ringden O, Tammik C, Zetterberg E, Westgren M, Le Blanc K. Immunologic properties of human fetal mesenchymal stem cells. *Am J Obstet Gynecol.* Jan 2004;190(1):239-245.

[101] Moffett A, Loke C. Immunology of placentation in eutherian mammals. *Nat Rev Immunol.* Aug 2006;6(8):584-594.

[102] Ljunggren HG, Karre K. In search of the 'missing self': MHC molecules and NK cell recognition. *Immunol* Today. Jul 1990;11(7):237-244.

[103] Manilay JO, Sykes M. Natural killer cells and their role in graft rejection. *Curr Opin Immunol.* Oct 1998;10(5):532-538.

[104] Rasmusson I, Ringden O, Sundberg B, Le Blanc K. Mesenchymal stem cells inhibit the formation of cytotoxic T lymphocytes, but not activated cytotoxic T lymphocytes or natural killer cells. *Transplantation.* Oct 27 2003;76(8):1208-1213.

[105] Sotiropoulou PA, Perez SA, Gritzapis AD, Baxevanis CN, Papamichail M. Interactions between human mesenchymal stem cells and natural killer cells. *Stem Cells.* Jan 2006;24(1):74-85.

[106] Spaggiari GM, Capobianco A, Becchetti S, Mingari MC, Moretta L. Mesenchymal stem cell-natural killer cell interactions: evidence that activated NK cells are capable of killing MSCs, whereas MSCs can inhibit IL-2-induced NK-cell proliferation. *Blood.* Feb 15 2006;107(4):1484-1490.

[107] Krampera M, Cosmi L, Angeli R, et al. Role for interferon-gamma in the immunomodulatory activity of human bone marrow mesenchymal stem cells. *Stem Cells.* Feb 2006;24(2):386-398.

[108] Moffett-King A. Natural killer cells and pregnancy. *Nat Rev Immunol.* Sep 2002;2(9):656-663.

[109] Amado LC, Saliaris AP, Schuleri KH, John M St, Xie J-S, Cattaneo S, Durand DJ, Fitton T, Kuang JQ, Stewart G, Lehrke S, Baumgartner WW, Martin BJ, Heldman AW, Hare JM: Cardiac repair with intramyocardial injection of allogeneic mesenchymal stem cells after myocardial infarction. *PNAS* 2005; 102:11474-11479.

[110] Dai W, Hale SL, Martin BJ, Kuang J-Q, Dow JS, Wold LE, Kloner RA: Allogeneic mesenchymal stem cell transplantation in postinfarcted rat myocardium: Short- and Long-term effects. *Circulation* 2005; 112:214-223.

[111] MacDonald DJ, Luo J, Saito T, Shum-Tiom D, Duong M, Bernier PL, Chiu RCJ: Persistence of marrow stromal cells implanted into acutely infarcted myocardium: observations in a xenotransplant model. *J Thorac Cardiovasc Surg* 2005; 130(4): 1114-21.

[112] Nian M, Lee P, Khaper N, Liu P: Inflammatory cytokines and postmyocardial infarction remodeling. *Circ. Res.* 2004; 94:1543-1553.

[113] Togel F, Hu Z, Weiss K, Isaac, J, Lange C, Westenfelder C: Administered mesenchymal stem cells protect against ischemic acute renal failure through differentiation-independent mechanisms. *Am J Physiol Renal Physio* 2005; 289: F31-F42.

[114] Kajstura J, Rota M, Whang B et al. Bone marrow cells differentiate in cardiac cell lineages after infarction independently of cell fusion. *Circ Res* 2005; 96:127-137.

[115] Anguera I, Miranda-Guardiola F, Bosch X et al.: Elevation of serum levels of the anti-inflammatory cytokine interleukin-10 and decreased risk of coronary events in patients with unstable angina. *Am Heart J* 2002; 144:811-817.

[116] Matzinger P. The danger model: a renewed sense of self. *Science* 2002; 296(5566):301-5.

[117] Chiu RC: "Stealth immune tolerance" in stem cell transplantation: potential for "universal donors" in myocardial regenerative therapy. *J Heart Lung Transplant* 2005; 24(5): 511-516.

[118] Prince JM, Levy RM, Yang R et al. Toll-like receptor-4 signaling mediates hepatic injury and systemic inflammation in hemorrhagic shock. *J Am Coll Surg* 2006;202: 407-17.

[119] Bianchi DW, Zickwolf GK, Weil GJ et al. Male fetal progenitor cells persist in maternal blood for as long as 27 years postpartum. *Proc Natl Acad Sci* USA 1996;93:705-708.

[120] Sethe S, Scutt A, Stolzing A. Aging of mesenchymal stem cells. *Ageing Research Review* 2006;5:91-116.

In: Immune Tolerance Research Developments
Editor: Emile B. Pontell, pp. 167-185

ISBN: 978-1-60456-209-5

Chapter 8

A Defect of Thymus-Dependent Self-tolerance to Insulin-Secreting β Cells in the Pathogenesis of Type 1 Diabetes

Isabelle Hansenne[1,*], Céline Louis and Vincent Geenen[1]
[1] University of Liege, Center of Immunology, Institute of Pathology CHU-B23, 4000 Liege-Sart Tilman, Belgium

Abstract

More and more evidence accumulates for a defect in thymus-dependent tolerance to islet β cells as a major factor in initiation and development of the diabetogenic autoimmune response. Type 1 diabetes (T1D) results from specific and progressive β-cell destruction by auto-reactive T cells directed against three auto-antigens: Insulin (as the primary and β-cell specific auto-antigen), the 65-kDa isoform of glutamic acid decarboxylase (GAD65), and the insulinoma-associated tyrosine phosphatase 2 (IA-2). The thymus plays a prominent role in T-cell education to recognize and tolerate neuroendocrine functions through transcription by thymic epithelial cells (TEC) of genes belonging to neuroendocrine families. All members of the Insulin gene family are transcribed in the thymus according a precise hierarchy and cell topography, whereby *IGF2* (cortical [c] and medullary [m] TEC) exceeds *IGF1* (macrophages), and is much higher than *INS* (subsets of mTEC). The autoimmune regulator gene (*AIRE*) encodes a transcription factor that controls the level of intrathymic expression of genes encoding T1D-related self-antigens (including *IGF2*, *INS*, and *GAD67*), as well as many – but not all - tissue-restricted antigens. The genetic locus *IDDM2* (VNTR) determines individual susceptibility to T1D through modulation of intrathymic *INS* transcription. A defect in thymus-dependent self-tolerance results both in a progressive enrichment of the T-cell repertoire with "forbidden" islet self-reactive T cells, as well as to a decrease in the thymic generation of T1D self-antigen specific regulatory T cells (T_{Reg}). Undoubtedly, further knowledge of the thymic mechanisms responsible for central tolerance of islet Insulin-

* E-mail address: Isabelle.Hansenne@ulg.ac.be; University of Liege, Center of Immunology, Institute of Pathology CHU B-23, B-4000 Liege-Sart Tilman, Belgium. (Corresponding author)

secreting β cells will lead to the development of novel therapies aiming to restore T-cell tolerance to T1D auto-antigens.

Introduction

Type 1 diabetes (T1D), previously known as juvenile diabetes or insulin-dependent diabetes mellitus (IDDM), is an organ-specific autoimmune disease characterized by a massive and selective destruction of pancreatic β cells which is mediated by both CD4+ and CD8+ T cells. T1D-related auto-antibodies are not pathogenic but exhibit a predictive value because they precede the time of clinical diagnosis which occurs when already up to 80% of β cells have been destroyed [1]. This disease can be divided into two phases. First, an "insulitis" develops and is characterized by the invasion of several leukocyte populations into the Langerhans' islets. This leukocyte infiltration initiates the destruction phase. The second phase is the overt clinical diabetes which appears when 60-80% of the β cells have been destroyed and when the residual Insulin production is not sufficient to preserve glucose homeostasis. Several genetic factors contribute to the susceptibility of T1D. Forty-two percent of T1D genetic risk resides within the major histocompatibility complex (MHC) locus (Reviewed in [2]). In human, this susceptibility is linked to the expression of MHC class II molecules, HLA-DR and HLA-DQ, for which a disequilibrium linkage exists between DR4 and DQ8 (DQB1*0302) alleles and between DR3 and DQ2 (DQB1*0201) alleles. These alleles are present in more than 90% of T1D patients, and the higher risk is encoded by the heterozygous genotype HLA DR4-DQ8/DR3-DQ2. Less than 1% of T1D patients possess the DR15-DQ6 allele that is then considered to be protective against the disease. Consequently, HLA typing has become an important research tool to identify subjects at genetic risk for T1D development. In recent years, whole genome screenings have identified at least 15 other loci associated with T1D, including several loci implied in control of the immune response such as *CTLA-4*, *PTPN22*, *ICAM1*, and *ILR2A* [3, 4].

Although many susceptibility loci are known in humans and mice, genetic factors alone are not sufficient to develop the disease. Some indirect observations (such as epidemiologic data and the incomplete concordance of T1D development in homozygotic twins) argue for the implication of environmental factors such as food components (*e.g.* bovine milk, presence of insulin in milk, deficiency of vitamin D), toxins, drugs, and viral infections (*e.g.* enteroviruses).

Two animal models [non-obese diabetic (NOD) mice and BioBreeding (BB) rats] have been very useful to dissect the very complex pathogenic mechanisms of human T1D. NOD mice were discovered in Japan in 1970, with a 70-80% of diabetes incidence in females and 20-30% in males. The emergence of the disease appeared around 12-14 weeks old in females and weakly later in males [5]. Both sexes of BB rats develop an insulitis around 4-weeks old in 80% of them, and the diabetes-prone BB rat strain is also characterized by a lymphopenia that affects the regulatory T cell (T_{Reg}) RT6+ subset. The drug cyclophosphamide (CY) accelerates diabetes incidence in NOD mice but is not diabetogenic in normal mice. Ten-weeks-old male NOD mice (40-60%) develop T1D within 14 days after CY injection [6]. Nowadays, the acceleration of T1D after CY administration in NOD mice is known to be associated with a decrease in CD4+ CD25+ FoxP3+ T_{Reg} [7]. Immunization studies were attempted to create an induced-T1D animal model mainly with the major and primary autoantigen, Insulin. Insulin immunization of normal mice does not lead to overt diabetes. Immunization with the B9-23 peptide of Insulin induces auto-antibodies in Balb/c mice, but not in C57BL/6 mice. In combination with Poly IC in Balb/c mice, the Insulin B9-23 peptide is able to promote auto-antibody induction and insulitis, but not complete autoimmune diabetes [8, 9]. Recently, genetic modifications were performed to evaluate the importance of self-antigen expression on T1D initiation and to analyze the developmental sequence of T1D. These studies included expression of transgenic auto-antigens under the rat Insulin promoter in mouse strains that are genetically resistant for the disease. TCR transgenic mice were also used to create mice with an increased number of auto-reactive T lymphocytes. The neo-antigen transgenic mice can be also crossed with mice expressing a T cell receptor (TCR) transgene specific of neo-antigen on circulating T-cells, and they develop autoimmune diabetes [10-16].

Major β-Cell Autoantigens of T1D (Table 1)

Many T-cell clones isolated from NOD mice and from T1D patients are specific for some auto-antigenic epitopes, which were originally identified from auto-antibodies. The major auto-antigens recognized by T1D auto-antibodies are the 65-kDa glutamic acid decarboxylase isoform (GAD65), the insulinoma-associated tyrosine phosphatase 2 (IA-2), and Insulin [17].

Table I. Autoantigens in type 1 diabetes and NOD mice

Autoantigens	Characteristics	Knockout NOD	Influence on T1D
GAD65	Catalyzes GABA production. Exists under two isoforms : 65kDa (GAD65) and 67kDa (GAD67)	*GAD65*$^{-/-}$ NOD →	Normal insulitis/diabetes
		GAD67$^{-/-}$ mouse →	Death
		GAD65 and GAD67: antisense transgene (insulin promoter) →	Suppression of diabetes
IA-2	Protein tyrosin phosphatase-like molecule. Two forms: IA-2 and IA-2β.	*IA-2*$^{-/-}$ NOD →	Normal insulitis/diabetes
		IA-2β$^{-/-}$ NOD →	Normal insulitis/diabetes
Insulin	Hypoglycemic hormone. Two genes present in mouse genome : *Insulin1* and *Insulin2*	*Ins1*$^{-/-}$ NOD →	Reduced progression of insulitis/diabetes.
		Ins2$^{-/-}$ NOD →	Normal auto-antibodies Increased progression of insulitis/diabetes.
		Ins1$^{-/-}$ and *Ins2*$^{-/-}$ NOD →	Amplified auto-antibodies No insulitis/diabtes No auto-antibody

GAD catalyzes the production of GABA from glutamic acid, and exists under two isoforms, 65kDa and 67kDa, which are encoded by two non-allelic genes in mammals [18, 19]. The function of GAD65 in islet β cells is still not known. GAD65 is post-translationally modified to be anchored to the membrane of synaptic vesicles. In contrast, GAD67 remains soluble [20]. Both human and rat islets predominantly express GAD65, whereas GAD67 is the major form in mouse islets. Human islets are significantly distinct from mouse and rat islets and from brain because they only express GAD65, which is consistent with the predominant role of this form as a target of auto-antibodies associated with β-cell destruction in humans [21]. A study using *Gad65*$^{-/-}$ NOD mice suggests that the 65-kDa isoform is not primary implicated in the initiation of disease since deletion of *Gad65* in NOD mice does not influence the emergence of diabetes [22]. It can be hypothesized that the normal expression of GAD67 in *Gad65*$^{-/-}$ mouse influences the development of the disease because mouse β islets preferentially express GAD67. *Gad67*$^{-/-}$ mice die within the first day of life due to the deficiency of *Gad67* expression in brain. A study based on anti-sense transgene expression of GAD65 and GAD67 under control of the Insulin promoter in NOD mice shows that the suppression of these antigens blocks the development of diabetes when the transgene is highly expressed clearly indicating that GAD expression is an essential element in the pathogenesis of NOD diabetes [23].

IA-2, also known as ICA512, is a transmembrane protein that belongs to the family of protein tyrosine phosphatase (PTP). Another molecule from the same family, which is 74% identical to IA-2, is also a T1D auto-antigen known as IA-2β (or phogrin) [24]. Auto-antibodies against both forms are detected in 60-80% of new diagnosed diabetic patients and in less than 2% of controls [25]. However, these auto-antibodies are not detected in NOD mice and BB rats [26]. Implication of this auto-antigen in the development of NOD diabetes is not confirmed since *Ia2*$^{-/-}$ NOD mice and *Ia2β*$^{-/-}$ NOD mice develop diabetes at the same rate and frequency than *Ia2*$^{+/+}$ NOD mice and *Ia2β*$^{+/+}$ NOD mice in a model of CY-induced diabetes [27, 28].

Insulin is the only T1D-related auto-antigen that is specific of β cells. In most species, a single gene encodes Insulin, except in mouse where two non-allelic genes [*Insulin 1(Ins1)* and *Insulin 2 (Ins2)*] have been identified. Auto-antibodies are present in 59% of diabetic patients, and are primarily directed to the B chain of human (pro)Insulin. The majority of T-cell clones isolated from islets of pre-diabetic NOD mice (CD4+ clones) react to Insulin. One major T-cell epitope is the amino acid sequence 9 to 23 of the B chain (Insulin B9-23) because more than 90% of Insulin-reactive clones isolated from NOD mice respond to this peptide [29, 30]. Deletion of *Ins1* in NOD mice prevents insulitis and progression of diabetes, but does not affect the auto-antibody production [31]. *Ins2*$^{-/-}$ NOD mice showed an acceleration of insulitis/diabetes with an amplified auto-antibody production [31, 32]. The low expression of *Ins1* in thymus may explain prevention of the disease in *Ins1*$^{-/-}$ NOD mice and acceleration of diabetes in *Ins2*$^{-/-}$ NOD mice. Thymic *Ins2* seems to be the major factor responsible for central tolerance to Insulin (Ins1 and Ins2), and *Ins2* defect in the thymus results in a defective thymus-dependent self-tolerance to Ins1 and Ins2, whereas persistence of *Ins1* expression in pancreatic islet β cells maintains presentation of the principal auto-antigen targeted by autoimmune diabetes. The deletion of *Ins1*, which is not or very less expressed in the thymus, does not affect immunological tolerance to islet β cells. Thus, in mouse, central self-tolerance to islet β cells is mainly mediated by *Ins2* that is predominantly expressed in the thymus [33].

Thymus Dysfunction in T1D (Figure 1)

To maintain homeostasis of the immune system, the thymus organ ensures the following functions: 1) development of competent and self-tolerant T cells; 2) deletion or developmental arrest of self-reactive T cells; and 3) generation of self-antigen specific T_{Reg}. The importance of a thymus defect in the development of autoimmune diabetes was first suggested in animal models of this disease. Spontaneous diabetes is prevented in BB rat after neonatal thymectomy [34], and is transferred by thymic transplantation from NOD mice in more than 50% of nude mice [35]. Athymic NOD mice and NOD.*scid* mice do not develop autoimmune diabetes [36]. Adoptive transfer studies demonstrate a role for CD4+ and CD8+ T cells in promoting T1D development [37-40]. Specific inactivation of CD4+ T cells in NOD mice treated with anti-CD4 antibodies leads to a decrease in lymphocyte infiltration and prevents the emergence of the disease [41]. This T-cell subset is sufficient to initiate T1D because the transfer of CD4+ islet-specific T-cell clones from NOD mice accelerates the development of diabetes in young NOD mice [42]. CD8+ T cells are also important effector cells since they are able to destroy β cells *in vitro* [43], and to transfer very rapidly the disease *in vivo* without any intervention of CD4+ T cells [44].

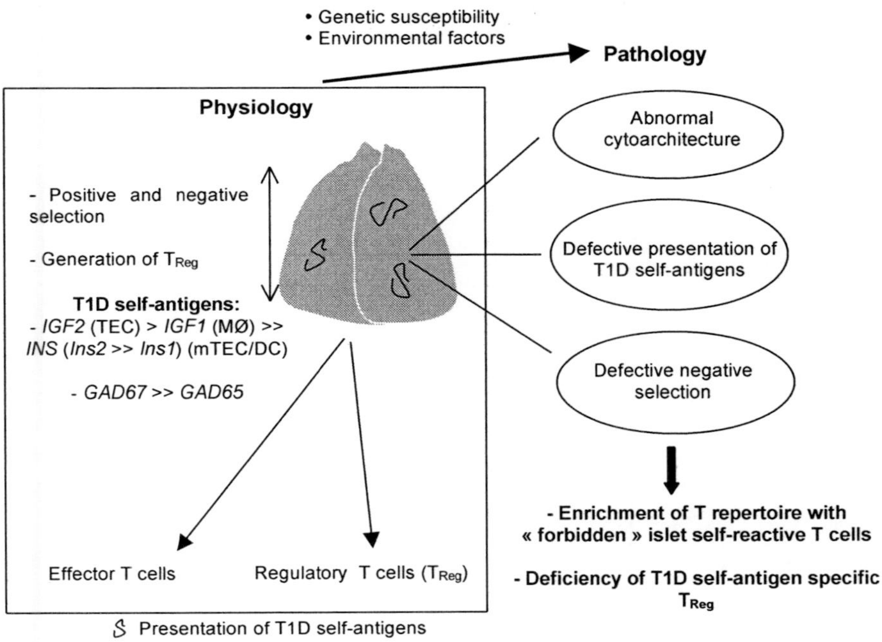

Figure 1. Thymus dysfunction in T1D. The thymus is responsible for establishment of central self-tolerance and generation of competent and self-tolerant naïve T cells. A defect of thymus-dependent self-tolerance may lead to the emergence of "forbidden" self-reactive effector T cells in periphery, as well as to the absence of self-antigen specific T_{Reg}. More and more evidence points to a defect of thymus tolerance to Insulin as a crucial event in the initiation of the autoimmune response selective of islet β cells.

A defect in intrathymic negative selection is also suggested by the emergence in periphery of a high number of auto-reactive T cells in NOD mice [14], and NOD thymocytes were shown to be resistant to intrathymic clonal deletion [45]. Both Fas-dependent and Fas-independent pathways of thymic apoptosis are defective in NOD mice [46]. Amongst the mechanisms implicated in a defective thymus-dependent self-tolerance in this species, a failure to induce Bim, a pro-apototic protein member of Bcl-2 family, was proposed to underline the generalized resistance to thymic deletion of self-reactive T cells as observed in the NOD model [47].

Presentation of self-antigens in the thymus can be affected by disturbed interactions between thymus T cells and thymic antigen presenting cells (APC) – thymic epithelial cells (TEC), dendritic cells (DC), and macrophages – that are essential for a normal function of this organ. In spontaneous animal models, the thymus shows an impaired cytoarchitecture that already suggests abnormal interactions between TEC and developing T cells [48]. In NOD mice, a disturbed organization of medullary (m) TEC precedes autoimmune diabetes development [49]. Variation in self-antigen presentation process by thymic MHC could also be implicated in β-cell autoimmunity development. The MHC of NOD mice (I-A^{g7}) is particular with two substitutions at position 56 and 57; a similar substitution is also observed in the susceptible HLA-DQ2 allele from T1D patients. Such substitutions might affect the binding of self-peptides to thymic MHC and lead to a less effective negative selection of self-reactive T cells [50, 51].

T1D-related Self-antigen Expression in Thymus

The extensive transcription by thymic stromal cells of genes encoding tissue-specific self-antigens has now been fully demonstrated. Jolicoeur and colleagues described expression of pancreas-specific genes (Insulin and GAD67) in C57Bl/6 thymus [52]. Insulin gene transcription in this organ was described from fetal period to post-natal period (few weeks after the birth). Mouse fetus at embryonic day 14, 18-19 and 4-week old mouse express *Ins2* but not *Ins1* in the thymus [53]. A higher expression of *Ins2* in the thymus has been confirmed by several studies [54-56]. A similar situation is also observed for GAD, whose the isoform GAD67 is preferentially expressed in the thymus [56]. *INS* expression in human thymus is also precociously detected [57, 58]. Insulin, GAD67, GAD65 and IA-2 are exclusively expressed in murine mTEC. Thymic DC, cTEC and macrophages do not display any expression of these antigens [59]. Moreover, intrathymic self-antigen expression is highly conserved between mouse and human.

The strength of thymus-dependent self-tolerance depends on the level of self-antigen expression in the thymus. Clonal deletion of self-reactive T cells is complete when a self-antigen is highly expressed by thymic APC, but is partial when this antigen is present in low level [60]. A mouse model was performed to study the influence of self-expression level on thymic selection. Crossing of *Ins1*- and *Ins2*-deficient mice induced a graded deficiency of Insulin expression correlated with Insulin gene copies number. In these mice, a low level of Insulin expression in the thymus promotes the presence in the periphery of T cells with a measurable activity against Insulin. By contrast, normal mice with a normal number of Insulin gene copies do not display any T-cell reactivity against the hormone [55]. Thymus overexpression of heat shock protein 60 (Hsp60), an auto-antigen also implicated in T1D, leads to clonal deletion of Hsp60 specific T cells and to inhibition of the disease. Transgenic overexpression of Hsp60 performed in NOD mice (under MHC class II promoter) decreased insulitis and diabetes [15]. A partial tolerance is already observed when the transgene is weakly expressed [52].

Expression of Insulin-related Genes in Thymus

Several studies in humans and mice have confirmed that Insulin is the primary auto-antigen implicated in early events of the disease. Deletion of both *Ins* genes in NOD mice promotes a 'metabolic diabetes' due to the absence of any insulin. To prevent diabetes in such mice, preproinsulin-transgenic strains with a mutated sequence were developed on a NOD background. The transgene directed the production of preproinsulin with an alanin residue at position B16 instead of native tyrosine. This mutation preserves insulin metabolic activity but abrogates T-cell reactivity against Insulin B9-23. These *Ins1*$^{-/-}$ *Ins2*$^{-/-}$ transgenic NOD mice failed to produce auto-antibodies, did not show any insulitis, and did not develop diabetes [61]. Kent and colleagues also showed that Insulin is a primary auto-antigen in human T1D; cloned T cells from T1D patients identified Insulin A1-15 as an important T-cell epitope [62]. Krishnamurthy and colleagues also studied the role of Insulin in the initiation of T1D [63]. They used two transgenic models, NOD-PI mice that overexpress *proinsulin2* in APC and NOD-IGRP mice that overexpress *IGRP* in their APC. IGRP (for islet-specific glucose-6-phosphatase catalytic subunits-related protein) is an auto-antigen implicated in diabetes. NOD-PI presented neither insulitis, nor diabetes, nor any immune response against IGRP, contrary to the situation in NOD-IGRP mice which developed diabetes despite IGRP tolerance. This research supports the "epitope spreading" concept in which Insulin is the primary auto-antigen promoting the first steps of the auto-immune diabetogenic response which then tackles other β-cell auto-antigens.

The Insulin gene/protein family includes three members in mammals: *Insulin (INS)*, *Insulin-like growth factor 1 (IGF1)* and *Insulin-like growth factor 2 (IGF2)*. Both *IGFs* participate in fetal and post-natal development, while *INS* encodes the hormone responsible for glucose homeostasis. In most species, *INS* is encoded by a single gene, except in mice in which two non-allelic genes (*Ins1* on chromosome 19 and *Ins2* on chromosome 7) exist. *IGF2* is contiguous on chromosome 11 with the gene for *tyrosine hydroxylase* and *INS (Ins2)*, whereas *IGF1* is located on chromosome 12 in humans and on chromosome 10 in mice. *IGF2* expression is paternally imprinted excepted in brain (choroid plexus and leptomeninges), as well as in thymus (mTEC) where a biallelic expression is observed [64]. An opposite situation is observed for *INS* which exhibits a biallelic expression in human and mouse pancreas, whereas a monoallelic *INS* expression has been reported in human thymus [57, 58]. IGF-1 and IGF-2 proteins are 70% homologous in mammals; with regard to their primary and ternary structure, a homology of 50% is observed between A and B chain from IGF and INS.

In the human thymus, there is a precise hierarchy and topography in the expression of the members of the insulin family: *IGF2* (all TEC) > *IGF1* (TEC/macrophages) >> *INS* (mTEC and/or dendritic cells) [52, 57, 65-67]. In murine thymus, the expression of *Ins2* is much higher than *Ins1* [54, 55]. Thymic IGF-2 is not secreted but is expressed at the outer surface of human TEC plasma membrane as shown by confocal microscopy [68].

The marked dominance of *IGF2* over *INS* expression in the thymus stromal network led us to advance the hypothesis that IGF-2 is more tolerized than Insulin and that, given their sequence homology, IGF-2 is implicated in the establishment of a full immunological tolerance to Insulin. This hypothesis was investigated through the help of *Igf2*-deficient mice. When compared to *Igf2*$^{+/+}$ mice, immunization of *Igf2*$^{-/-}$ mice with Insulin promotes a significantly higher humoral response against Insulin. The importance of intrathymic IGF-2 expression for diabetes protection was also supported by data collected in BB rats. A defect in *Igf2* transcription was demonstrated in the thymus of more than 80% of diabetes-prone BB rat, in close accordance with the incidence (86%) of autoimmune diabetes in this rat strain. This defect was not detected in diabetes-resistant BB rat, and was not found in any other organ studied [69]. Immunological tolerance to IGF-2 was indirectly evaluated by the measurement of auto-antibodies to IGF-2 in T1D patients. With the exception of 2 young T1D patients, there was no significant difference in the levels of these auto-antibodies between 100 healthy controls and 100 T1D patients (C. Louis et al., submitted for publication). Although this should be further confirmed in thymus biopsies, these data suggest that, contrary to the situation in diabetes-prone BB rats, there is no defect of central tolerance to IGF-2 in T1D patients. Our findings also confirm that, due to its high expression in the thymus, the immunological tolerance to IGF-2 is very strong and very hard to break. This is correlated with active tolerogenic/regulatory properties of IGF-2 which promotes *IL10* transcription and IL-10 secretion in PBMC cultures derived from healthy controls and from T1D patients (C. Louis et al., submitted for publication).

Control of the Intrathymic Expression of T1D-Related Self-antigens

AIRE Control

The AIRE protein, firstly identified in 1997 [70, 71], is a transcription factor as suggested by these different motifs (a nuclear localization signal at the N-terminus [71], two PHD-type zinc-finger domains [71], four LXXLL domains and an inverted LXXLL domain [72], a SAND domain in the C-terminus [73], and a proline rich region [74]). Its subcellular localization, mainly into nuclear dot-like structures supports such a role as a transcription factor. A mutation of this gene is responsible for a congenital polyautoimmune syndrome known as autoimmune polyendocrinopathy candidiasis and ectodermal dystrophy (APECED), or autoimmune polyendocrine syndrome type 1 (APS-1). This disease is a rare autosomal recessive disorder characterized by various immune responses against multiple peripheral tissues such as thyroid, parathyroid, adrenals, and pancreas... *Aire*$^{-/-}$ mice present several autoimmune disorders similar – but not identical to – those observed in APS-1 patients [75, 76]. In human, the highest level of *AIRE* expression is in the thymus, particularly in mTEC followed by thymic DC [77, 78]. More specifically, the AIRE protein is expressed by a specific subset of mature mTEC and is correlated with the expression of tissue-specific genes [64]. In addition to the thymus, *AIRE* is expressed at a lower level in many tissues such as lymph nodes, fetal liver, spleen and blood cells. In mouse, *Aire* expression seems to be more anarchic [79-81] but, in the thymus, it is exclusively located in the medulla and more specifically in mTEC [82]. Aire is responsible for activation of several tissue-specific genes, but also for repression of some other genes indicating both transcriptional activator and repressor properties [83]. Despite structural and functional differences, Aire-dependent genes are organized in cluster along chromosomes [77, 83].

A direct link between Aire and an autoimmune phenotype was evidenced in an autoimmune eye disease (uveitis), which appears when the single Aire-dependent auto-antigen implicated in this disease is lost [84]. An indirect relation between *Aire* expression and autoimmunity was also observed in animal models such as NOD mice and RelB-deficient mice which present a defect of *Aire* expression in the thymus leading to an abnormal thymus development and an ineffective negative selection [82]. The influence of Aire on thymic self-antigen expression and on central tolerance has been extensively studied. In mice, Anderson and colleagues have shown that the expression of a substantial number of tissue-specific genes (including *Ins2*, *Igf2*, *oxytocin* and *neuropeptide Y*) in thymus is significantly decreased by *Aire* deletion, but *Aire* does not control the whole set of tissue-specific genes expressed in the thymus [76] suggesting that several additional mechanisms are involved in thymus self expression [85]. In the thymus, but not in peripheral organs like testis, the expression of hen egg lysozyme (HEL) is significant reduced in *Aire*-deficient mice when this gene is expressed under control of the rat Insulin promoter. Deletion of HEL-specific CD4+ lymphocytes is reduced, indicating the emergence in periphery of self-reactive T cells and an increased susceptibility to diabetes. *Aire* mutation causes a failure to delete tissue-specific auto-reactive T cells in the thymus, suggesting a direct role for *Aire* in the control of negative selection [86, 87]. A recent study analyzing the cellular mechanisms implicated in *Aire* control shows that the emergence of autoimmune disease in *Aire*$^{-/-}$ mice is not due to a defect of positive selection of T_{Reg}, but to a defect of negative selection of effector auto-reactive T cells [88, 89]. Further implication of Aire in T_{Reg} development was seriously challenged by a recent study showing that *Aire*$^{+}$ mTEC are able and sufficient to generate specific-T_{Reg} [90]. Aire action seems to be dose-dependent because, in *Aire*$^{+/-}$ mice, the deletion of auto-reactive T cells is intermediate between *Aire*$^{+/+}$ and *Aire*$^{-/-}$ mice [86]. Contrary to Insulin-related genes, *Gad67* and *Ia2* transcription is *Aire*-independent because it was similar between the two kinds of mice [76, 91]. The *Ins2* and *Igf2* cluster is the highest Aire-regulated cluster [77, 83].

VNTR Control

Genetic susceptibility to T1D depends on the balance between susceptibility and protective alleles. As mentioned above, the first susceptibility locus in T1D is *IDDM1* including loci inside MHC (HLA in human and H2 in mouse). In human, *IDDM2* is constituted by a variable number of tandem repeats (VNTR) directly upstream of *INS* and *IGF2*, and is implicated for 8% of genetic transmission. *IDDM1* and *IDDM2* confer together around 50% of genetic susceptibility [92].

VNTR locus is constituted by a variable series of 14-15pb repeat elements of a consensus sequence (ACAGGGGTGTGGGG), from 25 to >300 repeat units [93, 94]. In Caucasians, a VNTR polymorphism has been divided into three distinct classes according to a correlation with the susceptibility of T1D. Short class I alleles (between 26 and 63 repeats) are predisposing to the disease, while long class III alleles (between 140 and 210 repeats) confer a dominant protective effect [95-97]. These two classes are the most common classes in

Europe where the intermediary class II alleles are very rarely distributed. This mini-satellite is not transcribed, but modulates the transcription of close genes such as *INS* and *IGF2*. In human fetal [98] and adult [99] pancreas, class III allele is associated with a decrease between 15% and 20% of *INS* mRNA levels, contrary to the class I allele. In the human thymus, *INS* mRNA concentration is 2-3 times higher in association with class III alleles compared to class I alleles [57, 58, 100]. This higher intrathymic *INS* expression, in association with class III allele, has been recently confirmed though no signification was found due to the large variability among samples. The same study also showed that the heterozygous classI/classIII and the homozygous classIII/classIII allele promote a 2-fold and more 10 ten-fold higher expression of *INS*, respectively, compared to homozygous classI/classI allele [91]. It has been suggested that the protective effect of class III alleles would result from higher *INS* transcripts in the thymus, resulting in a more effective central tolerance to Insulin. Concerning VNTR impact on *IGF2* transcription, no significant difference on *IGF2* mRNA levels was observed in human thymus and pancreas [101] but well on placental *IGF2* expression, suggesting that the role of VNTR on *IGF2* expression is tissue-specific [102].

The Interaction between Both Transcription Factors (VNTR and AIRE)

Thymic Insulin expression can be influenced by both factors (VNTR and AIRE) and two recent studies analyzed the interaction between these two factors and Insulin expression in the thymus [91, 100]. Analyzes of heterozygous classI/classIII alleles and homozygous classI/classI alleles showed a correlation between thymic *AIRE* and *INS* expression for both kind of alleles. However, for a determined *AIRE* expression level, thymic *INS* expression was higher in heterozygous classI/classIII allele compared to homozygous classI/classI allele. Therefore, these data show that AIRE and VNTR haplotypes interact to modulate *INS* transcription in the thymus [91].

Conclusion

A defect of thymus-dependent self-tolerance more and more appears as a crucial motor implicated in the pathogenesis of T1D. The deciphering of the precise mechanisms underlying such thymus-specific defect will greatly enhance our knowledge in the pathogenesis of autoimmunity, and will undoubtedly help the development of immunotherapies designed to specifically restore the immunological self-tolerance that is absent or broken in organ-specific autoimmune diseases like T1D.

Acknowledgments

Isabelle Hansenne was supported by the 'Fonds pour la Recherche en Industrie et en Agronomie' (FRIA, Belgium), by the 'Fonds Léon Fredericq pour la recherche biomédicale' (Liege Medical School and CHU), and by the Walloon Region (Project TOLEDIA – postdoctoral fellowship). These studies were supported by the National Fund of Scientific Research (NFSR, Belgium), by the 'Fondation Vaugrenier pour la recherche en tolérance'

(Geneva), by the European Association for the Study of Diabetes (EASD, Düsseldorf), and by the European Union FP6 Integrated Project Euro-Thymaide LSHB-CT-2003-503410.

Appendix

Current Abbreviations

APC	Antigen presenting cells
APECED	autoimmune polyendocrinopathy candidiasis and ectodermal dystrophy
APS-1	autoimmune polyendocrine syndrome type 1
BB	Bio-Breeding
CY	Cyclophosphamide
DC	Dendritic cell
GAD	Glutamic acid decarboxylase
HEL	Hen egg lysozyme
Hsp60	Heat shock protein of 60kDa
IA-2	Insulinoma-associated protein 2
IGF-1	Insulin-like growth factor-1
IGF-2	Insulin-like growth factor-2
INS	Human insulin
MHC	Major histocompatibility complex (HLA in human and H2 in mouse)
NOD	Non obese diabetic
PBMC	Peripheral blood mononuclear cells
TEC	Thymic epithelial cells
mTEC	Medullary thymic epithelial cells
T1D	Type 1 diabetes
TCR	T cell receptor
T_{Reg}	Regulatory T cell
VNTR	Variable number of tandem repeats

References

[1] Notkins, AL and Lernmark, A, Autoimmune type 1 diabetes: resolved and unresolved issues. *Journal of Clinical Investigation*, 2001 108(9): p. 1247-52.

[2] McDevitt, HO, The role of MHC class II molecules in susceptibility and resistance to autoimmunity. *Current Opinion in Immunology*, 1998 10(6): p. 677-81.

[3] Maier, LM and Wicker, LS, Genetic susceptibility to type 1 diabetes. *Current Opinion in Immunology*, 2005 17(6): p. 601-8.

[4] Jahromi, MM and Eisenbarth, GS, Genetic determinants of type 1 diabetes across populations. *Annals of The New York Academy of Sciences*, 2006 1079: p. 289-99.

[5] Anderson, MS and Bluestone, JA, The NOD mouse: a model of immune dysregulation. *Annual Review of Immunology*, 2005 23: p. 447-85.

[6] Harada, M and Makino, S, Promotion of spontaneous diabetes in non-obese diabetes-prone mice by cyclophosphamide. *Diabetologia*, 1984 27(6): p. 604-6.

[7] Brode, S; Raine, T; Zaccone, P and Cooke, A, Cyclophosphamide-induced type-1 diabetes in the NOD mouse is associated with a reduction of CD4+CD25+Foxp3+ regulatory T cells. *Journal of Immunology*, 2006 177(10): p. 6603-12.

[8] Abiru, N; Maniatis, AK; Yu, L; Miao, D; Moriyama, H; Wegmann, D and Eisenbarth, GS, Peptide and major histocompatibility complex-specific breaking of humoral tolerance to native insulin with the B9-23 peptide in diabetes-prone and normal mice. *Diabetes*, 2001 50(6): p. 1274-81.

[9] Moriyama, H; Wen, L; Abiru, N; Liu, E; Yu, L; Miao, D; Gianani, R; Wong, FS and Eisenbarth, GS, Induction and acceleration of insulitis/diabetes in mice with a viral mimic (polyinosinic-polycytidylic acid) and an insulin self-peptide. *Proceedings of National Academy of Sciences of U S A*, 2002 99(8): p. 5539-44.

[10] DiPaolo, RJ and Unanue, ER, The level of peptide-MHC complex determines the susceptibility to autoimmune diabetes: studies in HEL transgenic mice. *European Journal of Immunology*, 2001 31(12): p. 3453-9.

[11] von Herrath, M and Holz, A, Pathological changes in the islet milieu precede infiltration of islets and destruction of beta-cells by autoreactive lymphocytes in a transgenic model of virus-induced IDDM. *Journal of Autoimmunity*, 1997 10(3): p. 231-8.

[12] Yang, Y and Santamaria, P, T-cell receptor-transgenic NOD mice: a reductionist approach to understand autoimmune diabetes. *Journal of Autoimmunity*, 2004 22(2): p. 121-9.

[13] Byersdorfer, CA; Schweitzer, GG and Unanue, ER, Diabetes is predicted by the beta cell level of autoantigen. *Journal of Immunology*, 2005 175(7): p. 4347-54.

[14] Lesage, S; Hartley, SB; Akkaraju, S; Wilson, J; Townsend, M and Goodnow, CC, Failure to censor forbidden clones of CD4 T cells in autoimmune diabetes. *Journal of Experimental Medicine*, 2002 196(9): p. 1175-88.

[15] Birk, OS; Douek, DC; Elias, D; Takacs, K; Dewchand, H; Gur, SL; Walker, MD; van der Zee, R; Cohen, IR and Altmann, DM, A role of Hsp60 in autoimmune diabetes: analysis in a transgenic model. *Proceedings of National Academy of Sciences of U S A*, 1996 93(3): p. 1032-7.

[16] Jasinski, JM; Yu, L; Nakayama, M; Li, MM; Lipes, MA; Eisenbarth, GS and Liu, E, Transgenic insulin (B:9-23) T-cell receptor mice develop autoimmune diabetes dependent upon RAG genotype, H-2g7 homozygosity, and insulin 2 gene knockout. *Diabetes*, 2006 55(7): p. 1978-84.

[17] Lieberman, SM and DiLorenzo, TP, A comprehensive guide to antibody and T-cell responses in type 1 diabetes. *Tissue Antigens*, 2003 62(5): p. 359-77.

[18] Erlander, MG; Tillakaratne, NJ; Feldblum, S; Patel, N and Tobin, AJ, Two genes encode distinct glutamate decarboxylases. *Neuron*, 1991 7(1): p. 91-100.

[19] Bu, DF; Erlander, MG; Hitz, BC; Tillakaratne, NJ; Kaufman, DL; Wagner-McPherson, CB; Evans, GA and Tobin, AJ, Two human glutamate decarboxylases, 65-kDa GAD and 67-kDa GAD, are each encoded by a single gene. *Proceedings of National Academy of Sciences of U S A*, 1992 89(6): p. 2115-9.

[20] Christgau, S; Schierbeck, H; Aanstoot, HJ; Aagaard, L; Begley, K; Kofod, H; Hejnaes, K and Baekkeskov, S, Pancreatic beta cells express two autoantigenic forms of glutamic acid decarboxylase, a 65-kDa hydrophilic form and a 64-kDa amphiphilic form which can be both membrane-bound and soluble. *Journal of Biological Chemistry*, 1991 266(31): p. 21257-64.

[21] Kim, J; Richter, W; Aanstoot, HJ; Shi, Y; Fu, Q; Rajotte, R; Warnock, G and Baekkeskov, S, Differential expression of GAD65 and GAD67 in human, rat, and mouse pancreatic islets. *Diabetes*, 1993 42(12): p. 1799-808.

[22] Yamamoto, T; Yamato, E; Tashiro, F; Sato, T; Noso, S; Ikegami, H; Tamura, S; Yanagawa, Y and Miyazaki, JI, Development of autoimmune diabetes in glutamic acid decarboxylase 65 (GAD65) knockout NOD mice. *Diabetologia*, 2004 47(2): p. 221-4.

[23] Yoon, JW; Yoon, CS; Lim, HW; Huang, QQ; Kang, Y; Pyun, KH; Hirasawa, K; Sherwin, RS and Jun, HS, Control of autoimmune diabetes in NOD mice by GAD expression or suppression in beta cells. *Science*, 1999 284(5417): p. 1183-7.

[24] Lu, J; Li, Q; Xie, H; Chen, ZJ; Borovitskaya, AE; Maclaren, NK; Notkins, AL and Lan, MS, Identification of a second transmembrane protein tyrosine phosphatase, IA-2beta, as an autoantigen in insulin-dependent diabetes mellitus: precursor of the 37-kDa tryptic fragment. *Proceedings of National Academy of Sciences of U S A*, 1996 93(6): p. 2307-11.

[25] Lan, MS; Wasserfall, C; Maclaren, NK and Notkins, AL, IA-2, a transmembrane protein of the protein tyrosine phosphatase family, is a major autoantigen in insulin-dependent diabetes mellitus. *Proceedings of National Academy of Sciences of U S A*, 1996 93(13): p. 6367-70.

[26] DeSilva, MG; Jun, HS; Yoon, JW; Notkins, AL and Lan, MS, Autoantibodies to IA-2 not detected in NOD mice or BB rats. *Diabetologia*, 1996 39(10): p. 1237-8.

[27] Kubosaki, A; Gross, S; Miura, J; Saeki, K; Zhu, M; Nakamura, S; Hendriks, W and Notkins, AL, Targeted disruption of the IA-2beta gene causes glucose intolerance and impairs insulin secretion but does not prevent the development of diabetes in NOD mice. *Diabetes*, 2004 53(7): p. 1684-91.

[28] Kubosaki, A; Miura, J and Notkins, AL, IA-2 is not required for the development of diabetes in NOD mice. *Diabetologia*, 2004 47(1): p. 149-50.

[29] Daniel, D; Gill, RG; Schloot, N and Wegmann, D, Epitope specificity, cytokine production profile and diabetogenic activity of insulin-specific T cell clones isolated from NOD mice. *European Journal of Immunology*, 1995 25(4): p. 1056-62.

[30] Wegmann, DR; Norbury-Glaser, M and Daniel, D, Insulin-specific T cells are a predominant component of islet infiltrates in pre-diabetic NOD mice. *European Journal of Immunology*, 1994 24(8): p. 1853-7.

[31] Moriyama, H; Abiru, N; Paronen, J; Sikora, K; Liu, E; Miao, D; Devendra, D; Beilke, J; Gianani, R; Gill, RG and Eisenbarth, GS, Evidence for a primary islet autoantigen (preproinsulin 1) for insulitis and diabetes in the nonobese diabetic mouse. *Proceedings of National Academy of Sciences of U S A*, 2003 100(18): p. 10376-81.

[32] Thebault-Baumont, K; Dubois-Laforgue, D; Krief, P; Briand, JP; Halbout, P; Vallon-Geoffroy, K; Morin, J; Laloux, V; Lehuen, A; Carel, JC; Jami, J; Muller, S and Boitard, C, Acceleration of type 1 diabetes mellitus in proinsulin 2-deficient NOD mice. *Journal of Clinical Investigation*, 2003 111(6): p. 851-7.

[33] Pugliese, A, Central and peripheral autoantigen presentation in immune tolerance. *Immunology*, 2004 111(2): p. 138-46.

[34] Like, AA; Kislauskis, E; Williams, RR and Rossini, AA, Neonatal thymectomy prevents spontaneous diabetes mellitus in the BB/W rat. *Science*, 1982 216(4546): p. 644-6.

[35] Georgiou, HM and Mandel, TE, Induction of insulitis in athymic (nude) mice. The effect of NOD thymus and pancreas transplantation. *Diabetes*, 1995 44(1): p. 49-59.

[36] Makino, S; Harada, M; Kishimoto, Y and Hayashi, Y, Absence of insulitis and overt diabetes in athymic nude mice with NOD genetic background. *Jikken Dobutsu*, 1986 35(4): p. 495-8.

[37] Yagi, H; Matsumoto, M; Kunimoto, K; Kawaguchi, J; Makino, S and Harada, M, Analysis of the roles of CD4+ and CD8+ T cells in autoimmune diabetes of NOD mice using transfer to NOD athymic nude mice. *European Journal of Immunology*, 1992 22(9): p. 2387-93.

[38] Christianson, SW; Shultz, LD and Leiter, EH, Adoptive transfer of diabetes into immunodeficient NOD-scid/scid mice. Relative contributions of CD4+ and CD8+ T-cells from diabetic versus prediabetic NOD.NON-Thy-1a donors. *Diabetes*, 1993 42(1): p. 44-55.

[39] Bendelac, A; Carnaud, C; Boitard, C and Bach, JF, Syngeneic transfer of autoimmune diabetes from diabetic NOD mice to healthy neonates. Requirement for both L3T4+ and Lyt-2+ T cells. *Journal of Experimental Medicine*, 1987 166(4): p. 823-32.

[40] Wicker, LS; Miller, BJ and Mullen, Y, Transfer of autoimmune diabetes mellitus with splenocytes from nonobese diabetic (NOD) mice. *Diabetes*, 1986 35(8): p. 855-60.

[41] Shizuru, JA; Taylor-Edwards, C; Banks, BA; Gregory, AK and Fathman, CG, Immunotherapy of the nonobese diabetic mouse: treatment with an antibody to T-helper lymphocytes. *Science*, 1988 240(4852): p. 659-62.

[42] Haskins, K and McDuffie, M, Acceleration of diabetes in young NOD mice with a CD4+ islet-specific T cell clone. *Science*, 1990 249(4975): p. 1433-6.

[43] Nagata, M and Yoon, JW, Studies on autoimmunity for T-cell-mediated beta-cell destruction. Distinct difference in beta-cell destruction between CD4+ and CD8+ T-cell clones derived from lymphocytes infiltrating the islets of NOD mice. *Diabetes*, 1992 41(8): p. 998-1008.

[44] Wong, FS; Visintin, I; Wen, L; Flavell, RA and Janeway, CA, Jr., CD8 T cell clones from young nonobese diabetic (NOD) islets can transfer rapid onset of diabetes in NOD mice in the absence of CD4 cells. *Journal of Experimental Medicine*, 1996 183(1): p. 67-76.

[45] Zucchelli, S; Holler, P; Yamagata, T; Roy, M; Benoist, C and Mathis, D, Defective central tolerance induction in NOD mice: genomics and genetics. *Immunity*, 2005 22(3): p. 385-96.

[46] Kishimoto, H and Sprent, J, A defect in central tolerance in NOD mice. *Nature Immunology*, 2001 2(11): p. 1025-31.

[47] Liston, A; Lesage, S; Gray, DH; O'Reilly, LA; Strasser, A; Fahrer, AM; Boyd, RL; Wilson, J; Baxter, AG; Gallo, EM; Crabtree, GR; Peng, K; Wilson, SR and Goodnow, CC, Generalized resistance to thymic deletion in the NOD mouse; a polygenic trait characterized by defective induction of Bim. *Immunity*, 2004 21(6): p. 817-30.

[48] Takeoka, Y; Chen, SY; Boyd, RL; Tsuneyama, K; Taguchi, N; Morita, S; Yago, H; Suehiro, S; Ansari, AA; Shultz, LD and Gershwin, ME, A comparative analysis of the murine thymic microenvironment in normal, autoimmune, and immunodeficiency states. *Developmental Immunology*, 1997 5(2): p. 79-89.

[49] Atlan-Gepner, C; Naspetti, M; Valero, R; Barad, M; Lepault, F; Vialettes, B and Naquet, P, Disorganization of thymic medulla precedes evolution towards diabetes in female NOD mice. *Autoimmunity*, 1999 31(4): p. 249-60.

[50] Stratmann, T; Apostolopoulos, V; Mallet-Designe, V; Corper, AL; Scott, CA; Wilson, IA; Kang, AS and Teyton, L, The I-Ag7 MHC class II molecule linked to murine diabetes is a promiscuous peptide binder. *Journal of Immunology*, 2000 165(6): p. 3214-25.

[51] Carrasco-Marin, E; Shimizu, J; Kanagawa, O and Unanue, ER, The class II MHC I-Ag7 molecules from non-obese diabetic mice are poor peptide binders. *Journal of Immunology*, 1996 156(2): p. 450-8.

[52] Jolicoeur, C; Hanahan, D and Smith, KM, T-cell tolerance toward a transgenic beta-cell antigen and transcription of endogenous pancreatic genes in thymus. *Proceedings of National Academy of Sciences of U S A*, 1994 91(14): p. 6707-11.

[53] Heath, VL; Moore, NC; Parnell, SM and Mason, DW, Intrathymic expression of genes involved in organ specific autoimmune disease. *Journal of Autoimmunity*, 1998 11(4): p. 309-18.

[54] Brimnes, MK; Jensen, T; Jorgensen, TN; Michelsen, BK; Troelsen, J and Werdelin, O, Low expression of insulin in the thymus of non-obese diabetic mice. *Journal of Autoimmunity*, 2002 19(4): p. 203-13.

[55] Chentoufi, AA and Polychronakos, C, Insulin expression levels in the thymus modulate insulin-specific autoreactive T-cell tolerance: the mechanism by which the IDDM2 locus may predispose to diabetes. *Diabetes*, 2002 51(5): p. 1383-90.

[56] Pleau, JM; Esling, A; Geutkens, S; Dardenne, M and Homo-Delarche, F, Pancreatic hormone and glutamic acid decarboxylase expression in the mouse thymus: a real-time PCR study. *Biochemical and Biophysical Research Communications*, 2001 283(4): p. 843-8.

[57] Pugliese, A; Zeller, M; Fernandez, A, Jr.; Zalcberg, LJ; Bartlett, RJ; Ricordi, C; Pietropaolo, M; Eisenbarth, GS; Bennett, ST and Patel, DD, The insulin gene is transcribed in the human thymus and transcription levels correlated with allelic variation at the INS VNTR-IDDM2 susceptibility locus for type 1 diabetes. *Nature Genetics*, 1997 15(3): p. 293-7.

[58] Vafiadis, P; Bennett, ST; Todd, JA; Nadeau, J; Grabs, R; Goodyer, CG; Wickramasinghe, S; Colle, E and Polychronakos, C, Insulin expression in human thymus is modulated by INS VNTR alleles at the IDDM2 locus. *Nature Genetics*, 1997 15(3): p. 289-92.

[59] Derbinski, J; Schulte, A; Kyewski, B and Klein, L, Promiscuous gene expression in medullary thymic epithelial cells mirrors the peripheral self. *Nature Immunology*, 2001 2(11): p. 1032-9.

[60] Sprent, J and Webb, SR, Intrathymic and extrathymic clonal deletion of T cells. *Current Opinion in Immunology*, 1995 7(2): p. 196-205.

[61] Nakayama, M; Abiru, N; Moriyama, H; Babaya, N; Liu, E; Miao, D; Yu, L; Wegmann, DR; Hutton, JC; Elliott, JF and Eisenbarth, GS, Prime role for an insulin epitope in the development of type 1 diabetes in NOD mice. *Nature*, 2005 435(7039): p. 220-3.

[62] Kent, SC; Chen, Y; Bregoli, L; Clemmings, SM; Kenyon, NS; Ricordi, C; Hering, BJ and Hafler, DA, Expanded T cells from pancreatic lymph nodes of type 1 diabetic subjects recognize an insulin epitope. *Nature*, 2005 435(7039): p. 224-8.

[63] Krishnamurthy, B; Dudek, NL; McKenzie, MD; Purcell, AW; Brooks, AG; Gellert, S; Colman, PG; Harrison, LC; Lew, AM; Thomas, HE and Kay, TW, Responses against islet antigens in NOD mice are prevented by tolerance to proinsulin but not IGRP. *Journal of Clinical Investigation*, 2006 116(12): p. 3258-65.

[64] Derbinski, J; Gabler, J; Brors, B; Tierling, S; Jonnakuty, S; Hergenhahn, M; Peltonen, L; Walter, J and Kyewski, B, Promiscuous gene expression in thymic epithelial cells is regulated at multiple levels. *Journal of Experimental Medicine*, 2005 202(1): p. 33-45.

[65] Kecha, O; Martens, H; Franchimont, N; Achour, I; Hazee-Hagelstein, MT; Charlet-Renard, C; Geenen, V and Winkler, R, Characterization of the insulin-like growth factor axis in the human thymus. *Journal of Neuroendocrinology*, 1999 11(6): p.435-40.

[66] Geenen, V; Achour, I; Robert, F; Vandersmissen, E; Sodoyez, JC; Defresne, MP; Boniver, J; Lefebvre, PJ and Franchimont, P, Evidence that insulin-like growth factor 2 (IGF2) is the dominant thymic peptide of the insulin superfamily. *Thymus*, 1993 21(2): p. 115-27.

[67] de Mello Coelho, V; Villa-Verde, DM; Farias-de-Oliveira, DA; de Brito, JM; Dardenne, M and Savino, W, Functional insulin-like growth factor-1/insulin-like growth factor-1 receptor-mediated circuit in human and murine thymic epithelial cells. *Neuroendocrinology*, 2002 75(2): p. 139-50.

[68] Achour, I, Les facteurs de croissance apparentés à l'insuline (IGFs) dans le thymus humain et dans le thymus d'un modèle animal de diabète insulino-dépendant, in PhD Thesis. 1997, University of Liege: Liege.

[69] Kecha-Kamoun, O; Achour, I; Martens, H; Collette, J; Lefebvre, PJ; Greiner, DL and Geenen, V, Thymic expression of insulin-related genes in an animal model of autoimmune type 1 diabetes. *Diabetes and Metabolism Research Reviews*, 2001 17(2): p. 146-52.

[70] Nagamine, K; Peterson, P; Scott, HS; Kudoh, J; Minoshima, S; Heino, M; Krohn, KJ; Lalioti, MD; Mullis, PE; Antonarakis, SE; Kawasaki, K; Asakawa, S; Ito, F and Shimizu, N, Positional cloning of the APECED gene. *Nature Genetics*, 1997 17(4): p. 393-8.

[71] Consortium, TF-GA, An autoimmune disease, APECED, caused by mutations in a novel gene featuring two PHD-type zinc-finger domains. The Finnish-German APECED Consortium. Autoimmune Polyendocrinopathy-Candidiasis-Ectodermal Dystrophy. *Nature Genetics*, 1997 17(4): p. 399-403.

[72] Savkur, RS and Burris, TP, The coactivator LXXLL nuclear receptor recognition motif. *Journal of Peptides Research*, 2004 63(3): p. 207-12.

[73] Gibson, TJ; Ramu, C; Gemund, C and Aasland, R, The APECED polyglandular autoimmune syndrome protein, AIRE-1, contains the SAND domain and is probably a transcription factor. *Trends in Biochemical Sciences*, 1998 23(7): p. 242-4.

[74] Kay, BK; Williamson, MP and Sudol, M, The importance of being proline: the interaction of proline-rich motifs in signaling proteins with their cognate domains. *Faseb Journal*, 2000 14(2): p. 231-41.

[75] Ramsey, C; Winqvist, O; Puhakka, L; Halonen, M; Moro, A; Kampe, O; Eskelin, P; Pelto-Huikko, M and Peltonen, L, Aire deficient mice develop multiple features of APECED phenotype and show altered immune response. *Human Molecular Genetics*, 2002 11(4): p. 397-409.

[76] Anderson, MS; Venanzi, ES; Klein, L; Chen, Z; Berzins, SP; Turley, SJ; von Boehmer, H; Bronson, R; Dierich, A; Benoist, C and Mathis, D, Projection of an immunological self shadow within the thymus by the aire protein. *Science*, 2002 298(5597): p. 1395-401.

[77] Gotter, J; Brors, B; Hergenhahn, M and Kyewski, B, Medullary epithelial cells of the human thymus express a highly diverse selection of tissue-specific genes colocalized in chromosomal clusters. *Journal of Experimental Medicine*, 2004 199(2): p. 155-66.

[78] Heino, M; Peterson, P; Kudoh, J; Nagamine, K; Lagerstedt, A; Ovod, V; Ranki, A; Rantala, I; Nieminen, M; Tuukkanen, J; Scott, HS; Antonarakis, SE; Shimizu, N and Krohn, K, Autoimmune regulator is expressed in the cells regulating immune tolerance in thymus medulla. *Biochemical and Biophysical Research Communications*, 1999 257(3): p. 821-5.

[79] Halonen, M; Pelto-Huikko, M; Eskelin, P; Peltonen, L; Ulmanen, I and Kolmer, M, Subcellular location and expression pattern of autoimmune regulator (Aire), the mouse orthologue for human gene defective in autoimmune polyendocrinopathy candidiasis ectodermal dystrophy (APECED). *Journal of Histochemistry and Cytochemistry*, 2001 49(2): p. 197-208.

[80] Meriluoto, T; Halonen, M; Pelto-Huikko, M; Kangas, H; Korhonen, J; Kolmer, M; Ulmanen, I and Eskelin, P, The autoimmune regulator: a key toward understanding the molecular pathogenesis of autoimmune polyendocrinopathy-candidiasis-ectodermal dystrophy. *Keio Journal of Medicine*, 2001 50(4): p. 225-39.

[81] Adamson, KA; Pearce, SH; Lamb, JR; Seckl, JR and Howie, SE, A comparative study of mRNA and protein expression of the autoimmune regulator gene (Aire) in embryonic and adult murine tissues. *Journal of Pathology*, 2004 202(2): p. 180-7.

[82] Heino, M; Peterson, P; Sillanpaa, N; Guerin, S; Wu, L; Anderson, G; Scott, HS; Antonarakis, SE; Kudoh, J; Shimizu, N; Jenkinson, EJ; Naquet, P and Krohn, KJ, RNA and protein expression of the murine autoimmune regulator gene (Aire) in normal, RelB-deficient and in NOD mouse. *European Journal of Immunology*, 2000 30(7): p. 1884-93.

[83] Johnnidis, JB; Venanzi, ES; Taxman, DJ; Ting, JP; Benoist, CO and Mathis, DJ, Chromosomal clustering of genes controlled by the aire transcription factor. *Proceedings of National Academy of Sciences of U S A*, 2005 102(20): p. 7233-8.

[84] DeVoss, J; Hou, Y; Johannes, K; Lu, W; Liou, GI; Rinn, J; Chang, H; Caspi, RR; Fong, L and Anderson, MS, Spontaneous autoimmunity prevented by thymic expression of a single self-antigen. *Journal of Experimental Medicine*, 2006 203(12): p. 2727-35.

[85] Gotter, J and Kyewski, B, Regulating self-tolerance by deregulating gene expression. *Current Opinion in Immunology*, 2004 16(6): p. 741-5.

[86] Liston, A; Lesage, S; Wilson, J; Peltonen, L and Goodnow, CC, Aire regulates negative selection of organ-specific T cells. *Nature Immunology*, 2003 4(4): p. 350-4.

[87] Liston, A; Gray, DH; Lesage, S; Fletcher, AL; Wilson, J; Webster, KE; Scott, HS; Boyd, RL; Peltonen, L and Goodnow, CC, Gene dosage--limiting role of Aire in thymic expression, clonal deletion, and organ-specific autoimmunity. *Journal of Experimental Medicine*, 2004 200(8): p. 1015-26.

[88] Anderson, MS; Venanzi, ES; Chen, Z; Berzins, SP; Benoist, C and Mathis, D, The cellular mechanism of Aire control of T cell tolerance. *Immunity*, 2005 23(2): p.227-39.

[89] Kuroda, N; Mitani, T; Takeda, N; Ishimaru, N; Arakaki, R; Hayashi, Y; Bando, Y; Izumi, K; Takahashi, T; Nomura, T; Sakaguchi, S; Ueno, T; Takahama, Y; Uchida, D; Sun, S; Kajiura, F; Mouri, Y; Han, H; Matsushima, A; Yamada, G and Matsumoto, M, Development of autoimmunity against transcriptionally unrepressed target antigen in the thymus of Aire-deficient mice. *Journal of Immunology*, 2005 174(4): p. 1862-70.

[90] Aschenbrenner, K; D'Cruz, LM; Vollmann, EH; Hinterberger, M; Emmerich, J; Swee, LK; Rolink, A and Klein, L, Selection of Foxp3+ regulatory T cells specific for self antigen expressed and presented by Aire+ medullary thymic epithelial cells. *Nature Immunology*, 2007 8(4): p. 351-8.

[91] Taubert, R; Schwendemann, J and Kyewski, B, Highly variable expression of tissue-restricted self-antigens in human thymus: implications for self-tolerance and autoimmunity. *European Journal of Immunology*, 2007 37(3): p. 838-48.

[92] Davies, JL; Kawaguchi, Y; Bennett, ST; Copeman, JB; Cordell, HJ; Pritchard, LE; Reed, PW; Gough, SC; Jenkins, SC; Palmer, SM and et al., A genome-wide search for human type 1 diabetes susceptibility genes. *Nature*, 1994 371(6493): p. 130-6.

[93] Bell, GI; Selby, MJ and Rutter, WJ, The highly polymorphic region near the human insulin gene is composed of simple tandemly repeating sequences. *Nature*, 1982 295(5844): p. 31-5.

[94] Ullrich, A; Dull, TJ; Gray, A; Philips, JA, 3rd and Peter, S, Variation in the sequence and modification state of the human insulin gene flanking regions. *Nucleic Acids Research*, 1982 10(7): p. 2225-40.

[95] Undlien, DE; Bennett, ST; Todd, JA; Akselsen, HE; Ikaheimo, I; Reijonen, H; Knip, M; Thorsby, E and Ronningen, KS, Insulin gene region-encoded susceptibility to IDDM maps upstream of the insulin gene. *Diabetes*, 1995 44(6): p. 620-5.

[96] Lucassen, AM; Julier, C; Beressi, JP; Boitard, C; Froguel, P; Lathrop, M and Bell, JI, Susceptibility to insulin dependent diabetes mellitus maps to a 4.1 kb segment of DNA spanning the insulin gene and associated VNTR. *Nature Genetics*, 1993 4(3): p. 305-10.

[97] Julier, C; Hyer, RN; Davies, J; Merlin, F; Soularue, P; Briant, L; Cathelineau, G; Deschamps, I; Rotter, JI; Froguel, P and et al., Insulin-IGF2 region on chromosome 11p encodes a gene implicated in HLA-DR4-dependent diabetes susceptibility. *Nature*, 1991 354(6349): p. 155-9.

[98] Vafiadis, P; Bennett, ST; Colle, E; Grabs, R; Goodyer, CG and Polychronakos, C, Imprinted and genotype-specific expression of genes at the IDDM2 locus in pancreas and leucocytes. *Journal of Autoimmunity*, 1996 9(3): p. 397-403.

[99] Bennett, ST; Lucassen, AM; Gough, SC; Powell, EE; Undlien, DE; Pritchard, LE; Merriman, ME; Kawaguchi, Y; Dronsfield, MJ; Pociot, F and et al., Susceptibility to human type 1 diabetes at IDDM2 is determined by tandem repeat variation at the insulin gene minisatellite locus. *Nature Genetics*, 1995 9(3): p. 284-92.

[100] Sabater, L; Ferrer-Francesch, X; Sospedra, M; Caro, P; Juan, M and Pujol-Borrell, R, Insulin alleles and autoimmune regulator (AIRE) gene expression both influence insulin expression in the thymus. *Journal of Autoimmunity*, 2005 25(4): p. 312-8.
[101] Vafiadis, P; Grabs, R; Goodyer, CG; Colle, E and Polychronakos, C, A functional analysis of the role of IGF2 in IDDM2-encoded susceptibility to type 1 diabetes. *Diabetes*, 1998 47(5): p. 831-6.
[102] Paquette, J; Giannoukakis, N; Polychronakos, C; Vafiadis, P and Deal, C, The INS 5' variable number of tandem repeats is associated with IGF2 expression in humans. *Journal of Biological Chemistry*, 1998 273(23): p. 14158-64.

Index

A

B

C

D

G

H

I

J

K

L

N

O

P

Q

R

S

T

U

V

W

X

Y

Z